Infections and the Cardiovascular System
New Perspectives

Emerging Infectious Diseases of the 21st Century

Series Editor: I. W. Fong
Professor of Medicine, University of Toronto
Head of Infectious Diseases, St. Michael's Hospital

INFECTIONS AND THE CARDIOVASCULAR SYSTEM: New Perspectives
Edited by I. W. Fong

Infections and the Cardiovascular System
New Perspectives

Edited by

I. W. Fong

Professor of Medicine, University of Toronto
Head of Infectious Diseases, St. Michael's Hospital
Toronto, Ontario,
Canada

Kluwer Academic / Plenum Publishers
New York, Boston, Dordrecht, London, Moscow

Library of Congress Cataloging-in-Publication Data

Fong, I.W. (Ignatius W.)
    Infections and the cardiovascular system : new perspectives / I.W. Fong.
      p. cm. – (Emerging infectious diseases of the 21st century)
    Includes bibliographical references and index.
    ISBN 0-306-47404-2
    1. Cardiovascular system–Infections. I. Title. II. Series.
    RC678 .F665 2002
    616.1'07–dc21
                                                              2002028278

ISBN: 0-306-47404-2

© 2003 Kluwer Academic/Plenum Publishers
233 Spring Street, New York, NY 10013

http://www.wkap.nl/

10 9 8 7 6 5 4 3 2 1

Printed in the United States of America

Preface

Infectious agents have been recognized to involve the heart and vascular system for well over a century. Traditional concepts and teachings of their involvement in the pathogenesis of disease have been by a few established mechanisms. Bacterial and occasionally fungal microorganisms were known to invade and multiply on the endocardium of valves, vascular prostheses or shunts and aneurysm. Similarly viral, bacterial, mycobacterial, fungal, and parasitic pathogens could cause disease by invasion of the pericardium and muscles of the heart. Pathogenesis of some diseases of the endocardium, myocardium, and pericardium could involve indirect mechanisms with molecular mimicry inducing injury through an autoimmune process, such as in rheumatic heart disease and post viral cardiomyopathy.

It was recognized by the mid-20th century that *Treponema pallidum*, the etiology of syphilis, could cause cardiovascular damage (aortitis and aortic aneurysm) by obliteration of the vasa vasorum supplying the root of the aorta by endarteritis obliterans, and by then the connection between streptococcal infection and rheumatic heart disease was clear.

Since the last decade of the 20th century there has been renewed interest in the medical and public media on infectious diseases affecting the cardiovascular and cerebrovascular systems, through the relationship with development or acceleration of atherosclerosis. Atherosclerosis has traditionally been considered the consequence of certain lifestyle (smoking, obesity, inactivity), hyperlipidemia, and hypertension or genetic diseases (diabetes mellitus, familial hypercholesterolemia, etc.). However, the concept that infections could play a role in the pathogenesis of atherosclerotic heart disease is not new, and was in vogue in the later part of the 19th century in Europe when the germ theory of many diseases was popular, especially after Koch proved that consumption was due to *Mycobacteria tuberculosis*. In the early part of the

20th century, Osler and Billings were advocates of the infectious theory of atherosclerotic cardiovascular disease. Interest in this theory waned soon after Anitschkow in St. Petersburg published his landmark studies of cholesterol-induced atherosclerosis in the rabbit model in 1913.

However, we should learn from the lessons taught by the peptic ulcer and *Helicobacter pylori* saga in the pathogenesis of this common disease. It was just over two decades ago that the paradigm for peptic ulcer etiology was accepted as due to gastric acid hyper-secretion, with lifestyle factors such as stress playing a major precipitating factor. It should be remembered that around 1906, Billings speculated that some gastric and duodenal ulcers were caused by bacterial infection of the mucous membranes that rendered the cells prone to digestion by the gastric juices. He was concerned that long standing focal infection leading to chronic systemic disease was not appreciated. He wrote, "I think there can be no doubts that the insidious slow degenerative processes which occur in many patients who arrive at the meridian of life are due to slow intoxications from chronic focal infections variously located." The main purpose of this book is to highlight and review these new perspectives of infections on the cardiovascular system.

ACKNOWLEDGMENTS

This book would not have been be possible without the collaboration of my colleagues in various studies, especially Dr. Brian Chiu and Dr. James Mahony. I am also grateful to Dr. Maria Kolia for her assistance in compiling various literature and data; to Dawn Bajhan, Debbie Reid and my wife (Cheryl) for their assiduous secretarial and administrative assistance.

I. W. FONG

Contents

Chapter 4

Effect of Infection on Lipoproteins and the Coagulation System

Section II

Emerging Relationships of Infections and the Cardiovascular System

Chapter 5

***Chlamydia pneumoniae* and the Cardiovascular System**

Chapter 6

Periodontal Disease and the Cardiovascular System

Chapter 7

Cytomegalovirus and Herpes Simplex Virus in Cardiovascular Disease

Chapter 8

**Miscellaneous Infections and Atherosclerosis:
Cardiovascular and Cerebrovascular Disease**

Section I

Traditional Infections Affecting the Cardiovascular System

1

New Insights and Updates for Established Entities

1.1. INTRODUCTION

This chapter will deal with updates or new advances in the pathogenesis, epidemiology, diagnosis, or management of conditions such as infective endocarditis, rheumatic fever, myocarditis, and vascular device infections. Descriptive details of these conditions that are present in many textbooks of medicine will not be addressed here.

1.2. INFECTIVE ENDOCARDITIS

Invasion of the endocardium (valves, septal defects, mural endocardium, shunts such as patent ductus arteriosis) has been described with nearly all classes of microorganisms recognized to cause disease in humans. Although common bacteria that colonize humans are the most frequent culprits, other invaders include chlamydiae, rickettsiae, mycoplasmas, fungi, mycobacteria, and possible viruses. There has been no major shift in the prevalence of the various bacteria causing endocarditis in the past 10 years. For native valve endocarditis, the α hemolytic streptococci (viridans group) and *Staphylococcus aureus* remain the most frequent isolated pathogens. In prosthetic valve endocarditis, staphylococci, led by coagulase-negative species, are the most frequent isolates in the first 60 days after surgery. Fungal endocarditis have become rare entities following valve replacement, since the advent of shortened perioperative antibiotic prophylaxis.

Significant update in the microbiology of infective endocarditis includes the recognition of *Bartonella* spp. as important causes of "culture negative" endocarditis. *B. quintana* (formerly *Rochalimae quintana* and *Rickettsia quintana*), a fastidious gram-negative bacterium which caused trench fever in the Great World Wars, transmitted primarily by the body louse, is mostly implicated in endocarditis of the homeless with alcoholism[1-4], mainly in urban areas or cities. Cases have been recognized in such cities as Seattle, Paris, Lyon, Halifax, Washington DC, Marseille, Boston and we have diagnosed two cases in Toronto (unpublished).

Other Bartonella spp. have also been reported to cause endocarditis but are not associated with homelessness in the inner city. *B. henselae*, the putative cause of cat scratch fever, can produce endocarditis[5,6] (and may be associated with contact with cats), as well as *B. elizabethae*[7], and other undifferentiated species[4]. In the largest series of Bartonella endocarditis reported by Raoult et al.[4], 22 new cases were described in addition to 11 other previously reported cases. *Bartonella* spp. were estimated to cause 3% of the cases of endocarditis seen in three study centers. Five were infected with *B. quintana*, four with *B. henselae*, and thirteen with undetermined *Bartonella* spp.

Bartonella spp. may be isolated from blood with the BACTEC culture bottles (Becton Dickinson Diagnostic, Sparks, MD), but growth is slow, often requiring 20–40 days, and subculture onto fresh chocolate agar, followed by extended incubation under 5% carbon dioxide at 37 °C, or lysis centrifugation of blood culture systems which may improve the recovery. Serological techniques for diagnosing Bartonella infection are available and include indirect immunofluorescence assay and ELISA-based techniques. Serological cross-reaction between *B. quintana* and *B. henselae* does exist[8] and *Coxiella burnetii* may cause false positive serology for *B. quintana*[9]. Infection with *B. quintana* may also induce false positive cross-reactive antibodies to *Chlamydia pneumoniae*, and some culture negative endocarditis ascribed to *C. pneumoniae* were likely caused by *Bartonella*[4] spp. Endocarditis caused by *Bartonella* spp. is associated with very high antibody titers usually $\geq 1:1600$[4]. Valvular vegetations in cases requiring valve replacement, PCR amplification of the 16S r RNA or citrate synthase genes can confirm *B. quintana* infection[3]. Based on limited data, treatment of Bartonella endocarditis has been recommended with 4–6 months therapy with doxycycline (100 mg twice daily) or a macrolide such as azithromycin (500 mg once daily)[10]. However, currently the most effective treatment is unknown and aminoglycosides, ceftriaxone, ciprofloxacin, and rifampin have been used in various combinations with success[4]. The *Bartonella* spp. are very susceptible to the aminoglycosides[11,12] in vitro and the common combination of ampicillin and gentamicin used for culture negative endocarditis should provide adequate antimicrobial coverage.

1.2.1. Advances in the Diagnosis of Infective Endocarditis

Probably the most important advances in the field of infective endocarditis in the past two decades are in the area of diagnosis. Infective endocarditis is a syndrome based on the presence of multiple findings rather than on any single definitive test result. Improvement in the technology of ultrasonic imaging has paved the way for refinements in the diagnosis of endocarditis. Introduction of echocardiography in the 1970s led to the detection of vegetation on valves by non-invasive techniques. However, the sensitivity for detection of intracardiac vegetations with transthoracic echocardiography (TTE) varied from <50% to >90%, with an average sensitivity of 60–65%. The sensitivity of a TTE in detecting valvular vegetation is highest in right-sided infective endocarditis (reflecting closeness of the tricuspid and pulmonic valves to the chest wall), and lowest in prosthetic valve infection. The introduction of transesophageal echocardiography (TEE) has improved the diagnosis of suspected infective endocarditis. TEE is more sensitive than conventional TTE in the detection of intracardiac vegetations with a sensitivity varying from 82% to 100%[13,14] and averages 90–95% and with a specificity close to 98%. The TEE is particularly advantageous in the setting of prosthetic valves and for vegetations less that 10 mm in diameter. Although negative results from a TEE do not exclude infective endocarditis, it lowers the probability greatly and if the diagnosis is strongly suspected, it should be repeated in 7–10 days.

Previous diagnostic criteria for infective endocarditis were published by Von Reyn et al.[15] (Beth Israel criteria), but did not use echocardiographic findings in the case definition. The isolation of "typical pathogens" from blood cultures was not considered in the Beth Israel definition. Thus, many cases now classified as "definite" infective endocarditis were defined as "probable" endocarditis. A new set of diagnostic criteria were introduced by Durack et al.[16] and came to be known as the Duke criteria. The Duke criteria improved upon the Beth Israel criteria by including echocardiographic demonstration of vegetations or paravalvular complications of infective endocarditis, and isolation of typical infective endocarditis pathogens from blood cultures were now included as major criteria for diagnosis (See Tables 1.1 and 1.2). There have been over 11 studies comparing the Duke and Beth Israel criteria in over 1,400 patients for suspected infectious endocarditis, including patients with native or prosthetic valve involvement, and with or without intravenous drug abuse. The Duke criteria was more sensitive in diagnosing

Table 1.1
Duke Criteria for Diagnosis of Infective Endocarditis

Definite infective endocarditis

Pathologic criteria

 Microorganisms demonstrated by culture or histology in a vegetation, or in a vegetation that has embolized, or in an intracardiac abscess, or Pathologic lesions; vegetation or intracardiac abscess present, confirmed by histology showing active endocarditis.

 Clinical criteria using specific definitions listed in Table 1.2:

- 2 major criteria, or
- 1 major and 3 minor criteria, or
- 5 minor criteria.

Possible infective endocarditis

Findings consistent with infective endocarditis that fall short of "definite" but not "rejected"

Rejected

 Firm alternate diagnosis for manifestation of endocarditis, or resolution of manifestation of endocarditis with antibiotic therapy for 4 days or less, or

 no pathologic evidence of infective endocarditis at surgery or autopsy, after antibiotic therapy for 4 days or less.

Note. Adapted from Durack et al.[16] with the permission of the publisher.

infectious endocarditis and in identifying definite cases[17]. Using pathologically confirmed cases as the gold standard, the Duke criteria collective sensitivity was >80% with a high specificity and negative predictive value[18–21]. Despite these data, the Duke criteria have short comings. The group classified as "possible infective endocarditis" may be too broad and nonspecific, as the presence of only one minor criterion without meeting the rejected criteria is enough for this diagnostic label. Further issues that remain include assessment of the relative risk of endocarditis in the presence of *S. aureus* bacteremia, poor diagnostic sensitivity in suspected cases of Q fever endocarditis, and the relative role of nonspecific findings of a TEE in the diagnosis of infective endocarditis. These issues were recently addressed by Li et al.[22] from Duke University with proposed modification of the original Duke criteria. The proposed changes were based on the analysis of prospectively collected data on >800 cases of definite and possible infective endocarditis since 1984. The proposed modifications of Duke criteria include that the category "possible infective endocarditis" be defined as having at least one major criterion and one minor criterion or three minor criteria. The minor criterion "echocardiogram consistent with infective endocarditis but not meeting major criterion" should be eliminated. Bacteremia due to *S. aureus* should be considered a major criterion regardless of whether the infection is nosocomically acquired or whether a removable source of infection is present. Positive Q fever serology, an antiphase-1 IgG titer ≥1:800, or a single blood culture positive for *C. burnetii* should be considered a major criterion (See Tables 1.3 and 1.4).

Table 1.2
Definitions of Terminology Used in the Duke Criteria

Major criteria

Positive blood culture for infective endocarditis

Typical microorganism for infective endocarditis from two separate blood cultures:

   V. streptococci, S. bovis, HACEK group, or community-acquired *S. aureus* or enterococci, in the absence of a primary focus, or

   Persistently positive blood culture, defined as recovery of a microorganism consistent with endocarditis from:

- Blood cultures drawn more than 12 hr apart, or
- all three or a majority of four or more separate blood cultures, with first and the last drawn at least 1 hr apart.

Evidence of endocardial involvement

Positive echocardiogram for infective endocarditis:

- Oscillating intracardiac mass on valve or supporting structures, or in the path of regurgitant jets, or in implanting material, in the absence of an alternative explanation, or
- abscesses, or
- new partial dehiscence or prosthetic valve or new valular regurgitation (increase or change in preexisting murmur not sufficient).

Minor criteria

- Predisposing heart condition or intravenous drug use
- Fever $\geq$ 38.0 °C (100.4 °F)
- *Vascular phenomena*: major arterial emboli, septic pulmonary infarcts, mycotic aneurysm, intracranial hemorrhage, conjuctival hemorrhages, Janeway lesions
- *Immunologic phenomena*: glomerulonephritis, Osler's nodes, Roth spots, rheumatoid factor
- *Microbiologic evidence*: positive blood culture[*] but not meeting major criterion as noted previously or serologic evidence of active infection with organisms consistent with infective endocarditis
- *Echocardiogram*: consistent with infective endocarditis, but not meeting major criterion as noted previously.

Note. HACEK—*Hemophilus* spp., *Actinobacillus* spp., *Cardiobacterium* spp., *Eikenella* spp., and *Kingella kingase.* Adapted from Durack et al.[16]

[*] Exclude single positive cultures for coagulase-negative staphylococci and organism that do not usually cause endocarditis.

1.2.2. Update on Prevention of Infective Endocarditis

For many years it has been accepted conventional practice to use antibiotic perioperative prophylaxis before dental and genito-urinary invasive procedures in subjects with abnormal cardiac valves and shunts, in order to prevent infective endocarditis. These recommendations were based on limited anecdotal reports of association with these procedures and development of endocarditis in subjects with underlying significant valvular abnormalities as well as studies in animal models. This has been a contentious and controversial

Table 1.3
Definition of Infective Endocarditis According to the Proposed Modified Duke Criteria

---

Definite infective endocarditis
- Pathologic criteria ⎫
- Clinical criteria   ⎬ No change from original Duke criteria.
                      ⎭

Possible infective endocarditis
- 1 major criterion and 1 minor criterion, or
- 3 minor criteria.

Rejected
- Same as previous criteria, but now include
- Does not meet criteria for possible infective endocarditis, as above

---

Note. Adapted from Li et al.[22] with the permission of the publisher.

Table 1.4
Definitions of Terms Used in the Modified Duke Criteria for Infective Endocarditis

---

Major criteria

Blood culture positive for infective endocarditis
    Same as original Duke criteria but now include:

- *S. aureus* as typical organism irrespective of source
- Single positive blood cultures for *C. burnetii* or antiphase IgG antibody titer $> 1:800$.

Evidence of endocardial involvement
    Echocardiogram positive for infective endocarditis—same as original Duke criteria except:

- TEE recommended in patients with prosthetic valves rated at least "possible endocarditis" by clinical criteria or complicated endocarditis (suspected paravalvular abscess)
- TTE as first test in other patients.

Minor criteria

Same as original Duke criteria except:

- Echocardiographic minor criteria eliminated.

Note.   TEE: transesophageal echocardiography; TTE: transthoracic echocardiography. Adapted from Li et al.[22] with the permission of the publisher.

issue in the medical literature for the past 20 years, as there was no randomized prospective study that proved the value of antibiotic prophylaxis in preventing infective endocarditis. Many experts felt that the transient bacteremia occurring after these surgical procedures posed minuscule risk for infective endocarditis as compared with daily transient bacteremia in our lives from brushing our teeth, eating hard candies, and defecation with hard stools. On the other hand, others point to the fact that infective endocarditis is a serious infection and potentially fatal, and that relatively high grade bacteremia has been shown after dental and other procedures. The low incidence of the disease has also made randomized human trails of antibiotic prevention impractical.

Previous case series had found that 15% of patients with infection caused by mouth organisms had a recent dental procedure[23], but the risk in the general population is unknown. Furthermore, a hospital-based case control study did not find an elevated risk associated with dental therapy, except for a slight increase associated with dental scaling[24].

In a recent population-based case control study, involving 54 hospitals in the Philadelphia area, persons with community-acquired infective endocarditis (not associated with intravenous drug abuse), were compared with community residents, matched by age, sex, and neighborhood of residence[25]. During the preceding 3 months before the diagnosis of infective endocarditis, dental treatment was no more frequent among case patients than controls (adjusted odds ratio, 0.8 [95% CI, 0.4–1.5]). Of 273 case-patients, 104 (38%) knew of previous cardiac lesions compared with 17 controls (6%) adjusted odds ratio, 16.7. Among case-patients with known cardiac lesions, dental therapy was significantly less common than among controls over 3 months, adjusted odds ratio 0.2, $p = 0.03$. The authors concluded that dental treatment does not seem to be a risk factor for infective endocarditis in patients with cardiac valvular abnormalities. Even with 100% effectiveness of antibiotic prophylaxis, few cases of infective endocarditis would be preventable. Two other major studies[26,27] have presented substantial grounds on which to challenge the value of the usual practice of antibiotic prophylaxis before dental procedures. In the accompanying editorial by Durack[28] it was suggested that the time has come to scale back on prophylaxis against endocarditis before dental treatment. He suggested that antibiotic prophylaxis for most dental procedures not be recommended except for extractions, gingival surgery, implant placement, and for most cardiac conditions except prosthetic valves and previous endocarditis. When any one or more of these four high risk factors is present, prophylaxis should follow the present American Heart Association (AHA) guidelines. Mitral valve prolapse is not included among the conditions requiring antibiotic prophylaxis because the number of susceptible persons are large and the risk for the individual is lower than for prosthetic valves or previous endocarditis[25]. The proposed changes would eliminate most of the prophylactic doses currently given to dental patients. This would result in less antibiotic use, fewer side effects, and may potentially reduce the risk for antibiotic resistance, and lower the cost for patients or third party payers.

A potential problem to the practicing physician would be malpractice claims if a patient does develop infective endocarditis after a dental procedure without prophylaxis. The standard of care is evolving in many areas of medicine with our increasing knowledge from clinical trials. It is about time leading authorities or bodies such as the AHA make recommendations or guidelines primarily on the principle of evidence-based medicine. It would appear that the primary means of reducing endocarditis in patients with underlying valvular abnormalities should be aimed at educating the public in maintaining healthy gums and oral hygiene through the supervision of their dental practitioners.

1.2.3. Advances in the Treatment of Infective Endocarditis

Infective endocarditis is associated with high morbidity and mortality. For a good outcome it is essential to make a rapid diagnosis, institute effective treatment, and recognize and promptly treat any complications. Guidelines for therapy of infective endocarditis for the more commonly encountered organisms, including streptococci, enterococci, staphylococci, and the HACEK organisms (*Hemophilus parainfluenzae, Hemophilus aphrophilus, Actinobacillus actinomycetemcomitans, Cardiobacterium hominis, Eikenella* spp., and *Kingella* spp.) were published in 1995[29] and more recent guidelines on atypical microorganisms were addressed in 1998[30]. Since infective endocarditis is relatively uncommon there has been a paucity of randomized clinical trails, and these guidelines are not evidence-based but largely opinion-based by "experts," depending largely on in vitro susceptibility and animal data. However, even the animal data does not reflect the human infective endocarditis model and therefore may be of questionable significance.

Right-sided endocarditis caused by *S. aureus* generally has a more favorable prognosis than does left-sided endocarditis. Because most of these infections occur in drug abusers who have poor intravenous access and refuse prolonged hospitalization, it has become standard practice to use a β-lactamase resistant penicillin with an aminoglycoside for only 2 weeks, with cure rates over 90%[31]. However, in patients allergic to penicillin, 2 weeks of vancomycin and aminoglycoside may not be effective. In a recent small randomized trail of *S. aureus* right-side endocarditis, 31 drug abusers were allocated to receive intravenous cloxacillin or vancomycin or teicoplainin plus gentamicin for 14 days[32]. The cure rate was 100% in the cloxacillin group, 60% and 70% in the vancomycin and teicoplainin arms, respectively, $p=0.03$, for cloxacillin versus the combined glycopeptide groups[32]. It is postulated that aminoglycosides enhance the killing effect of the β-lactamase resistant penicillin and allow rapid sterilization of the valves. However, the aminoglycoside may cause adverse reactions such as ototoxicity, vestibular disturbance, and renal impairment. In a previous study from Spain, 74 drug abusers were randomized to receive cloxacillin alone or combined with gentamicin for 14 days, and the results were similar: 34 of 38 (89%) receiving cloxacillin alone and

31 of 36 (86%) receiving combined therapy were cured[33]. Thus, suggesting that a short course of β-lactamase resistant penicillin alone is sufficient for right-sided endocarditis with methicillin sensitive *S. aureus*.

It has also been shown that endocarditis caused by *Viridans streptococci* can be cured with combined penicillin and aminoglycoside for only two weeks. However, for enterococcal endocarditis the traditional recommendation has been to use the aminoglycoside (combined with penicillin or ampicillin) for as long as 4–6 weeks. The main drawback of such a treatment is the high risk of aminoglycoside toxicity, especially in older patients where the risk of enterococcal endocarditis is greatest. However, in a recent 5-year prospective nationwide study from Sweden, the results of a shortened aminoglycoside course produced cure rates similar to an experience with traditional 4–6 weeks course[34]. In this study from 1995 to 1999 in Sweden from a national registry of infective endocarditis, 93 episodes of enterococcal endocarditis was diagnosed (the largest series so far presented), where shortened aminoglycoside course is usually used to minimize toxicity. The median duration of cell wall active agent (penicillin or vancomycin) was 42 days and the aminoglycoside 15 days, resulting in a cure rate of 81%, with 16% mortality and 3% relapse rate[34]. Thus, in many enterococcal endocarditis episodes, duration of amioglycoside therapy could probably be shortened to 2–3 weeks.

Economy pressures that dictate shorter hospital stays have resulted in greater popularity of home or outpatient parenteral antibiotic therapy for infective endocarditis in the past 5–10 years. The literature on this outpatient therapy reports excellent patient outcomes in carefully selected patients[35]. However, concerns raised include development of complications such as valve ring abscess with conduction disturbance, sudden severe heart failure, or systemic embolization, which require immediate medical attention and may not be recognized promptly with home parenteral therapy or could lead to delayed management and increased mortality[36]. Thus, proposed guidelines have been published for outpatient therapy of native valve infective endocarditis, with a conservative approach (inpatient or daily outpatient follow up) during the critical phase (0–2 weeks of treatment) when complications are more likely, and outpatient management for the continuation phase (2–4 or 6 weeks) when life threatening complications are less likely[36].

Surgical management (valve replacement or drainage of an abscess) plays an important role in the complicated cases of infective endocarditis (both native or prosthetic valve), and can be life saving for those with severe heart failure, ring abscesses, dehiscence of the prosthetic valve, failure of medical therapy on adequate antimicrobials, recurrent visceral emboli and other mechanical complications, and fungal endocarditis. However, the appropriate timing of surgical intervention is not always clear and the need for valve replacement without the usual indications has been controversial. Early surgical intervention (even in those without evidence of cardiac complications) may reduce the mortality in *S. aureus* prosthetic valve endocarditis based on retrospective observations[37]. In a more recent series of 252 patients with infective endocarditis (47 or 19% due to *S. aureus*), early surgical intervention (without the standard indications) improved long-term survival rates mainly in patients with *S. aureus* infections ($p=0.04$)[38]. This trend existed even when prosthetic endocarditis cases were excluded; the median duration for survival after early surgery was >150 months versus 61.5 months in the medically treated groups ($p=0.1$)[38]. These data indicate that a prospective randomized study is needed to determine the safety and efficacy of early surgical intervention, especially in patients with *S. aureus* endocarditis.

1.3. UPDATES ON RHEUMATIC FEVER AND RHEUMATIC CARDITIS

Rheumatic fever and rheumatic heart disease are still major causes of diseases, and the most important cause of valvular heart abnormalities in developing countries. Rheumatic fever had declined in most developed countries in the past several decades and had become a rarity to most physicians practicing in North America. The incidence of acute rheumatic fever in the early 1900s was 100–200 cases per 100,000 in the United States[39]. The incidence of rheumatic fever in North America and Western Europe progressively declined over the years until it reached 0.5 cases per 100,000 in the early 1980s[39]. However, evidence suggests that there is little if any decline in the occurrence of rheumatic fever in the developing world over the past few decades. It is estimated that the incidence rates of rheumatic fever is as high as 206 per 100,000 and rheumatic heart disease prevalence as high as 18.6 per 100,000 in developing countries. A resurgence of rheumatic fever in the United States have been seen since the 1980s with eight documented outbreaks[40–42]. The first and largest of the outbreaks was reported from Salt Lake City, Utah in 1985[40]. Other outbreaks have been reported in Pennsylvania, Ohio, Tennessee, West Virginia, and in San Diego, California[42]. Unlike previous outbreaks which mainly occurred in children from low-income inner city families, these recent outbreaks were in the children from high to middle income families. The main risk factor recognized were large families with crowding. The precise reason for a resurgence of rheumatic fever and invasive streptococcal disease in North America is unknown.

1.3.1. Update on the Diagnosis of Rheumatic Fever

The original Jones criteria have been modified four times and the updated revised criteria were published in 1992[43]. Major manifestations include carditis, polyarthritis, chorea, erythema marginatum, and subcutaneous nodules. Minor manifestations include fever, arthralgia, and laboratory findings of elevated erythrocyte sedimentation rate, C-reactive protein, and prolonged PR interval on electrocardiogram. For making a diagnosis of acute rheumatic fever, two major or one major and two minor manifestations must be accompanied by supporting evidence of antecedent Group A streptococcal infection in the form of positive throat culture or elevated or rising anti-streptolysin titer. The updated guidelines also highlighted a subgroup of "exceptions to Jones criteria" for patients with chorea, indolent carditis, and previous history of rheumatic fever or rheumatic heart disease. The role of echocardiography has not been defined in these modifications but may be important, as clinical detection of soft murmurs may be difficult in the presence of tachycardia. Several studies have confirmed that the yield of carditis with valvular regurgitation increases with the use of echocardiography in patients with acute rheumatic fever.

1.3.2. Advances in the Pathogenesis of Rheumatic Fever and Carditis

The relationship of *Streptococcus pyogenes* and rheumatic fever is well established but the precise pathogenesis of rheumatic fever and rheumatic heart disease is less well elucidated or established. Advances in molecular biology and technology in the past two decades have provided revealing insight into the immunologic aspects of the disease.

The association of certain M protein serotypes of Group A streptococci with rheumatic fever over the past several decades suggest that M proteins play a role in the development of disease in susceptible hosts. The serotypes involved with new and previous outbreaks of rheumatic fever include M types 1, 3, 5, 6, and 18[44]. The epidemiological data has led to the proposal that Group A streptococci associated with acute rheumatic fever outbreaks harbor a unique antigen or epitope that is associated with the development of acute rheumatic fever and carditis in the susceptible host. Serotype-specific M protein, attached to the bacterial cell wall and membrane (and considered a virulence factor with anti-phagocytic properties) is the major candidate antigen. The α-helical coiled-coil structure of the M proteins are similar to α-helical coiled-coil structure in host tissue proteins such as tropomyosin[45,46].

The M proteins have been divided into Class I and Class II molecules based on their reaction with antibodies against the C repeat region of the M protein. In studies of streptococcal isolates there was a strong correlation between serotypes known to produce rheumatic fever and the presence of the Class I epitopes[47]. Antibodies against heart in rheumatic fever were associated with the M-associated protein I antigen[48].

The current hypothesis is that rheumatic fever and carditis are autoimmune diseases which occur in genetically predisposed individuals exposed to Group A streptococcal antigens resulting in cross-reactive antibodies to the host cardiac tissues through molecular mimicry. The streptococcal M protein[49,50] and the streptococcal membranes[51] were shown to contain heart and myosin cross-reactive epitopes that were recognized by antimyosin antibodies in acute rheumatic fever and by murine and human antistreptococcal monoclonal antibodies.

Other earlier studies suggest that the Group A streptococcal polysaccharide and the glycoproteins of heart valves containing N-acetyl-glucosamine were responsible for the antistreptococcal antibody cross-reactivity with heart[52]. Another study reported that hyaluronic acid in the streptococcal capsule might induce immune responses against the joint tissues[53]. Thus, several group A streptococcal antigens may be involved in the process.

Recently, a streptococcal gene was cloned for a 60 kDa protein associated with hyper-responsiveness and reactivity with antimyosin antibodies in acute rheumatic fever[54]. Upon sequence the gene was found to have sequence homology with Class II HLA antigens such as DR, DP, and DQ in humans.

Using newer techniques such as two-dimensional immunoblotting and N-terminal sequence analysis, other cross-reactive antigens for streptococcal-induced antibodies have been identified. In a recent study[55] of 56 patients with acute rheumatic heart disease, analysis identified creatinine kinase, two mitochondrial proteins and, at a low level, various stress proteins as cross-reactive myocardial antigens. Therefore, in addition to myosin and creatinine kinase, the mitochondrial proteins may be major antigens for auto-reactive antibodies in rheumatic heart disease. Using another approach preferential recognition of human myocardial antigens by T lymphocytes from rheumatic heart disease patients have been investigated[56]. Peripheral blood mononuclear cells (PBMC) from these patients were examined for in vitro proliferative responses to myocardial proteins in a T-cell western Assay. PBMC from a significant percentage of patients (40%) versus none of controls responded to discrete bands of myocardial protein (50–54 kDa in molecular mass). This increased to 90% in rheumatic heart disease patients versus none in controls after priming of the patients cells with opsonized Group A streptococci. Antibodies generated to the partially purified 50–54 kDa myocardial proteins did not cross react with either streptococcal homogenates, purified M protein, myosin, laminin, or vimentin, suggesting a lack of cross reactivity at the humoral level. This study suggests that 50–54 kDa myocardial proteins contain a putative antigen that is preferentially recognized by T-cells from patients with rheumatic carditis, and exposure to streptococcal antigen enhances the ability of patients' PBMC to recognize these proteins[56].

1.3.3. Host Susceptibility to Rheumatic Fever and Carditis

Antigen processing among individuals of different HLA phenotypes may differ, and individuals with rheumatic fever may respond differentially from normal subjects with uncomplicated streptococcal infection. Hyper-responsiveness to streptococcal antigens is characteristic of the patient with rheumatic fever. Higher frequencies of HLA-DR2 expression in black patients with rheumatic fever and HLA-DR4 in Caucasian patients with rheumatic fever have been described[57]. In black South Africans with rheumatic fever, HLA-DR1 and DRW6 were observed more frequently[58]. In Turkish patients with chronic rheumatic heart disease, the HLA phenotypes B16, DR3, and DR7 were encountered in a significantly higher frequency than in the control population, and DR5 was significantly less in patients than controls (possible conferring protection)[59]. The association of different HLA phenotypes with rheumatic fever in various ethnic groups indicates that the immunogenetics of host susceptibility is very complex.

1.3.4. Update on Rheumatic Fever Prophylaxis

Subjects with previous rheumatic fever are prone to recurrent episodes with repeated infections with group A streptococci. Moreover, recurrent episodes of rheumatic fever are more likely to lead to significant cardiac valvular damage than a single episode. For North America and most countries, secondary prevention of recurrent rheumatic fever is best achieved by a single injection of 1.2 million units of benzathine penicillin every four weeks. However, in a recent 12-year controlled study of 249 patients with rheumatic fever in Taiwan, prevention of recurrent episodes was better with a 3-week than a 4-week prophylaxis regimen[60]. Prophylaxis failed in 2 patients (0.25 per 100 patient-years) receiving the 3-week regimen versus 10 (1.29 per 100 patient-years) receiving the 4 week regimen, $p=0.015$. Thus, in developing countries with high incidence of rheumatic fever, the 3-week regimen should be recommended. Alternate regimens such as oral penicillin V 250 mg

Table 1.5

Duration of Secondary Rheumatic Fever Prophylaxis

Duration	Category
Rheumatic fever with carditis and residual valvular disease	At least 10 years since last episode and at least until age 40 years
Rheumatic fever with carditis but no residual valvular disease	10 years or well into adulthood, whichever is longer
Rheumatic fever without carditis	5 years or until age 21, whichever is longer

Note. Reproduced with permission from *Pediatrics, 96,* 758–764, table 2, Copyright 1995.

twice daily and for penicillin allergic patients, sulfadiazine 0.5 gm ($<$60 pounds weight) or 1 gm ($>$60 pounds) once daily, or erythromycin 250 mg twice daily have not changed. The optimum duration of secondary prophylaxis remains controversial, but prophylaxis should never be discontinued until the patient has reached his twenties or at least five years have elapsed since the most recent rheumatic attack[61]. Current recommendations of the AHA are shown in Table 1.5[62].

1.3.5. Progress in Myocarditis

Myocarditis, inflammation of the heart muscle, may present as an acute, subacute, or chronic illness and a large proportion of afflicted individuals may be asymptomatic. The insidious nature of the disease and the epidemiology has been recognized through post mortem studies. Prospective and retrospective studies have identified myocardial inflammation in 1–9% of routine post mortem examinations[63–65]. Myocarditis is a major cause of sudden, unexpected death (up to 20% of cases) in adults less than 40 years of age, young athletes, and Air Force recruits[66–68]. Endomyocardial biopsy, introduced in the early 1980s has been used in living patients for suspected myocarditis. The incidence of myocarditis in these biopsy studies have been very variable, ranging from 0 to 80%[69]. The variability in results in different studies may be related to differences in diagnostic criteria, patient selection, and inherent insensitivity of the biopsy. In 1986, the Dallas criteria for the histologic diagnosis of myocarditis was introduced[70]. The endomyocardial biopsy was considered diagnostic of active myocarditis if histology revealed infiltrating lymphocytes and myocytolysis. Borderline or ongoing myocarditis was considered if there were no myocytolysis, despite lymphocytic infiltration. The biopsy was considered negative if both were absent. Less than 10% of the patients with suspected myocarditis had positive biopsies assessed by the

Dallas criteria[71], thus, raising the issue of insensitivity and interobserver variability. A second clinico-pathological classification system was proposed in 1991[72] but has not been widely accepted.

1.3.6. Causation of Myocarditis

There has not been any major advances in the recognition of the etiology of myocarditis in recent years, except that new molecular techniques such as PCR and genomic hybridization have allowed for confirmation of the etiology in some cases which would have remain unknown. Previous diagnostic tests using serology and cultures were very insensitive. The cause of myocarditis may include a variety of infectious diseases (see Table 1.6), systemic diseases, toxins, and drugs. Viruses, especially enteroviruses are the most important causes of myocarditis in developed countries. The enterovirus genome has been identified in the myocardium of patients with myocarditis and subjects with dilated cardiomyopathy[73–75]. Viral genome has been identified in less than 20% of patients with presumed myocarditis[76] and in 10–34% of patients with dilated cardiomyopathy[77], but the insensitivity may be due to

Table 1.6
Infectious Causes of Myocarditis

Viruses

Enteroviruses—primarily Coxsackie B virus	Human immunodeficiency virus
Adenovirus	Hepatitis C virus
Cytomegalovirus	Influenza A and B
Epstein–Barr virus	Dengue virus
Measles virus	Mumps virus
Parvovirus	Others

Bacteria

Mycoplasma pneumoniae	*C. pneumoniae*
Cornybacterium diphtheriae	*Treponema pallidum*
Tropheryma whippelii	*Borrelia burgdorferi*
Leptospira spp.	Others

Rickettsia	Parasites	Fungi
C. burnetti	*Trypanosoma cruzi*	*Candida* spp.
R. rickettsii	*Toxplasma gondii*	*Aspergillosis*
R. tsutsugamushi	*Trichenells spiralis*	*Histoplasmosis*
	Others	*Blastomycosis*
		Others

sampling error with a single, tiny endomyocardial-biopsy sample. To overcome this problem of sampling error, Japanese investigators [78] have analyzed large myocardial specimens from partial ventrilectomy in 26 patients with dilated cardiomyopathy. PCR and strand-specific detection of enteroviral RNA to differentiate between active enteroviral replication and latent persistence were used in this study. More than one third of the patients tested positive for plus-strand enteroviral RNA. In 78% of these patients, minus-strand enteroviral RNA was also detected, indicating active infection. The only viral sequences detected in the patients came from Coxsackie B viruses such as B3 and B4. Genomic materials of other potentially cardiotropic viruses were not demonstrated. However, another previous report suggests that adenovirus may also be important in causing myocarditis[79]. Recent studies have also suggested that hepatitis C virus may be involved in dilated cardiomyopathy and the presence of both positive and negative strand RNA in the myocardium suggests active replication[80,81]. However, further larger studies are needed to confirm the relationships between myocarditis and hepatitis[82].

The human immunodeficiency virus Type I (HIV-1) has also been implicated in cardiac disease, with pericardial and myocardial involvement. HIV-1 RNA has been detected in heart tissue in patients with acquired immunodeficiency syndrome (AIDS)[83]. Dilated cardiomyopathy has been reported in up to 8% of asymptomatic HIV positive patients over 60 months (1.6% per year)[84]. The incidence of dilated cardiomyopathy was higher in patients with CD4 count less than 400 cells/mm^3 and compared to those with higher CD4 cell count. A histologic diagnosis of myocarditis was made in 83% of the patients with dilated cardiomyopathy and HIV nucleic acid sequences were detected by in situ hybridization in 58 patients (36 or 62% had active myocarditis). Among the 36 patients with active myocarditis, six (17%) were also infected with Coxsackie virus group B, two with cytomegalovirus virus (6%), and one with Epstein–Barr virus (3%). However, other recent studies have failed to identify HIV proviral DNA in myocardial samples obtained post mortem from HIV infected children with histological evidence of myocarditis, but immunohistochemical evidences of adenovirus and cytomegalovirus were present[85]. In vitro studies also showed that HIV-1 did not infect fetal cardiomyocytes [86]. Thus, it remains unclear whether the HIV-1 itself or co-infection with other viruses that account for the higher incidence of myocarditis and dilated cardiomyopathy in HIV infected patients.

1.3.7. Pathobiology of Myocarditis

The pathophysiology of myocarditis has been elucidated mainly by animal studies. Cardiotropic virus, such as Coxsackie virus B are taken into cells by receptor mediated endocytosis and are translated into the cells to produce viral protein[87]. The virus then replicates in the cytoplasm of the myocytes, released into the interstitium where it undergoes phagocytosis by macrophages[88]. Death can occur within 4 days in susceptible mice, but surviving mice develop marked myocarditis between 4 and 14 days after infection[89]. The second phase is characterized by infiltration by inflammatory cells, including natural killer cells and macrophages, with subsequent release of pro-inflammatory cytokines[88]. Viral clearance is mediated through activation of interferon-γ and interleukin-2 by natural killer cells, and by activated T helper cells and cytotoxic T-cells. Activated cytotoxic T lymphocytes are able to lyse virus-infected cardiocytes, and viral clearance is also enhanced by development of neutralizing antibodies[90].

There is a delicate balance between clearing the viral infection by the immune response, and continued overactive immunologic activation causing further tissue damage (see Figure 1.1). In some strains of mice, inadequate immune response can lead to persistent viral infection of the myocytes, resulting in chronic viral disease with dilated cardiomyopathy[91]. Alternatively, persistent activation of infiltrating T-cells can cause long-term tissue damage, leading to dilated cardiomyopathy[92]. The pro-inflammatory cytokines induced by the inflammatory cells have significant negative inotropic effects,

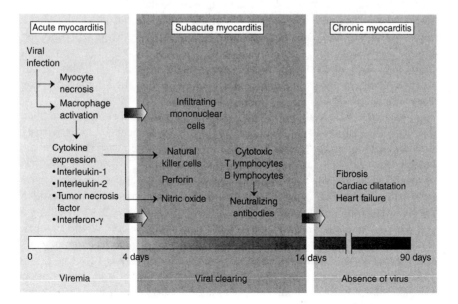

Figure 1.1. Time course of experimental viral myocarditis in mice. Adapted from Kawai[88] with the permission of the publisher.

and products of natural killer cells such as perforin and granzymes can exacerbate disease by injuring the cardiomyocytes[93].

Human studies in patients with dilated cardiomyopathy have supported the infectious-immune hypothesis derived from murine models. In patients with myocarditis or cardiomyopathy, an imbalance exists between helper and cytotoxic T-cells[94], and circulating organ-specific auto-antibodies are present in the serum[95]. However, in patients with histologically proved myocarditis, auto-antibodies varies from 25% to 73%[95,96], compared to 5% in ischemic heart disease. Idiopathic dilated cardiomyopathy has been postulated to develop as a result of myocarditis in a subgroup of patients with genetic predisposition. In a prospective study, nearly one third of asymptomatic relatives of patients with cardiomyopathy had echocardiographic evidence of left ventricular dysfunction[97] and first degree relatives had higher incidence of auto-antibodies than the normal population[98].

1.3.8. Treatment of Myocarditis

Besides supportive care and treatment of underlying heart failure, there has been no significant advances made in the therapy of myocarditis. Although there is plausible reason to use immunosuppressive therapy, to modify cellular and humoral excessive activation, controlled, randomized trials have failed to confirm any benefit of immunosuppressive therapy or intravenous immoglobulin[99–101]. Patients with acute fulminant myocarditis may benefit from short-term circulatory support with left ventricular assist devices[102,103]. Although the early mortality is higher in acute fulminant myocarditis the longer term prognosis appears to be better than acute non-fulminant myocarditis[104].

Since it is believed that most myocarditis and dilated cardiomyopathy in developed countries are related to viral infection, especially enteroviruses, then antiviral agents may be of benefit. There are isolated case reports of successful treatment with antiviral agents in myocarditis[105–107], but the benefit of treatment is questionable as most patients with myocarditis will recover spontaneously. Pleconaril, a novel compound that integrates into the capsid of picornaviruses, including enteroviruses, preventing the virus from attaching to cellular receptors and uncoating to release RNA into the cell, would be a candidate agent for further study in myocarditis. However, antiviral agents would likely be only beneficial in the early phase (within 2 weeks of illness) during viral replication. The European Study of Epidemiology and Treatment of Cardiac Inflammatory Disease is now assessing interferon-α in a randomized, placebo controlled trial[108].

1.4. CARDIAC DEVICE INFECTION—UPDATES

In the past few decades there has been a proliferation in the use of implantable cardiac electrophysiologic devices as the population of the elderly increases. Worldwide there are approximately 3.25 million functioning pacemakers and 180,000 functioning implantable cardioverter defibrillators[109]. Infection rates for these devices range from 1% to 7%[110–113]. There are two main types of clinical manifestations: (i) presence of local inflammation with erythema, swelling, pain and discharges from the device pocket, pocket infection, usually without fever or bacteremia; (ii) lead infection or device-associated endocarditis, presenting mainly with fever and continuous bacteremia, often with lead or valvular vegetation on TEE.

Infection can occur early within the first month, approximately 25%, late between 1 and 12 months (approximately 33%), or delayed after one year (approximately 42%)[109]. Sixty nine percent of patients presented with symptoms localized to the pulse generator pocket, 20% presented with a combination of local and systemic symptoms and 11% with systemic symptoms and signs alone in a recent series[109].

The most common pathogens are coagulase-negative staphylococci (68%), *S. aureus* (24%), enteric gram-negative bacilli (17%), and polymicrobial (13%)[109].

Foreign body implants are highly susceptible to microbial infection, even with agents of low pathogenicity and our understanding of the pathogenesis of these infections have improved in the past decade. The most important mechanisms in the development of these infections include the deposition of host proteins over the surface of the devices immediately after implantation. These proteins modulate host cell response that promote bacterial adhesion to the biomaterial. Neutrophils and other cells such as fibroblasts adhere to several extracellular matrix proteins such as fibronectin, fibrinogen, collagen, vitronectin, via specific cell surface receptor[110]. Adherence of the bacteria to the foreign body is a first and critical step. Several genes and gene products have been identified that enhanced staphylococcal adherence to biomaterials[111]. Adherence is followed by accumulation and the microorganisms organize themselves into a complex multilayer of cells covered with polysaccharide, called biofilm. Several organisms are capable of forming biofilms on biomaterial surfaces, namely *S. epidemidis, S. aureus* and some gram-negative bacilli, such as *Pseudomonas aeuroginosa*. The bacteria (best studied with coagulase negative staphylococci) undergo complex and as yet undefined metabolic changes that in combination with biofilm formation allow them to persist on the foreign body and become less susceptible to antibiotics and evade the immune defense mechanisms[111,112].

Optimal treatment of infected pacemaker and implantable defibrillator devices involves complete removal of all hardware, followed by antibiotic therapy and early reimplantation at a new site[109,113–116]. Patients with lead infection or device associated endocarditis should receive intravenous therapy for 28 days. Conservative treatment without removal of all hardware is frequently unsuccessful[109]. Infected devices should be removed as soon as possible as delayed removal would result in further morbidity and cost. Conservative therapy may be tried for a short time but should be reserved for patients who are unsuitable for surgical procedures[117]. Reimplantation should be done only after the continued need for such has been documented as a substantial number of patients may no longer require such devices.

There are no randomized studies comparing pacemaker lead extraction with a conservative strategy aimed at salvaging the leads and the generator. However, retrospective and observational studies have provided the basis for the above recommendation. Lewis et al.[118] described 75 patients (including 10 with epicardial systems) including 17 patients with positive blood cultures. From 32 patients treated conservatively (antibiotics, limited debridement, and irrigation or aspiration of the infected site) only one patient was cured. In the remaining 43 patients, primary removal of all hardware led to successful resolution of infection in all patients. Similarly, Molina[119] reported the outcome of infection in 21 pacemaker and 17 defibrillator patients. Infection persisted in all 12 cases treated with antibiotics only (including two deaths). Primary removal of leads and generator in 26 patients cured all of them. Brodman et al.[120] had successful outcome in 41 of 42 patients for whom all hardware was removed, and the single death occurred in a patient with persistent sepsis from a retained lead segment. However, in lead related endocarditis, surgical mortality occurred in 2 of 52 patients, and recurrence of infection occurred in two more patients with three late mortality after the surgical procedure from infection in one study[121].

Successful conservative treatment have only been reported in a few studies with substantial number of cases. Hurst et al.[122] described successful eradication in 19 patients with infection limited to the pacemaker pocket or skin erosion. Treatment consisted of extensive debridement and generous enlargement of the pocket to ensure adequate closure without tension, plus a closed irrigation system containing antibiotics and tyloxapol. Successful relocation of the generator to deeper subfascial plane in the abdominal wall was accomplished in 10 patients with exposed pacemaker without gross signs of infection[123].

In conclusion total removal of the pacemaker system or defibrillator is the most reliable way of eradicating these biomaterial-related infections. Attempts at conservative treatment should be limited to patients with skin erosion with no obvious pocket infection. If chosen, relocation to a deeper plane along with careful attention to prevent further erosion by hardware is advisable. Complete removal of the entire pacing system is recommended as failure to extract the lead may result in persisting infection. Persistence of infection has been described in 17–77% of patients in whom only the generator was removed, and mortality of 5.6–19% have been reported with retained leads[124,125].

REFERENCES

1. Spach, D. H., Callis, K. P., Paauw, D. S., Houze, Y. B., Schoenknecht, F. D., Welch, D. F., Rosen, H., & Brenner, D. J. (1993) Endocarditis caused by *Rochalimae quintana* in a patient infected with Human Immunodeficiency Virus, *J. Clin. Microbiol.*, *31*, 692–694.
2. Spach, D. H., Kanter, A. S., Daniels, N. A., Nowowiejski, D. J., Larson, A. M., Schmidt, R. A., Swaminathan, B., & Brenner, D. J. (1995) *Bartonella* (*Rochalimaea*) species as a cause of apparent "Culture-negative" endocarditis, *Clin. Infect. Dis.*, *20*, 1044–1047.
3. Dramcourt, M., Mainardi, J. L., Brouqui, P., Vandenesch, F., Carda, A., Lehnert, F., Etienne, J., Goldstein, F., Acar, J., & Raoult, D. (1995) *Bartonella* (*Rochalimaea*) *quintana* endocarditis in three homeless men, *N. Engl. J. Med.*, *332*, 419–423.
4. Raoult, D., Fournier, P. E., Dramcourt, M., Marrie, T. J., Etienne, J., Crosserat, J., Cacoub, P., Poinsignon, Y., Leclercq, P., & Sefton, A. M. (1996) Diagnosis of 22 new cases of Bartonella endocarditis [published erratum appears in *Ann. Intern. Med.* (1997) *127*, 249], *Ann. Intern. Med.*, *125*, 646–652.
5. Hadfield, T. L., Warren, R., Kass, M., Brun, E., & Levy, C. (1993) Endocarditis caused by *Rochalimaea henselae*, *Hum. Pathol.*, *24*, 1140–1141.
6. Holmes, A. H., Greenough, T. C., Balady, G. J., Regnery, R. L., Anderson, B. E., O'Keane, J. C., Fonger, J. D., & McCrone, E. L. (1995) *Bartonella henselae* endocarditis in an immunocompetent adult, *Clin. Infect. Dis.*, *21*, 1004–1007.
7. Daly, J. S., Worthington, M. G., Brenner, D. J., Moss, C. W., Hollis, D. G., Weyant, R. S., Steigerwalt, A. G., Weaver, R. E., Daneshvar, M. I., & O'Connor, S. P. (1993) *Rochalimaea elizabethae* sp. Nov. isolated from a patient with endocarditis, *J. Clin. Microbiol.*, *31*, 872–881.
8. Jackson, L. A., Spach, D. H., Kippen, D. A., Sugy, N. K., Regnery, R. L., Sayers, M. H., & Stamm, W. E. (1996) Seroprevalence to *Bartonella quintana* among patients at a community clinic in downtown Seattle, *J. Infect. Dis.*, *173*, 1023–1026.
9. La Scola, B., & Raoult, D. (1996) Serological cross-reactions between *Bartonella quinanta*, *Bartonella henselae*, and *Coxiella burnettii*, *J. Clin. Microbiol.*, *34*, 2270–2274.
10. Ohl, M. E., & Spach, D. H. (2000) *Bartonella quintana* and urban trench fever, *Clin. Infect. Dis.*, *31*, 131–135.

11. Maurin, M., & Raoult, D. (1993) Antimicrobial susceptibility of *Rochalimae quintana, Rochalimae vinsonii* and the newly recognized *Rochalimae henselae, J. Antimicrobial Chemother.*, *32*, 587–594.
12. Musso, D., Dramcourt, M., & Raoult, D. (1995) Lack of bactericidal effect of antibiotics except aminoglycosides on *Bartonella (Rochaelimae) henselae, J. Antimicrobial Chemother.*, *36*, 101–108.
13. Erbel, R., Rohmann, S., Drexler, M., Mohr-Kahaly, S., Gerharz, C. D., Iversen, S., Oelert, H., & Meyer, J. (1988) Improved diagnostic value of echocardiography in patients with infective endocarditis by transesophageal approach. A prospective study, *Eur. Heart J.*, *9*, 43–53.
14. Mügge, A., Daniel, W. G., Frank, G., & Lichtlen, P. R. (1987) Echocardiography in infective endocarditis: Reassessment of prognostic implications of vegetation size determined by the transthoracic and transesophageal approach, *J. Am. Coll. Cardiol.*, *14*, 631–638.
15. Von Reyn, C. F., Levy, B. S., Arbeit, R. D., Friedland, G., & Crumpacker, C. S. (1982) Infective endocarditis: An analysis based on strict case definitions, *Ann. Intern. Med.*, *94*, 505–518.
16. Durack, D. T., Lukes, A. S., Bright, D. K., & Duke Endocarditis Service (1994) New criteria for diagnosis of infective endocarditis: utilization of specific echocardiographic findings, *Am. J. Med.*, *96*, 200–209.
17. Bayer, A. S., Bolger, A. F., Taubert, K. A., Wilson, W., Steckelberg, J., Karchmer, A. W., Levison, M., Chambers, H. F., Dajani, A. S., Gewitz, M. H., Newburger, J. W., Gerber, M. A., Shulman, S. T., Pallasch, T. J., Gage, T. W., & Ferrieri, P. (1988) Diagnosis and management of infective endocarditis and its complications, *Circulations*, *98*, 2936–2948.
18. Cecci, E., Parrini, I., Chinaglia, A., Pomari, F., Brusasco, G., Bobbio, R., Trinchero, R., & Brusca, A. (1997) New diagnostic criteria for infective endocarditis, a study of sensitivity and specificity, *Eur. Heart J.*, *18*, 1149–1156.
19. Sekeres, M. A., Abrutyn, E., Berlin, J. A., Kaye, D., Kinman, J. L., Korzeniowski, O. M., Levison, M. E., Feldman, R. S., & Strom, B. L. (1997) An assessment of the usefulness of the Duke criteria for diagnosing acute infective endocarditis, *Clin. Infect. Dis.*, *24*, 1185–1190.
20. Hoen, B., Beguinot, I., Rabaud, C., Jaussaud, R., Selton-Suty, C., May, T., & Canton, P. (1996) The Duke criteria for diagnosing infective endocarditis are specific: analysis of 100 patients with acute fever or fever of unknown origin, *Clin. Infect. Dis.*, *23*, 298–302.
21. Dodds, G. A., Sexton, D. J., Durack, D. T., Bashore, T. M., Carey, G. R., & Kisslo, J. (1996) Negative predictive value of the Duke criteria for infective endocarditis, *Am. J. Cardiol.*, *77*, 403–407.
22. Li, J. S., Sexton, D. J., Mick, N., Nettles, R., Fowler, V. G. Jr., Ryan, T., Bashore, T., & Corey, G. R. (2000) Proposed modifications to the Duke criteria for the diagnosis of infective endocarditis, *Clin. Infect. Dis.*, *30*, 633–638.
23. Weinstein, L., & Brusch, J. L. (1996) *Infective endocarditis*, New York: Oxford University Press.
24. Locassin, F., Hoen, B., Lepert, C., Selton-Suty, C., Delahaye, F., Goulet, V. E. J., & Briancon, S. (1995) Procedures associated with infective endocarditis in adults. A case control study, *Eur. Heart J.*, *16*, 1968–1974.

25. Strom, B. L., Abrutyn, E., Berlin, J. A., Kinman, J. L., Feldman, R. S., Stolley, P. D., Levison, M. E., Korzeniowski, O. M., & Kaye, D. (1998) Dental and cardiac risk factors for infective endocarditis: a population-based case control study, *Ann. Intern. Med.*, *129*, 761–769.
26. van der Meer, J. T., Thompson, J., Valkenburg, H. A., & Michel, M. F. (1992) Epidemiology of bacterial endocarditis in the Netherlands II. Antecedent procedures and use of prophylaxis, *Arch. Intern. Med.*, *152*, 1869–1873.
27. van der Meer, J. T., Van Wijk, W., Thompson, J., Vandenbroucke, J. P., Valkenburg, H. A., & Michel, M. F. (1992) Efficacy of antibiotic prophylaxis for prevention of native-value endocarditis, *Lancet*, *339*, 135–139.
28. Durack, D. T. (1998) Antibiotics for prevention of endocarditis during dentistry. Time to scale back? *Ann. Intern. Med.*, *129*, 829–831.
29. Wilson, W. R., Karchmer, A. W., Dajani, A. S., Taubert, K. A., Bayer, A., Kaye, D., Bisno, A. L., Ferrieri, P., Shulman, S. T., & Durack, D. T. (1995) Antibiotic treatment of adults with infective endocarditis due to streptococci, enterococci, staphylococci, and HACEK microorganisms: American Heart Association, *JAMA*, *274*, 1706–1713.
30. Bayer, A. S., Bolger, A. F., Taubert, K. A., Wilson, W., Steckelberg, J., Karchmer, A. W., Levison, M., Chambers, H. F., Dajani, A. S., Gewitz, M. H., Newburger, J. W., Gerber, M. A., Shulman, S. T., Pallasch, T. J., Gage, T. W., & Ferreri, P.: American Heart Association (1998) Diagnosis and management of infective endocarditis and its complications, *Circulation*, *98*, 2936–2948.
31. Chambers, H. F., Miller, R. T., & Newman, M. D. (1988) Right-sided *Staphylococcus aureus* endocarditis in intravenous drug abusers: two week combination therapy, *Ann. Intern. Med.*, *109*, 619–624.
32. Fortún, J., Navas, E., Martinez-Beltrán, J., Pérez-Molina, Martin-Davila, P., Guerrero, A., & Moreno, S. (2001) Short-course therapy for right-side endocarditis due to *Staphylococcus aureus* in drug abusers: cloxacillin versus glycopeptides in combination with gentamicin, *Clin. Infect. Dis.*, *33*, 120–125.
33. Riberia, E., Gómez-Jimenez, Cortes, E., del Valle, O., Planes, A., Gonzalez-Alujas, T., Almirante, B., Ocaña, I., & Pahissa, A. (1996) Effectiveness of cloxacillin with and without gentamicin in short-term therapy for right-sided *Staphylococcus aureus* endocarditis, *Ann. Intern. Med.*, *125*, 969–974.
34. Olaison, L., & Schaclewitz, K. for the Swedish Society of Infectious Disease Quality Assurance Study Group (2002) Enterococcal endocarditis in Sweden, 1995–1999: Can shorter therapy with aminoglycoside be used? *Clin. Infect. Dis.*, *34*, 159–166.
35. Rehm, S. J. (1998) Outpatient intravenous antibiotic therapy for endocarditis, in A. D. Tice (Ed.) *Infectious disease clinics of North America* (pp. 879–901), Philadelphia: W.B. Saunders.
36. Andrews, M. M., & von Reyn, C. F. (2001) Patient selection criteria and management guidelines for outpatient parenteral antibiotic therapy for native valve infective endocarditis, *Clin. Infect. Dis.*, *33*, 203–209.
37. John, M. D., Hibberd, P. L., Karchmer, A. W., Sleeper, L. A., & Calderwood, S. B. (1998) *Staphylococcus aureus* prosthetic valve endocarditis: Optimal management and risk factors for death, *Clin. Infect. Dis.*, *26*, 1302–1309.

38. Bishara, J., Leibovici, L., Gartman-Isreal, D., Sagie, A., Kazakov, A., Miroshnik, E., Ashkenazi, S., & Pitlik, S. (2001) Long term outcome of infective endocarditis: the impact of early surgical intervention, *Clin. Infect. Dis.*, *33*, 1636–1643.

39. Homer, C., & Shulman, S. T. (1991) Clinical aspects of acute rheumatic fever, *J. Rheumatol.*, *18*, 2–13.

40. Veasy, L. G., Weidmeier, S. E., & Orsmond, G. S. (1987) Resurgence of acute rheumatic fever in the intermountain area of the United States, *N. Engl. J. Med.*, *316*, 421–427.

41. Kaplan, E. L. (1991) The resurgence of group A Streptococcal infections and their sequelae, *Eur. J. Clin. Microbiol. Infect. Dis.*, *10*, 55–57.

42. Ayoub, E. M. (1992) Resurgence of rheumatic fever in the United States, *Post Grad. Med.*, *92*, 133–142.

43. Dajani, A. S. (1992) Guidelines for the diagnosis of rheumatic fever (Jones criteria, 1992 Update), *JAMA*, *268*, 2069–2073.

44. Kaplan, E. L., Johnson, D. R., & Cleary, P. P. (1989) Group A. Streptococcal serotypes isolated from patients and sibling contacts during the resurgence of rheumatic fever in the United States in the mid-1980s, *J. Infect. Dis.*, *159*, 101–103.

45. Manjula, B. N., & Fischetti, V. A. (1980) Tropomyosin-like seven residue periodicity in three immunologically distinct streptococcal M proteins and its implications for the antiphagocytic property of the molecule, *J. Exp. Med.*, *151*, 695–708.

46. Manjula, B. N., Trus, B. L., & Fischetti, V. A. (1985) Presence of two distinct regions in the coiled-coil structure of the streptococcal PeP M 5 protein: Relationship to mammalian coiled-coil proteins and implications to its biological properties, *Proc. Natl Acad. Sci. USA*, *82*, 1064–1068.

47. Bessen, D., Jones, K. F., & Fischetti, V. A. (1989) Evidence for two distinct classes of streptococcal M protein and their relationship to rheumatic fever, *J. Exp. Med.*, *169*, 269–283.

48. Widdowson, J. P. (1980) The M-associated protein antigens of group A streptococci, in S. E. Read and J. B. Zabriskie (eds) *Streptococcal diseases and the immune response*, New York: Academic Press, Inc., pp. 125–147.

49. Dale, J. B., & Beachey, E. H. (1986) Epitopes of streptococcal M protein shared with cardiac myosin, *J. Exp. Med.*, *162*, 583–591.

50. Cunningham, M. W., & Swerlick, R. A. (1986) Polyspecificity of antistreptococcal murine monoclonal antibodies and their implications in autoimmunity, *J. Exp. Med.*, *164*, 998–1012.

51. Barrett, L. A., & Cunningham, M. W. (1990) A new heart cross reactive antigen in *Streptococcus pyogenes* is not M protein, *J. Infect. Dis.*, *162*, 875–882.

52. Goldstein, I., Halperin, B., & Robert, L. (1967) Immunological relationship between streptococcus A polysaccharide and the structural glycoproteins of heart value, *Nature*, *213*, 44–47.

53. Sandson, J., Hamerman, D., & Janis, R. (1968) Immunologic and chemical similarities between the streptococcus and human connective tissues, *Trans. Assoc. Am. Physician*, *81*, 249–257.

54. Kil, K. S., Cunningham, M. W., & Barrett, L. A. (1994) Cloning and sequence analysis of a gene encoding a 60 kilodalton myosin cross reactive antigen of

Streptococcus pyogenes reveals its homology with Class II major histocompatibility antigens, *Infect. Immuno.*, *62*, 2440–2449.

55. Tontsch, D., Pankuweit, S., & Maisch, B. (2000) Autoantibodies in the sera of patients with rheumatic heart diseases: characterization of myocardial antigens by two-dimensional immunoblotting and N-terminal sequence analysis, *Clin. Exp. Immunol.*, *121*, 270–274.

56. El-Demellawy, M., El-Ridi, R., Guirguis, N. I., Abdel Alim, M., Kotby, A., & Kotb, M. (1997) Preferential recognition of human myocardial antigens by T-lymphocytes from rheumatic heart disease patients, *Infect. Immuno.*, *65*, 2197–2205.

57. Ayoub, E. (1986) Association of Class II human histocompatibility leucocyte antigens with rheumatic fever, *J. Clin. Invest.*, *77*, 2019–2026.

58. Massharaj, B., Hammond, M. G., & Appadov, B. (1987) HLA-A B, DR and DQ antigens in black patients with severe rheumatic chronic rheumatic heart disease, *Circulation*, *76*, 259–261.

59. Ozkan, M., Carin, M., Sonmez, G., Senocak, M., Ozdemir, M., & Yakut, C. (1993) HLA antigens in Turkish race with rheumatic heart disease, *Circulation*, *87*, 1974–1978.

60. Lue, H. C., Wu, M. H., Wang, J. K., Wu, F. F., & Wu, Y. N. (1994) Long term outcome of patients with rheumatic fever receiving benzathine penicillin G prophylaxis every three weeks versus every four weeks, *J. Pediatr.*, *125*, 812–816.

61. Berrios, X., del Campo, E., Guzman, B., & Bisro, A. L. (1993) Discontinuing rheumatic fever prophylaxis in selected adolescents and young adults: a prospective study, *Ann. Intern. Med.*, *118*, 401–406.

62. Dajani, A., Taubert, K., Ferrierci, P., Peterm, G., & Shulman, S. (1995) Treatment of acute, streptococcal pharyngitis and prevention of rheumatic fever: a statement for health professionals. Committee on rheumatic fever, endocarditis, and Kowaski Disease of the council on Cardiovascular disease in the young, American Heart Association, *Pediatrics*, *96*, 758–764.

63. Saphir, O. (1941) Myocarditis: A general review with an analysis of two hundred and forty cases, *Arch. Pathol.*, *32*, 1000–1051.

64. Gore, I., & Saphir, O. (1947) Myocarditis: a classification of 1402 cases, *Am. Heart J.*, *34*, 827–830.

65. Blankenhorn, M. A., & Gall, E. A. (1956) Myocarditis and myocardosis: A clinicopathologic approach, *Circulation*, *13*, 217–223.

66. Drory, Y., Turetz, Y., Hiss, Y., Lev, B., Fisman, E. Z., & Kramer, M. R. (1991) Sudden unexpected death in persons less than 40 years of age, *Am. J. Cardiol.*, *68*, 1388–1392.

67. McCaffrey, F. M., Braden, D. S., & Strong, W. B. (1991) Sudden cardiac death in young athletes: A review, *Am. J. Dis. Child.*, *145*, 177–183.

68. Phillips, M., Robinowicz, J., Higgins, J. R., Boron, K. J., Reed, T., & Virmani, R. (1986) Sudden cardiac death in Air Force recruits: a 20-year review, *JAMA*, *256*, 2696–2699.

69. Lie, J.T. (1988) Myocarditis and endomyocardial biopsy in unexplained heart failure: a diagnosis in search of a disease, *Ann. Intern. Med.*, *109*, 525–528.

70. Aretz, H. T., Billingham, M. E., Edwards, W. D., Factor, S. M., Fallion, J. T., Fengolis, J. J. Jr., Olsen, E. G., & Schoen, F. J. (1987) Myocarditis: a histopathologic definition and classification, *Am. J. Cardiovasc. Pathol.*, *1*, 3–14.

71. Mason, J. W., O'Connell, J. B., Herskowitz, A., Rose, N. R., McManus, B. M., Billingham, M. E., & Moon, T. E. (1995) A clinical trial of immunosuppressive therapy for myocarditis, *N. Engl. J. Med.*, *308*, 12–18.

72. Lieberman, E. B., Hutchins, G. M., Herskowitz, A., Rose, N. R., & Baughman, K. (1991) Clinico-pathologic description of myocarditis, *J. Am. Coll. Cardiol.*, *18*, 1617–1626.

73. Bowles, N. E., Richardson, P. J., Olsen, E. G. J., & Archard, L. C. (1986) Detection of Coxsackie-B virus specific RNA sequences in myocardial biopsy samples from patients with myocarditis and dilated cardiomyopathy, *Lancet*, *1*, 1120–1123.

74. Jin, O., Sole, M. J., Buttany, J. W., Chia, W. K., McLaughlin, P. R., Liu, P., & Liew, C. C. (1990) Detection of enterovirus RNA in myocardial biopsies from patients with myocarditis and cardiomyopathy using gene amplification by polymerase chain reaction, *Circulation*, *82*, 8–16.

75. Schwaiger, A., Umlauft, F., Weyner, K., Larcher, C., Lyons, J., Muhlberger, V., Dietze, D., & Grunewald, K. (1993) Detection of enteroviral ribonucleic acid in myocardial biopsies from patients with idiopathic dilated cardiomyopathy by polymerase chain reaction, *Am. Heart J.*, *126*, 406–410.

76. Fujioka, S., Koide, H., Kitaura, Y., Deguchi, H., Kawamura, K., & Kirai, K. (1996) Molecular detection and differentiation of enteroviruses in endomyocardial biopsies and pericardial effusions from dilated cardiomyopathy and myocarditis, *Am. Heart J.*, *131*, 760–765.

77. Why, H. J., Meany, B. T., Richardson, P. J., Olsen, E. G., Bowles, N. E., Cunningham, L., Freeke, C. A., & Archard, L. C. (1994) Clinical and prognostic significance of detection of enteroviral RNA in the myocardium of patients with myocarditis or dilated cardiomyopathy, *Circulation*, *89*, 2582–2589.

78. Fujioka, S., Kitaura, Y., Ukimua, A., Deguchi, H., Kawamura, K., Isomura, T., Suma, H., & Shimizu, A. (2000) Escalation of viral infection in the myocardium of patients with idiopathic dilated cardiomyopathy, *J. Am. Coll. Cardiol.*, *36*, 1920–1926.

79. Grumbach, I. M., Heim, A., Pring-Akerblom, P., Vanhof, S., Hein, W. J., Muller, G., & Figuella, R. R. (1999) Adenovirus and enteroviruses as pathogens in myocarditis and dilated cardiomyopathy, *Acta Cardiol.*, *54*, 83–88.

80. Matsumoni, A., Matoba, Y., & Sasayoma, S. (1995) Dilated cardiomyopathy associated with hepatitis (virus infection), *Circulation*, *92*, 2519–2525.

81. Okabe, M., Fukuda, K., Arakawa, K., & Kikuchi, M. (1997) Chronic variation of myocarditis associated with hepatitis C virus infection, *Circulation*, *96*, 22–24.

82. Grumbach, I. M., Heermann, K., & Figulla, H. R. (1998) Low prevalence of hepatitis C virus antibodies and RNA in patients with myocarditis and dilated cardiomyopathy, *Cardiology*, *90*, 75–78.

83. Rodriquez, E. R., Nasim, S., Hsia, J., Sandin, R. L., Ferreira, A., Hilliard, B. A., Ross, A. M., & Garrett, C. T. (1991) Cardiac myocytes and dendritic cells harbour human immunodeficiency virus in infected patients with and without cardiac

dysfunction: Detection of multiplex nested, polymerase chain reaction in individually microdissected cells from right ventricular endomyocardial biopsy tissue, *Am. J. Cardiol.*, *68*, 1511–1520.

84. Barbaro, G., Di Lorenzo, G., Grisorio, B., & Barbarini, G. for The Gruppo Italiano per Lo Stuchio Cardiologico ei Pazienti Affectti Da AIDS (1998) Incidence of dilated cardiomyopathy and detection of HIV in myocardial cells of HIV positive patients, *N. Engl. J. Med.*, *339*, 1093–1099.

85. Bowles, N. E., Kearney, D. L., Ni, J., Perez-Atayde, A. R., Kline, N. W., Bricker, J. T., Ayres, N. A., Lipshultz, S. E., Shearer, N. T., & Towbin, J. A. (1999) The detection of viral genomes by polymerase chain reaction in the myocardium of pediatric patients with advanced HIV disease, *J. Am. Coll. Cardiol.*, *34*, 857–865.

86. Rebolledo, M. A., Krogstad, P., Chen, F., Shannon, K. M., & Klitzer, T. S. (1998) Infection of human fetal cardiac myocytes by a human immunodeficiency virus-I-derived vector, *Circ. Res.*, *83*, 738–742.

87. Huber, S. A. (1993) Animal models: immunological aspects, in J. E. Banatvala (ed.) *Viral infections of the heart*, London: Edward Arnold, pp. 82–109.

88. Kawai, C. (1999) From myocarditis to cardiomyopathy: mechanisms of inflammation and cell death: learning from the past for the future, *Circulation*, *99*, 1091–1100.

89. Matsumori, A., & Kawai, C. (1982) An animal model of congestive (dilated) cardiomyopathy: Dilation and hypertrophy of the heart in the chronic state in DBA/2 mice with myocarditis caused by encephalomyocarditis virus, *Circulation*, *66*, 355–360.

90. Tomioka, N., Kishimoto, C., Matsumori, A., & Kawai, C. (1986) Effects of prednisone on acute viral myocarditis in mice, *J. Am. Coll. Cardiol.*, *7*, 868–872.

91. Knowlton, K. U., & Bardorff, C. (1999) The immune system in viral myocarditis: maintaining the balance, *Cir. Res.*, *85*, 559–561.

92. Opavsky, M. A., Penninger, J., Aitken, K., Wen, W. H., Dawood, F., Mak, T., & Liu, P. (1999) Susceptibility to myocarditis is dependent on the response of alpha β T-lymphocytes to Coxsackie viral infection, *Circ. Res.*, *85*, 551–558.

93. Gebhard, J. R., Perry, C. M., Harkins, S., Lane, T., Mena, I., Arsenio, V. C., Campbell, I. L., & Whitton, J. L. (1998) Coxsackie virus B$_3$ induced myocarditis: perforin exacerbates disease but plays no detectable role in viral clearance, *Am. J. Pathol.*, *153*, 417–428.

94. Sanderson, J. E., Koech, D., Iha, D., & Ojiambo, H. P. (1985) T-lymphocyte subsets in idiopathic dilated cardiomyopathy, *Am. J. Cardiol.*, *55*, 755–758.

95. Carforio, A. L. P., Goldman, J. H., Baig, M. K., Haven, A. J., Dalla Libera, L., Keeling, P. J., & McKennar, W. J. (1997) Cardiac autoantibodies in dilated cardiomyopathy become undetectable with disease progression, *Heart*, *77*, 62–67.

96. Pankuweit, S., Portig, I., Lottspeich, F., & Maisch, B. (1997) Autoantibodies in sera of patients with myocarditis: characterization of the corresponding proteins by isoelectric focusing and N-terminal sequence analysis, *J. Mol. Cell. Cardiol.*, *2*, 77–84.

97. Baig, M. K., Goldman, J. H., Caforio, A. L. P., Coonar, A. S., Keeling, P. J., & McKenna, W. J. (1998) Familial dilated cardiomyopathy: cardiac abnormalities are common in asymptomatic relative and may represent early disease, *J. Am. Coll. Cardiol.*, *31*, 195–201.

98. Caforio, A. L. P., Keeling, P. J., Zachara, E., Mestroni, L., Camerini, F., Mann, J. M., Bottazzo, G. F., & McKenna, W. J. (1994) Evidence from family studies for autoimmunity in dilated cardiomyopathy, *Lancet*, *344*, 773–777.

99. Parrillo, J. F., Cunnion, R. E., Epstein, S. E., Parker, M. M., Suffredini, A. F., Brenner, M., Schaer, G. L., Palmeri, S. T., Cannon, R. O. 3rd, & Alling, D. (1989) A prospective randomized controlled trial of Prednisone for dilated cardiomyopathy, *N. Engl. J. Med.*, *321*, 1061–1068.

100. McNamara, D. M., Starling, R. L., Dec, G. W., Torre-Amione, G., Gass, A., Janosko, K. M., Tokarczyk, T., Holubkov, R., & Feldman, A. M. (1999) Intervention in myocarditis and acute cardiomyopathy with immune globulin: results from the randomized placebo-controlled IMAC trial, *Circulation*, *100* (Suppl. I), 1–21 [Abstract].

101. Latham, R. D., Mulrow, J. P., Virmani, R., Robinowitz, M., & Moody, J. M. (1989) Recently diagnosed idiopathic cardiomyopathy: incidence of myocarditis and efficacy of prednisone therapy, *Am. Heart J.*, *117*, 876–882.

102. Reiss, N., el-Banayosy, A., Povisal, H., Morshuis, M., Minami, K., & Korfer, R. (1996) Management of acute fulminant myocarditis using circulatory support systems, *Artif. Organs*, *20*, 964–970.

103. Martin, J., Sarai, K., Schindler, M., van de Loo, A., Yoshitake, M., & Beyersdorf, F. (1997) MEDOS HIA-VAD biventricular assist device for bridge to recovery in fulminant myocarditis, *Ann. Thorac. Surg.*, *63*, 1145–1146.

104. McCarthy, R. E. III, Boehmer, J. P., Hruban, R. R. H., Hutchins, G. M., Kasper, E. K., Hare, J. M., & Baughman, K. L. (2000) Long term outcome of fulminant myocarditis as compared with acute (nonfulminant) myocarditis, *N. Engl. J. Med.*, *342*, 690–695.

105. McCormack, J. G., Bowler, S. D., Donnelly, J. E., & Steadman, C. (1998) Successful treatment of severe cytomegalovirus infection with ganciclovir in an immunocompetent host, *Clin. Infect. Dis.*, *26*, 1007–1008.

106. Bagkurt, C., Caglar, K., Ceviz, N., Akyug, C., & Secmeer, G. (1999) Successful treatment of Epstein–Barr virus infection associated with myocarditis, *Pediatr. Int.*, *41*, 389–391.

107. Rotbert, H. A., Webster, D. A., & for the Pleconaril Treatment Registry Group (2001) Treatment of potentially life-threatening enterovirus infections with pleconaril, *Clin. Infect. Dis.*, *32*, 228–235.

108. Maisch, B., Hufnagel, G., Schonian, U., & Hengstengberg, C. (1995) The European Study of Epidemiology and Treatment of Cardiac Inflammatory Disease (ESETCID), *Eur. Heart J.*, *16*, 173–175.

109. Chua, J. C., Wilkoff, B. L., Lee, I., Juratli, N., Longworth, D. L., & Gordon, S. M. (2000) Diagnosis and management of infections involving implantable electrophysiologic cardiac devices, *Ann. Intern. Med.*, *133*, 604–608.

110. Vaudaux, P., Francois, P., & Lew, P. D. (1998) Role of plasma and extracellular matrix proteins, in the physiopathology of foreign body infection, *Ann. Vasc. Surg.*, *12*, 34–40.

111. Vandecasteele, S. J., Van Wijngaerden, E., Van Elene, J., & Peetermans, W. E. (2000) New insights in the pathogenesis of foreign body infections with coagulase negative staphylococci, *Acta Clinica Belgica*, *55*, 148–153.

112. Janatova, J. (2000) Activation and control of complement, inflammation, and infection associated with the use of biomedical polymers, *ASAIO J.*, *46*, S53–62.
113. Frame, R., Brodman, R. F., Furman, S., Andrews, C. A., & Gross, J. N. (1993) Surgical removal of infected transvenous pacemaker leads, *Pacing Clin. Eletrophysiol.*, *16*, 2343–2348.
114. Kearney, R. A., Eisen, H. J., & Wolf, J. E. (1994) Non-valvular infections of the cardiovascular system, *Ann. Intern. Med.*, *121*, 219–230.
115. Lai, K. K., & Fontecchio, S. A. (1998) Infections associated with implantable cardioverter defibrillators placed transversely and via thoracotomies: epidemiology and infections control and management, *Clin. Infect Dis.*, *27*, 265–269.
116. Trappe, H. J., Pfitzner, P., Klein, H., & Werzlaff, P. (1995) Infections after cardioverter-defribrillation implantation: observation in 335 patients over 10 years, *Br. Heart J.*, *73*, 20–24.
117. O'Nunain, S., Perez, I., Roelke, M., Osswald, S., McGovern, B. A., Brooks, D. R., Torchiana, D. F., Vlahakes, G. J., Rushkin, J., & Garan, H. (1997) The treatment of patients with infected implantable-defibrillator systems, *J. Thorac. Cardiovasc. Surg.*, *113*, 121–129.
118. Lewis, A. B., Hayes, D. L., Holmes, D. R. Jr., Vlietstra, R. E., Pluth, J. R., & Osborn, M. J. (1985) Update on infections involving permanent pacemakers. Characterization and management, *J. Thorac. Cardiovasc. Surg.*, *89*, 758–763.
119. Molina, J. E. (1997) Undertreatment and overtreatment of patients with infected antiarrhythmic implantable devices, *Ann. Thorac. Surg.*, *63*, 504–509.
120. Brodman, R., Frame, R., Andrews, C., & Furman, S. (1992) Removal of infected transvenous leads requiring cardiopulmonary bypass or inflow occlusion, *J. Thorac. Cardiovasc. Surg.*, *103*, 649–654.
121. Klug, D., Lacroix, D., Savoye, C., Goullard, L., Grandmougin, D., Hennequin, J. L., Kacet, S., & Lekieffre, J. (1997) Systemic infection related to endocarditis on pacemaker leads: clinical presentation and management, *Circulation*, *95*, 2098–2107.
122. Hurst, L. N., Evans, H. B., Windle, B., & Klein, G. J. (1986) The salvage of infected cardiac pacemaker pockets using a closed irrigation system, *Pacing Clin. Electrophysiol.*, *9*, 785–792.
123. Garcia-Rinaldi, R., Revuetta, J. M., Bonnington, L., & Soltero-Harrington, L. (1985) The exposed cardiac pacemaker. Treatment by subfascial pocket relocation, *J. Thorac. Cardiovasc. Surg.*, *89*, 136–141.
124. Parry, G., Goudevenous, J., Jameson, S., Adams, P. C., & Gold, R. G. (1991) Complications associated with retained pacemaker leads, *Pacing Clin. Electrophysiol.*, *14*, 1251–1257.
125. Rettig, G., Doenecke, P., Sen. S., Volkmer, I., & Bette, L. (1979) Complications with retained transvenous pacemaker electrodes, *Am. Heart J.*, *98*, 587–594.

2

Atherosclerosis and Inflammation

2.1. INTRODUCTION

Atherosclerosis is the major underlying disease leading to most cases of myocardial infarction, cerebrovascular accidents (strokes), aneurysms of the aorta and peripheral gangrene of the lower limbs. Atherosclerotic heart disease is the leading cause of morbidity and mortality in the Western Hemisphere and developed countries[1-3]. More than 50 million people in the United States alone have cardiovascular disease, with prevalence rates exceeding 61 per 1,000 of middle-aged people. There were 2.3 million deaths attributed to myocardial infarction worldwide in 1997. Based on trends in 47 countries worldwide it has been projected that atherosclerotic cardiovascular disease will be the leading cause of disability and death in the world by the year 2020[4].

In the past two decades, major advances have been made in understanding the pathogenesis of atherosclerosis, especially at the cellular and molecular levels, and new risk factors have been implicated or associated with the disease. Suffice it to say that even after nearly a century of extensive studies on atherosclerosis there remains much to be elucidated. At present 40–50% of patients with myocardial infarction do not have any of the known traditional risk factors for cardiovascular disease. Therefore, it is important to investigate and explore potential new risk factors that may predispose to atherosclerosis in general.

It is well accepted that atherosclerotic cardiovascular disease is multifactorial in etiology and pathogenesis. The mechanisms leading to the development of atherosclerosis are complex active processes and not just passive deposition of lipids in the arterial wall.

2.2. PATHOLOGY OF ATHEROSCLEROSIS

Pathologists in Europe had recognized in the early part of the 19th century that atherosclerosis was an inflammatory disease[5]. The concept that the mild chronic inflammatory reaction was a response to injury was proposed well over a century ago by Von Rokitansky (1852)[6], and Virchow (1856)[7], and more recently reviewed by Ross (1999)[8].

The lesions of atherosclerosis occur mainly in large and medium-sized elastic and muscular arteries and progress slowly throughout a person's lifetime. The earliest lesion of atherosclerosis is the fatty streak, which is common in infants and early childhood[9].

Since it is impossible to follow changes in histology of a lesion by studying the same lesion over its lifetime, the sequence in the evolution of lesions was deduced by studying the lesions of many persons of different ages, from infancy to old age.

Recent evidence indicates that the initial event is endothelial dysfunction that results from injury, which alters the normal homeostatic properties and leads to denudation of the endothelium. There are many possible causes of the inciting injury leading to endothelial dysfunction and these include hypertension, elevated cholesterol (low-density lipoprotein [LDL]), free radicals caused by cigarette smoking, diabetes mellitus, elevated plasma homocysteine concentrations, infectious microorganisms, genetic alterations, and a combination of these or other factors[8]. The initial insult to the endothelium results in increased adhesiveness of the endothelium to leukocytes and platelets, and also increases the permeability. In response to injury vasoactive molecules, cytokines and growth factors are stimulated leading to the procoagulant environment. The inflammatory response is to neutralize any noxious agents, but continued stimulation may eventually lead to stimulation of migration and proliferation of smooth-muscle cells that become integrated with the area of the inflammation in the intima of the artery to form an intermediate lesion. Continuation of this process leads to thickening and remodeling of the arterial wall.

Further inflammation causes more accumulations of macrophages and lymphocytes, which migrate from the blood to the intima and subendothelial area. Release of cytokines, chemokines, growth factors, and hydrolytic enzymes result from activation of the inflammatory cells, leading to further damage and eventually to focal necrosis[10–12]. Repeated cycles of accumulation of inflammatory cells, proliferation of smooth-muscle cells and formation of fibrous tissue result in enlargement and restructuring of the lesion to form a complicated lesion, with a fibrous cap and a lipid-filled necrotic core. This advancement and growth of the complicated atheroma may then impinge on the lumen of the vessel and impair blood flow.

2.2.1. Inflammatory Response

The earliest changes in the arteries occur where there is increased turbulence and decreased shear stress caused by alterations of blood flow, such as those that occur at branches, bifurcations, and curvatures[13]. Interaction then occurs between the endothelium and leukocytes in an active complex process, leading to adherence, migration, and accumulation of monocytes and T-lymphocytes in the intima. The leukocytes–endothelial interactions are regulated by a cascade of molecular steps—tethering, triggering, strong adhesion, and migration—mediated by selectins, chemokine or integrins (intercellular adhesion molecule-1 [ICAM-1 & 2], vascular cell adhesion molecule [VCAM-1][14]). After strong adhesion to endothelium, leukocytes migrate under the influence of promigratory factors (cytokines). Monocyte chemoattractant protein-1 (MCP-1), macrophage inflammatory protein-1α (MIP-1α), MIP-1β, and regulated on activation normal T expressed and secreted (RANTES) act on monocytes and subsets of T-cells[15–17] in conjunction with platelet-endothelial cell adhesion molecules[18], osteopontin[19], and modified LDL to attract leukocytes to the arterial wall across the endothelium (see Figure 2.1, adapted

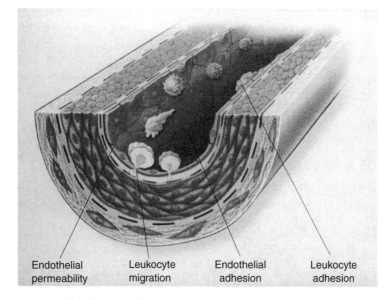

| Endothelial permeability | Leukocyte migration | Endothelial adhesion | Leukocyte adhesion |

Figure 2.1. Endothelial dysfunction or injury in atherosclerosis. The above figure depicts the interaction of the leukocyte and the endothelial as a result of stimulation of adhesion molecules; and migration of leukocytes into the arterial wall mediated by various cytokines and growth factors. Reproduced from Ross[8] with the permission of the publishers.

from Ross (1999)[8]). These chemoattractant molecules are generated by the endothelium, smooth-muscle cells, and monocytes and their expression is increased by reduced shear stress[20,21]. Rolling and adherence of monocytes and T-cells occur at these sites of turbulence and reduced shear stress as an upregulation of adhesion molecules on the endothelium and leukocytes. Chemokines through stimulation of chemotaxis then lead to accumulation of macrophages in fatty streaks.

2.2.2. Components of Atherosclerotic Lesion

The monocyte, a precursor of macrophages in all tissues, plays a pivotal role in the pathogenesis of atherosclerosis. The earliest lesion contains an influx of macrophages and T-cells, and the foam cells, hallmark of early atherosclerosis or fatty streak, are foamy macrophages laden with lipid or oxidized LDL. Monocyte-derived macrophages and T-cells replication and smooth-muscle cell proliferation are equally important in the expansion of atherosclerotic lesions[22] (see Figure 2.2). The ability of macrophages to

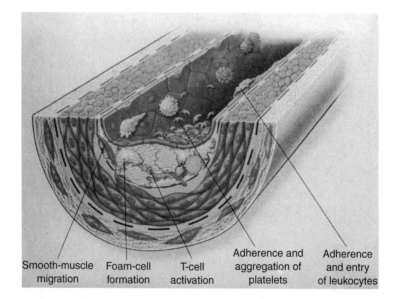

| Smooth-muscle migration | Foam-cell formation | T-cell activation | Adherence and aggregation of platelets | Adherence and entry of leukocytes |

Figure 2.2.   Fatty streak formation in atherosclerosis. The figure shows accumulation of lipid rich macrophages (foam cells) together with T-lymphocytes, and later migration of smooth-muscle cells. Reproduced from Ross[8] with permission of the publishers.

produce cytokines (such as tumor necrosis factor-α (TNF-α), interleukin-1
(IL-1) and transforming growth factor-β [TGF-β]), proteolytic enzymes
(metalloproteinases), and growth factors (platelet-derived factor and insulin-
like growth factor-1) leads to damage and repair of the arterial wall as the
lesions progress. The entry, survival, and replication of mononuclear cells in
the lesions may be stimulated by macrophage colony-stimulating factor and
IL-2. Inflammatory cytokines may both stimulate and enhance cell death of
macrophages, which make up the characteristic necrotic core of the advanced
atheroma, with lipids (see Figure 2.3). Cell mediated immune responses are
likely involved in atherogenesis as both CD4 and CD8 T-cells are present in
the lesions at all stages[23,24].

Both activated macrophages and activated T-cells result in the secretion
of cytokines that amplify the inflammatory response. Potential antigens that
activate the inflammatory response include oxidized LDL[25], heat shock
protein, through an autoimmune response, and infectious agents. Heat shock
proteins (a family of stress response proteins) may be elevated on endothelial cells and participate in the immune responses[26], and may play a role in
atherogenesis.

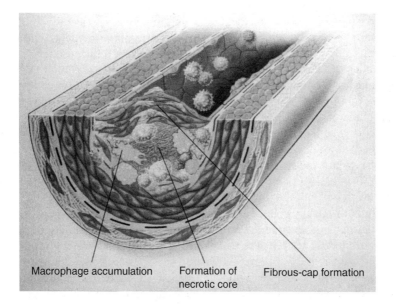

| Macrophage accumulation | Formation of necrotic core | Fibrous-cap formation |

Figure 2.3. Advanced atheroma. With progression of fatty streaks to intermediate and advanced
lesion, a fibrous cap is formed with a well-defined necrotic core, consisting of leukocytes, lipid, and
cellular debris. Reproduced from Ross[8] with permission of the publishers.

Platelets and their products may play an important role in the initiation and progression of the lesions of atherosclerosis[3] (see Figure 2.2). Initially platelets will adhere to the dysfunctional or denuded endothelium. Activation of platelets causes release of cytokines and growth factors from their granules, contributing to migration and proliferation of monocytes and smooth-muscle cells[27], transformation of prostaglandins (thromboxane A_2) via the arachidonic acid pathway, leading to vasoconstriction and amplification of the inflammatory response through formation of leukotrienes. Activated platelets also play a critical role in precipitating acute ischemic events, when an advanced atheroma rupture or ulcerate, by stimulating the formation of an acute thrombus to compromise the blood flow.

An important component of the platelet is the glycoprotein IIb/IIIa receptor that appears on the surface of platelets during activation and thrombus formation. Antagonists to these receptors have been used in clinical trials to prevent thrombus formation in myocardial infarction[28].

The inflammatory reaction leading to atherosclerosis is a chronic inflammatory fibro-proliferative disease, with mainly mononuclear cell interaction, as granulocytes are rare in atherosclerosis. The smooth-muscle cells play a principal role in the fibro-proliferative phase of the disease process. At least two different phenotypes of smooth-muscle cells have been described, based on the distribution of myosin filaments and the formation of secretory protein apparatus, such as the Golgi and rough endoplasmic reticulum[3]. Smooth-muscle cells of contractile phenotype respond to agents with vaso-constriction or vasodilation (through prostaglandins and nitric oxide (NO) stimulations). In contrast, cells in the synthetic state are capable of expressing genes for a number of growth-regulatory molecules and cytokines[29], can express appropriate receptors in response to growth factors, and synthesize extracellular matrix. Smooth-muscle cells in a lesion can change from a contractile to a synthetic phenotype. At sites where cell injury and necrosis occur, damaged smooth-muscle could secrete platelet-derived growth factor (PDGF), which activate neighboring cells to replicate and migrate, and release fibroblast growth factor (FGF) which also stimulate smooth-muscle cells, overlying endothelium or vascular channels within the lesion[30].

Smooth-muscle cells in atheromatous lesions and the media of arteries are supported and surrounded by different types of connective tissue (matrix). In atherosclerotic lesions, the matrix consists largely of proteoglycan, intermingled with loosely scattered collagen fibrils, whereas, the media connective tissue consists of Type I and III fibrillar collagen. The matrix not only acts as a cytoskeletal support but also plays an active role in cell matrix interaction. A number of the cytokines and growth regulatory factors can be affected by molecules in the connective tissue such as α_2-macroglobulin, fibronectin, and heparin sulfate. Thus, the milieu of the matrix can influence the inflammatory and fibro-proliferative response[31].

2.3. HISTOLOGICAL CLASSIFICATION OF ATHEROSCLEROTIC LESIONS

The histological classification of atherosclerosis based on Stary's definition[32] are divided into early lesions (Types I, II, and III), that are small lipid enriched deposits that do not disorganize the normal structure of the intima or affect blood flow but precede advanced lesions. Type III lesions forebode the probability of future clinical disease. Advanced atherosclerotic lesions (Types IV–VII, see Table 2.1) cause disorganization of the structure of the intima and change in the inner contour of the arterial segment.

Type I lesions are frequent in infants and children and are the initial, minimal changes without thickening of the arterial wall. The histological changes in the intima consist of small, isolated groups of macrophages, T-cells and foam cells (macrophage laden with lipid droplets). These changes occur preferentially at or near branches where adaptive intimal thickening normally occurs. Chemical and immunochemical data from laboratory animals indicate that the intimal macrophage increase and the formation of foam cells are sequels to and cellular markers of pathological accumulation of LDL in the same locations[33]. In the first 8 months of life, up to 45% of infants have macrophage foam cells in their coronary arteries[32].

Type II lesions are known as fatty streaks, visible flat, yellowish-colored streaks or patches seen on the inner surface of arteries. However, a Type II lesion may be below the endothelial surface and may not be visible as a fatty streak. These lesions increase the thickness of the intima by less than a milliliter and do not obstruct blood flow.

Microscopically, Type II lesions are more distinctly defined as lesions than Type I and consist of macrophage foam cells stratified in layers rather than isolated groups of a few cells. Macrophages with and without lipids and

Table 2.1
Histological Classification of Atherosclerotic Lesions and Associated Terms

Type I lesion	Initial lesion	}	Early lesions
Type II lesion	Fatty streak		
Type III lesions	Pre-atheroma	}	Intermediate or transitional lesion.
Type IV lesions	Atheroma	}	Fibrolipid plaque
Type V lesion	Fibroatheroma		
Type VI lesion	Complicated lesion	}	Advanced raised lesions
Type VII	Calcified plaque		
Type VIII	Fibrotic plaque		

Note. Adapted from Stary[32] with permission of publishers.

T-lymphocytes are more numerous than a Type I lesion. Intimal smooth-muscle cells may contain lipid droplets to form foam cells, but most lipid is in the macrophage foam cells. The extracellular space may contain smaller amounts of lipid droplets. Chemically the lipid of Type II lesions consists of cholesterol ester, cholesterol, and phospholipids. The arteries of children generally contain Type II lesions as the only visible lesions. Progression of Type II lesions will depend on the presence of risk factors for atherosclerosis and are more prominent at progression-prone lesions due to mechanical forces.

Type III lesions are also known as pre-atheroma or as in intermediate lesions. They thicken the intima only slightly more than Type II lesions and do not obstruct blood flow. Microscopically extracellular lipid accumulates below the layers of macrophage foam cells, replaces the proteoglycans and fibers that are normally present, separating the smooth cells and expanding the extracellular matrix. The differences in fatty acids between Type II and advanced lesions are by the overall increase in lipids and the change from intracellular to predominantly extracellular storage. However, Type III lesions have not developed a well-delineated accumulation of extracellular lipid core. Young adults commonly have Type III lesions and the presence indicates development of future clinical disease. However, Type I–III lesions can completely disappear if risk factors are drastically reduced.

Accumulation of extracellular lipid in a well-demonstrated lipid core is the hallmark of a Type IV lesion, known as the atheroma. This is an advanced lesion with disruption and disorganization of the arterial structure caused by large accumulation of extracellular lipid. The lipid core consists of extracellular lipids, cell debris, and dead cells in the deep part of the intima and the smooth-muscle cells are dispersed within and in the outer margin of the lipid core. There is a dense concentration of macrophages, foam cells, and lymphocytes on the periphery of the lipid core with capillaries on the outer border. The area between the lipid core and the lumen of the artery contains macrophages and smooth-muscle cells (with and without lipid droplets), lymphocytes and mast cells, and at this stage is collagen poor. The Type IV lesions are crescent-shaped increases in the thickness of the half of the arterial wall opposite the flow divider or bifurcation. The greatest thickness is just beyond a bifurcation (see Figure 2.4). The atheroma may not narrow the lumen of the artery except in persons at high risk, and in many persons may not be visible on angiography but can be detected by ultrasonography and magnetic resonance imaging. Although Type IV lesions are generally silent, they have the potential to develop symptoms from fissuring, hematoma, and thrombus formation. These lesions begin to appear around the third decade of life and may narrow the arterial lumen minimally.

Progressive lesion types that occur after about the fourth decade represent more advanced stages, with additional pathogenic mechanisms than lipid accumulation. A main additional mechanism involves collagen formation.

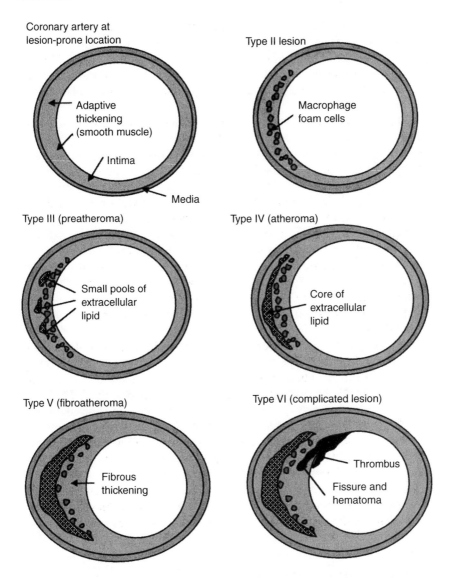

Figure 2.4. Diagnostic cross-section of a proximal coronary artery showing the progression from adaptive intimal thickening (normally present) to advanced Type VI complicated lesions. Adapted from Stary[32] with permission of the publishers.

Intimal smooth-muscle cells may synthesize increased collagen after dis-organization by lipid accumulation. After substantial collagen has been deposited in layers, mainly between the lumen and lipid core, replacing exist-ing proteoglycan matrix, the lesion is referred to as fibroatheroma or Type V lesions. Increased collagen is associated with increase in smooth-muscle cells, accounting for more of the thickness of the lesion than the underlying lipid accumulation. Capillaries may be more numerous than Type IV lesions and microhemorrhages within the lesion may occur. Lipid may also accumulate in the adjacent media and the medial smooth-muscle cells may also be disarranged.

The ischemic complications of atherosclerosis usually occur largely from complicated or Type VI lesions. The Type VI lesion consists of disruptions of the surface such as fissures, erosions, ulcerations, hematoma or hemorrhage, and thrombotic deposition (see Figure 2.4). Although complicated Type VI lesions usually have the underlying morphology of a Type V or IV lesion, occasionally they can be superimposed on a Type II lesion (fatty streak). The thrombotic deposits on the surface of the lesion often occur as a consequence of disruption of the surface endothelium, or rupture of the fibrous cap with release of lipid core, or after expansion of a lesion from lipid accumulation or hematoma, or with procoagulant systemic environment. The acute thrombus may compromise the already partially narrowed lumen of the artery and precipitate an ischemic event.

Thrombus formation on Type V or IV lesions are frequently found after the fourth decade of life in the aorta or coronary arteries at autopsy. In a previous study of a population aged 30–59 years, 38% of advanced lesions of the aorta had thrombi on the surface[34].

Some advanced atherosclerotic lesions neither contain a lipid core nor much-accumulated lipid as seen with others previously described. The intima of such lesions consists of layers of collagen, often hyalinized or with deposits of calcium or a combination. A Type VII lesion is predominantly calcified and a Type VIII (fibrotic lesions) consists of mainly collagen. In both these lesions the arterial wall is thickened and the lumen reduced. Some of these lesions may represent end stages of atherosclerotic lesions, where large accumulation of calcium may replace lipid accumulation, or after the lipid has diminished. Large lipid accumulation is associated with increased deposition of collagen which persists when lipid regresses or becomes calcified.

2.4. SYSTEMIC MARKERS OF INFLAMMATION AND CARDIOVASCULAR DISEASE

Inflammation plays an essential role in the initiation and progression of atherosclerosis as previously discussed, and also in erosion or fissure and eventually rupture of plaques. Several recent studies in the past decades have shown that various markers of systemic inflammation can predict future

Table 2.2

Systemic Inflammatory Markers in Atherosclerosis

Acute phase reactants
- Fibrinogen
- C-reactive protein
- Serum amyloid-A protein
- Albumin.

Cytokines
- Interleukin-6
- Interleukin-1β
- Tumor necrosis factor α.

Vascular adhesion molecules
- ICAM-I: intercellular adhesion molecule I
- VCAM-I: vascular cell adhesion molecule I
- E-selectin
- P-selectin.

Phospholipases
- Lipoprotein-associated phospholipase A_2
- Secretory phospholipase A_2.

Blood count
Leukocyte count

cardiovascular events including myocardial infarction, stroke, and the progression of peripheral vascular disease in men or women regardless of whether they are known to have atherosclerosis. The list of acute phase reactants or markers of inflammation associated with complications of atherosclerosis is growing (see Table 2.2), and the source of these markers is shown in Figure 2.5[35]. However, the largest body of data is on the classic acute phase reactants such as blood levels of fibrinogen, C-reactive protein (CRP), and albumin and leukocyte counts.

2.4.1. Fibrinogen

Many of the acute phase reactants are believed to modulate inflammation and tissue repair. Most of the data is on the role of fibrinogen, an acute phase reactant produced by the liver, in coronary heart disease (CHD). Plasma fibrinogen is directly related to homeostasis and the risk for thrombosis, and strongly affects serum viscosity and the erythrocyte sedimentation rate. Plasma fibrinogen is associated with a variety of other risk factors for

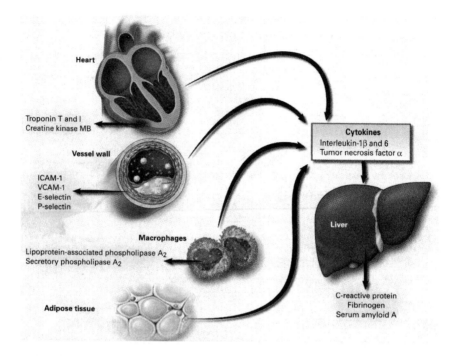

Figure 2.5. Sources of inflammatory markers and cytokines. This figure shows the interactions and sources of various markers of inflammation related to atherosclerosis, infection, and autoimmune processes. Reproduced from Rader[35] with permission of the publishers.

CHD including age, smoking, LDL-cholesterol, physical activity, and blood pressure[36]. Fibrinogen concentrations have also been consistently found to be associated with risk for CHD.

In a recent meta-analysis of prospective studies[37], 18 studies were identified involving a total of 4,018 cases with CHD with a mean age at a baseline of 56 years and a mean follow up of 8 years. Most studies made adjustments for smoking, blood lipid levels, and other standard vascular risk factors such as blood pressure. Fibrinogen is a large glycoprotein with a major role in homeostasis and increases viscosity and leukocyte adhesion. Different studies used different methods to measure fibrinogen levels, including clotting assays, nephelometry, and immunologic assays. Overall, comparison of individuals with fibrinogen levels in the top third with those in the bottom third at the baseline, yielded a combined risk ratio for CHD of 1.8 (95% CI, 1.6–2.0), and the estimated mean fibrinogen levels in these two groups were 10.3 and 7.4 μmol/L (0.35 and 0.25 g/dL). This risk ratio of 1.8 was similar to a previous meta-analysis[36], but since it involved five times as many cases, it would be more reliable.

The association of fibrinogen levels and CHD is thus firmly established, and a causal association is suggested by the consistency of findings from various prospective and other studies, as well as biological plausibility. Fibrinogen is the main coagulation protein in the plasma, important in blood viscosity[38], and acts as a co-factor for platelet aggregation[39]. However, fibrinogen levels are correlated with other known vascular risk factors such as age, smoking, LDL-concentration, physical inactivity, social class, alcohol abstinence[37], and inflammation. It is possible that fibrinogen is an end common pathway of these other factors, plus an independent co-factor, that plays a role in the thrombotic stage of precipitating acute coronary events.

2.4.2. C-Reactive Protein

CRP is another acute phase reactant produced by the liver that is less extensively studied than fibrinogen in cardiovascular disease. A major function of CRP is presumed to involve binding of phosphocholine on pathogenic microorganisms as well as phospholipid constituents on damaged or necrotic host cells. Through such a binding, CRP might both activate the complement system and promote phagocytic adherence, thereby initiating the process by which pathogenic microbes or necrotic cells are cleared by the host. These activities are most likely potentiated by CRP-induced production of inflammatory cytokines and tissue factors by monocytes. Although the exact function of CRP is uncertain, it does appear to have anti-inflammatory properties.

The association of increased serum concentration of CRP above the usual accepted reference of <10 mg/L with active CHD is well known. The interest in the involvement of low-grade chronic inflammation prompted studies of variation of CRP concentrations within the usually accepted interval and their relationship to CHD risk. CRP varies in response to more subtle influences than those found in major acute disease and smoking. A study of experimental inflammation demonstrated that CRP may increase but remain within the reference interval[40]. The variability of CRP within the individuals appears to be less than among populations. The assessment of CRP concentration epidemiological risk requires a more sensitive immunoassay than those generally available for more significant disease activity. Evaluation of concentrations in the range of 0.01–10 mg/L are possible using these "highly sensitive" CRP assays.

Seven prospective studies were included in Danesh et al.[37] meta-analysis involving a total of 1,053 cases with CHD and a mean age of 61 years at baseline and a mean follow up of 6 years. All but one of the studies reviewed used ultra-sensitive CRP assay methods, and all made adjustments for smoking and lipids, but only three studies adjusted for fibrinogen. Overall, comparison of individuals with CRP values in the top third with those in the bottom third at baseline yielded a combined risk ratio for CHD of 1.7 (95% CI, 1.4–2.1). The estimated mean CRP values in these two groups were 2.4 and 1.0 mg/L, a difference of 1.4 mg/L. Other studies of short-term design not included in this analysis, also showed correlation with CRP and cardiac complication in hospitalized patients for acute coronary syndromes such as the need for coronary revascularization[41–44]. These short-term complications, however, may be partly attributable to residual confounding by the severity of the disease that caused hospitalization.

In a more recent prospective, nested-case control study of 28,263 healthy postmenopausal women (mean age 59.3 years) followed for 3 years, 12 markers of cardiovascular risk were measured at baseline[45]. Measurements of highly sensitive CRP, serum amyloid A (SAA), soluble intercellular adhesion molecule Type I (sICAM-I), and IL-6 were predictive of the risk of future cardiovascular events. Of the 12 measures, the level of CRP was the most powerful predictor of risk in the univariate analysis (relative risk for women in the highest quartile, 4.4, 95% CI, 2.2–8.9, $p < 0.001$). Levels of several markers of inflammation were highly correlated, but correlations between lipid measures and markers of inflammation were low. After controlling for the various measures by using a series of logistic regression analyses, only the level of CRP and the ratio of total cholesterol to HDL cholesterol were found to be independent predictors of risk in women, matched for smoking, age, body-mass index (BMI), hypertension, diabetes, and parenteral history of premature CHD. In similar models that were limited to markers of inflammation, CRP remained an independent predictor of the risk of future cardiovascular events. Although a variety of mechanisms by which CRP might promote thrombosis and atherosclerosis have been proposed[46–48] there is no proven relevance for any of these putative mechanisms. Thus, it is possible that signs of inflammation detected in apparently healthy subjects at risk for future cardiovascular events may be an indirect marker of enhanced cytokine response to a variety of inflammatory stimuli that ultimately proved critical at the time of acute plaque rupture[49]. Postulated pathophysiologic role of CRP includes prothrombotic effects by increasing expression of tissue factors, activation of complement and directly related to IL-6 levels, a cytokine that promotes leukocyte adhesion to the vasculature.

2.4.3. Leukocyte Count

The peripheral blood leukocyte count is a well-established marker of inflammation and infection. Prospective studies have consistently identified an association between the leukocyte count and development of CHD. The Framingham study of 1,393 men and 1,401 women free of CHD demonstrated a significant association of onset of CHD with leukocyte count[50]. A rise of 1×10^9/L was associated with a 32% increase in CHD risk in men and 17% in women smokers. The total leukocyte count did correlate with smoking in this cohort and the changes in leukocyte count occurred within the usual normal range of values. In the National Health and Nutrition Examination Survey (NHANES-1), Epidemiological Follow-up Study, males without CHD at baseline were found to have a relative risk of 1.55 for CHD if their leukocyte count was $> 8,100$ compared to those whose counts were in the lowest fifth of distribution[51]. The relative risk remained significant (1.31) after adjustment for other risk factors such as diabetes, blood pressure, smoking, total cholesterol, and BMI. In females, the relative adjusted risk was the same. In elderly men, randomly selected and aged 64–84, the adjusted relative risk for onset of CHD was still significant (1.32) for an 1×10^9/L increase in total leukocyte count[52].

In a recent meta-analysis[37], 19 prospective studies of leukocyte count and CHD were analyzed, involving a total of 7,229 cases with a mean age of 55 years and mean follow up of 8 years. Most studies made adjustments for smoking, blood pressure, and obesity and several also adjusted for fibrinogen. Overall, comparison of individuals with a single baseline leukocyte count in the top third with those in the bottom third yielded a risk ratio of 1.5 (95% CI, 1.4–1.6). When the analysis was restricted to the seven largest studies (> 400 cases per study) and adjusted for smoking and other standard risk factors, the combined risk ratio was similar: 1.4 (95% CI, 1.3–1.5). The estimated mean usual leukocyte counts in the two groups were 8.4 and 5.6×10^9/L (upper third and the lower third, respectively), and the difference was 2.8×10^9/L.

2.4.4. Albumin

Albumin, a plasma protein produced by the liver, is a negative acute phase reactant, as CHD risk decreases with increasing albumin. In the NHANES-I follow-up study (9–16 years), there was a significant reduction in risk associated with serum albumin concentrations in middle-aged (45–64) men and women[53]. The adjusted relative risks for men and women with albumin values > 44.0 g/L compared with lower values were 0.51 and 0.70, respectively. Albumin concentrations greater than 47 g/L were also associated with an odds ratio of 0.45 for subsequent CHD-related death or myocardial infarction compared with values less than 44 g/L[54].

In the recent meta-analysis by Danesh et al. (1998)[37], eight prospective, population-based studies of albumin and CHD were analyzed, involving a total of 3,770 cases, with a mean age of 64 years and a mean follow up of 11 years. All adjusted for smoking and lipid levels, and several also adjusted for blood pressure, obesity, and socioeconomic status. Overall, comparison of individuals with albumin levels in the bottom third with those in the top third at baseline yielded a combined risk ratio of 1.5 (95% CI, 1.3–1.7). The mean albumin levels in the two groups were 38 and 42 g/L. The mechanism by which low albumin may act as a marker for future CHD is poorly understood.

2.4.5. Serum Amyloid A Protein

There are fewer studies on other markers of inflammation or indicators of acute phase response as predictors of cardiovascular disease. SAA protein is another acute phase reactant produced by the liver. SAA has been reported to potentiate adhesiveness and chemotaxis of phagocytic cells and lymphocytes[55]. There is also evidence that macrophages bear specific binding sites for SAA and that SAA-rich high density lipoprotein (HDL) mediate the transfer of cholesterol to macrophages at sites of inflammation[56], and that SAA enhances LDL oxidation in arterial wall[57]. SAA is also present in mouse and human atherosclerotic lesions and can be produced by cells of the artery wall[58]. In genetic studies in mice, the induction of SAA expression cosegregates with the development of aortic fatty streak lesions[59].

The first clinical study to show an association between elevations in SAA protein and the development of CHD in human was reported by Fyfe et al. (1997)[60]. SAA levels were analyzed in 76 sera from 36 patients after cardiac transplantation and in 346 other individuals, 85 patients with CHD and 261 of their relatives. The mean SAA level was fivefold higher in transplant patients compared with normal subjects without CHD, $p < 0.005$. SAA concentrations were also elevated in patients with spontaneous atherosclerotic CHD ($49 \pm 31\,\mu g/ml$), compared with unaffected relatives ($39 \pm 36\,\mu g/ml$), $p = 0.02$. There was no evidence for a genetic contribution to SAA levels.

A previous study had also shown that acute coronary syndrome was associated with an increase in CRP and SAA levels[61], probably associated with an increase in inflammatory activity within the plaque. In a more recent study by Ridker et al. (2000)[45], in a large cohort of postmenopausal women, SAA relative risk for cardiovascular events for the highest as compared with the lowest quartile was 3.0. The levels of CRP and SAA were significant predictors of risk event even in the subgroup of women with LDL cholesterol levels below 130 mg/dl (3.4 mmol/L), the target for primary prevention established by the National Cholesterol Education Program. In the series of logistic regression analyses that simultaneously controlled for increasing quartiles of other markers, the beta coefficients associated with SAA decreased substantially and were no longer statistically significant.

In a population-based cross-sectional study of 704 individuals without a history of CHD, plasma levels of CRP and SAA protein were strongly associated with each other ($p < 0.00001$) and inversely related to levels of serum albumin[62]. Serum albumin levels were strongly associated with blood pressure and plasma lipids and concentrations of SAA protein were strongly associated with obesity ($p < 0.0001$). The authors speculate that the study cross-sectional associations found between levels of these proteins with each other and with the concentrations of SAA suggest that some underlying inflammatory process is relevant to the causation of disease[62].

2.4.6. Phospholipase-A_2

A_2 phospholipase are a family of enzymes that can hydrolyze phospholipids to generate lysophospholipids and fatty acids. Lipoprotein-associated phospholipase-A_2 (LAPA-2) also hydrolyzes the proinflammatory phospholipid platelet-activating factor[63] and injection of this enzyme into mice reduces local inflammatory[64] and, thus, has been thought to inhibit inflammation and possibly atherogenesis[65]. However, secretory phospholipase-A_2 levels are elevated in acute and chronic inflammatory states and may predict the risk of events in patients with CHD[66]. LAPA-2 is also produced by the macrophages and could be included in this group of inflammatory markers. Several recent reports link Type II secretory phospholipase-A_2 to atherogenesis and the risk for CHD[66–68]. LAPA-2, also known as platelet activating factor acetylhydrolase, is regulated by mediators of inflammation[69] and in a small case control study was found to be a potential predictor of the risk of CHD[70]. In a more recent prospective study with a nested case control design, West of Scotland Coronary Prevention Study, LAPA-2 was assessed along with CRP, fibrinogen and leukocyte as predictors of CHD[71]. A total of 580 men with coronary events were each matched for age and smoking status with two control subjects (1,160) from the same cohort who had not had a coronary event. Levels of CRP, leukocyte count, and fibrinogen were strong predictors of the risk for coronary events; the risk in the highest quintile for each variable was approximately twice that in the lowest quintile. However, the association of these variables with risk was markedly attenuated when age, systole blood pressure, and lipoprotein levels were included in the multivariate models. LAPA-2 levels had a strong positive association with risk that was not confounded by other factors. It was associated with almost a doubling of the risk in the highest quintile compared with the lowest quintile[71].

2.4.7. Cytokines

Cytokines play a major role in mediating and modifying the inflammatory response and are important regulators of the acute phase reactants. Specific cytokines, particularly IL-1β, IL-6, and TNF-α, are largely responsible for the increased expression of inflammatory markers by the liver. The atherosclerotic plaque itself may be a source of cytokines as they can be produced by the macrophages and endothelial and vascular smooth-muscle cells. Increased levels of cytokines could also represent a systemic response to chronic infection, providing a potential link between infection and cardiovascular disease. Increased concentrations of IL-6 in blood have been detected in 60% of patients with unstable angina, but not detectable in patients with stable angina[72]. In a population-based cross-sectional study, electrocardiogram abnormalities were significantly associated independently with increases in IL-6 and TNF-α[73]. TNF-α was associated with increased IL-6 and triglycerides, while IL-6 was associated with increased fibrinogen, sialic acid, and triglycerides[73]. In a recent population-based prospective study in 1,293 healthy, non-disabled elderly subjects followed for 4.6 years, IL-6 and CRP were used as predictors for all-cause and cause-specific mortality[74]. Higher IL-6 levels were associated with twofold greater risk of death for the highest quartile (≥ 3.9 pg/ml) compared with the lowest quartile of 1.9 pg/ml (95% CI, 1.2–3.1). Higher CRP (≥ 2.98 mg/L) levels were also associated with increased risk (RR = 1.6, 95% CI, 1.0–2.6). Subjects with elevations of both IL-6, and CRP were 2.6 times more likely to die during follow up than those with low levels for both measurements. Similar results were found for cardiovascular and non-cardiovascular causes of death, as well as when subjects were stratified for sex, smoking status, and prior cardiovascular disease. Results were independent of age, sex, BMI, history of smoking, diabetes, cardiovascular disease, and markers such as fibrinogen, albumin, and leukocyte count.

In another prospective study involving 14,916 apparently healthy men, followed up for 6 years, 202 participants subsequently developed myocardial infarction and 202 matched controls, for age and smoking status, and those who remained free of vascular disease were selected for analysis[75]. Median IL-6 concentrations at baseline were higher among men who subsequently had a myocardial infarction than among those who did not (1.81 vs. 1.46 pg/ml, $p = 0.002$). The risk of future myocardial infarction increased with increasing quartiles of baseline IL-6 concentration, men in the highest quartile had a relative risk 2.3 times higher than those in the lowest quartile (95% CI, 1.3–4.3, $p = 0.005$); and for each quartile increase there was a 38% increase in risk ($p = 0.001$). This relationship remained significant after adjustment for other cardiovascular risk factors, including CRP, and was present in all low-risk subgroups including non-smokers[75].

Elevation of CRP may be a surrogate of IL-6 activity[76], and IL-6 may just be another marker rather than a cause of disease as preclinical atherosclerosis is itself an inflammatory stimulus. IL-6 is also raised in autoimmune and other inflammatory diseases and also increases with infection[77,78]. On the other hand, IL-6 may play a direct role in atherogenesis, as macrophages, which can produce IL-6 are abundant in atherosclerotic plaques, and IL-6 genes transcripts are expressed in human atheroma[79].

IL-6 concentrations in coronary sinus blood immediately after percutaneous transluminal coronary angioplasty (PTCA) also has been reported to have a positive correlation with late restenosis after 6 months ($r = 0.73$, $p < 0.001$)[80].

IL-6 is a pleotropic cytokine with a broad range of humoral and cellular immune effects relating to inflammation, host defense, and tissue injury. It is usually produced in response to stimulation by TNF-α, IL-1, and interferon-γ. Increasing levels of IL-1 receptor antagonist (Ra) and IL-6 during the first 2 days of hospitalizations in unstable angina are associated with increased risk in hospital of coronary events[81]. Interestingly, the IL-1 receptor antagonist genotype IL-RNA has been found to be significantly associated with single vessel coronary artery disease[82]. Mean serum IL-1β concentrations are also significantly higher in patients with angina with or without $>50\%$ stenosis compared with age-matched controls and did not correlate with leukocyte count, fibrinogen, or CRP[83]. Plasma concentrations of TNF-α have been found to be persistently elevated at 8.9 months after acute myocardial infarction in patients at increased risk for recurrent coronary events, compared to age, sex-matched controls free of these events, $p = 0.02$[84].

2.4.8. Adhesion Molecules

These cell surface molecules are expressed and upregulated by cytokines, and proteolysis results in soluble fragments—the portions of these molecules that are actually measured in blood. The endothelial cell adhesion molecules play an important role in the development of atherosclerosis and inflammatory disease, and the source of these markers is the arterial wall itself, particularly the endothelial and smooth-muscle cells. Markers in this category include soluble ICAM-1, VCAM-1, E-selectin, and P-selectin. Most of the studies so far on these markers were with ICAM-1, which mediates adhesion and transmigration of monocytes to the vessel wall[85]. Increased levels likely indicate endothelial cell activation and inflammation.

Soluble ICAM-1 levels were independently predictive of the risk of cardiovascular events; the risk of future myocardial infarction was 80% higher in men with the highest baseline quartile compared with men in the lowest quartile[86]. Although soluble ICAM-1 levels were associated with fibrinogen, HDL, homocysteine, triglycerides, and CRP, adjustment for these risk factors did not substantially decrease the relative risk associated with elevated concentrations of ICAM-1. In another study by the same group in women, ICAM-1 levels were also significantly associated with the cardiovascular events, relative risk for the highest compared to the lowest quartile 2.6, but the association was not significant after adjustment for the quartile of CRP[45]. Serum concentrations of soluble ICAM-1 have also been shown to be significantly higher in patients with stable angina, unstable angina and myocardial infarction compared with healthy controls[87]. Similar findings were found in another study when soluble ICAM-1 levels were measured in blood from the coronary sinus and aortic root of patients with unstable angina (20), stable exertional angina (19), and control subjects (16)[88]. The ICAM-1 levels were significantly higher in patients with unstable angina compared to those with stable angina or controls.

However, when 100 men with angiographically documented coronary stenosis ($>50\%$ obstruction) were compared to 100 age, sex, and smoking-matched controls with no history of CHD, plasma ICAM-1 was not significantly different between the groups, but CRP, SAA, and IL-6 were increased in patients with CHD[89]. A limitation of this study is that the control group could have had significant coronary artery stenosis without symptoms. In a similar study of cross-sectional design, 60 patients with angiographically proven CHD were compared with 60 controls with no evidence of stenosis on angiogram[90]. Of the markers examined, TNF-α receptor II (RII), IL-2 receptor, ICAM-1, VCAM-1, and E-selectin, only ICAM-1 and soluble TNF-α RII were independently correlated with the presence of CHD after multivariate logistic regression analysis[90]. In patients with familial hypercholesterolemia compared to healthy controls and using carotid artery intima media thickness (IMT), VCAM, ICAM, or E-selectin was not predictive of the presence or severity of atherosclerosis[91].

Endothelial dysfunction correlates with increased risk of atherothrombosis and cardiovascular disease. Determinants of endothelium-dependent vascular dysfunction include CRP levels and CD8 lymphocyte expression of ICAM-1 ($p = 0.001$), in 31 men with angiographical evidence of CHD[92]. However, in another study of 52 patients with uncomplicated hypercholesterolemia compared with 43 healthy controls, ICAM-1, VCAM-1, and E-selectin levels were not correlated with endothelium-dependent vasodilation[93], indicating that these adhesion molecules levels could not detect early hypercholesterolemic atherosclerosis. These latter studies imply that the adhesion molecules are not elevated in early, asymptomatic stages of atherosclerosis, counterintuitive to what is expected since the adhesion molecules are involved in the early initiation of atherogenesis. Alternatively, since the negative studies were in subjects with familial hypercholesterolemia, there may be differences in the pathogenesis or inflammatory response between populations with different risk factors.

Other studies have found that soluble VCAM-1 and E-selectin, but not ICAM-1 discriminate endothelium injury (assessed angiographically) in patients with documented CHD[94]. VCAM-1 was also increased in patients with unstable angina compared with healthy controls[95]. Although both increased ICAM-1 and VCAM-1 were increased in men with CHD, premenopausal or postmenopausal women with CHD taking estrogen demonstrate only increased VCAM[96]. This may be related to a recent observation that hormone replacement in postmenopausal women with CHD can reduce ICAM-1 levels but does not affect the concentrations of VCAM-1 and E-selectin[97]. Interestingly, although simvastatin reduced the total LDL cholesterol, it had no effect on any of the adhesion molecule levels[97].

2.5. CONCLUSION

There is conclusive evidence that atherosclerosis is a complex inflammatory process that begins early in life. Inflammatory reaction has been demonstrated in various stages of the atheromatous lesions in human and animal models. Furthermore, systemic markers of inflammation can predict future cardiovascular events in healthy populations. The process of initiation of atherosclerosis is not unlike that of the clotting cascade and similar to the inflammatory cascade in chronic infection. The differences may be only in the degree and extent of stimulation of the various reactions, and to specific types of cytokines stimulated which may dictate the type of cellular response. Whatever the nature of the initial insult that leads to endothelial injury, there follows a cascade of events—increased expression of adhesion molecules that stimulate adhesion, aggregation, and migration of leukocytes; upregulation of proinflammatory cytokines that causes further accumulation of leukocytes, foam cells, and lipids and at the same time stimulate hepatocytes to increase acute phase reactants; continued stimulation of cytokines and various tissue growth factors that influence migration and proliferation of smooth-muscle cells, fibroblasts, and leukocytes. It has been postulated that IL-6, an end product of TNF-α and IL-1β upregulation, is the central mediator of cardiovascular risk associated with chronic inflammation, smoking, diabetes, and visceral obesity[98,99]. IL-6 is a powerful inducer of the hepatic acute phase response, such as fibrinogen, CRP, and SAA, which are strong risk factors for

CHD, and is associated with increased blood viscosity, platelet number, and activity. Furthermore, raised SAA lowers HDL-cholesterol levels (which are protective against atherosclerosis). IL-6 also decreased lipoprotein lipase (LPL) activity and monomeric LPL levels in plasma, which increases macrophage uptake of lipids. In fatty streaks and the fibrous caps and shoulder regions of atheroma, macrophage foam cells and smooth-muscle cells express IL-6, along with IL-1β and TNF-α, indicating that the cytokines play a role in atherogenesis. Furthermore, circulating IL-6 stimulates the hypothalmic-pituitary-adrenal axis, activation of which is associated with central obesity, hypertension, and insulin resistance[99].

REFERENCES

1. McMillan, G. (1995) Historical review of research or atherosclerosis, *Adv. Exp. Med. Biol.*, *369*, 1–6.
2. Ross, R. (1986) The pathogenesis of atherosclerosis—an update, *N. Engl. J. Med.*, *314*, 488–500.
3. Ross, R. (1993) The pathogenesis of atherosclerosis: a perspective for the 1990s, *Nature*, *362*, 801–809.
4. Murray, C. J., & Lopez, A. D. (1997) Alternative projections of mortality and disability by cause, 1990–2020: global burden of disease study, *Lancet*, *349*, 1498–1504.
5. Nieto, J. F. (1998) Infections and atherosclerosis. New clues from an old hypothesis? *Am. J. Epidemiol.*, *148*, 937–948.
6. Von Rokitansky, C. A. (1852) Manual of pathological anatomy [Trans. G. I. Day], (Vol. 4, pp. 201–208), London: The Sydenham Society.
7. Virchow, R. (1856) Gesammelte Abhandlungen zur Wissen-Schaftilichen medium: phlogose ung thrombose in Yefussystem (pp. 458–463), Berlin: Meidinger Sohn and Co.
8. Ross, R. (1999) Mechanisms of disease: atherosclerosis—an inflammatory disease [review], *N. Engl. J. Med.*, *340*, 115–126.
9. Napoli, C., D'Armiento, F. P., Mancini, F. P., Postiglione, A., Witztum, J. L., Palumbo, G., & Palinski, W. (1997) Fatty streak formation occurs in human fetal aortas and is greatly enhanced by maternal hypercholesterolemia: intimal accumulation of low density lipoprotein and its oxidation precede monocyte recruitment into early atherosclerotic lesions, *J. Clin. Invest.*, *100*, 2680–2690.
10. Libby, P., & Ross, R. (1996) Cytokines and growth regulatory molecules, in V. Fuster, R. Ross, & E. J. Topol (Eds.) *Atherosclerosis and coronary artery disease* (Vol. I, pp. 585–594), Philadelphia: Lippincott-Raven.
11. Raines, E. W., Rosefeld, M. E., & Ross, R. (1996) The role of macrophages, in V. Fuster, R. Ross, & E. J. Topol (Eds.) *Atherosclerosis and coronary artery disease* (Vol. I, pp. 539–555), Philadelphia: Lippincott-Raven.

12. Falk, E., Shah, P. K., & Fuster, V. (1996) Pathogenesis of plaque disruption, in V. Fuster, R. Ross, & E. J. Topol (Eds.) *Atherosclerosis and coronary artery disease*, (Vol.1, pp. 492–510), Philadelphia: Lippincott-Raven.

13. Gotlieb, A. I., & Languille, B. L. (1996) The role of rheology in atherosclerotic coronary artery disease, in V. Fuster, R. Ross, & E. J. Topol (Eds.) *Atherosclerosis and coronary artery disease* (Vol. 1, pp. 595–606), Philadelphia: Lippincott-Raven.

14. Adams, D. H., & Shaw, S. (1994) Leucocyte-endothelial interactions and regulations of leucocyte migration (review), *Lancet, 343*, 831–836.

15. Tanaka, Y., Adams, D. H., Hubscher, S., Hirano, H., Sieberlist, U., & Shaw, S. (1993) T-cell adhesion induced by proteoglycan-immobilized cytokine MIP-1β, *Nature, 361*, 79–82.

16. Taub, D. D., Conlon, K., Lloyd, A. R., Oppenheim, J. J., & Kelvin, D. J. (1993) Preferential migration of activated human CD4+ and CD8+ T-cells in response to MIP-1α and MIP-1β, *Science, 260*, 355–358.

17. Schall, T. J. (1991) Biology of the RANTES/SIS cytokine family, *Cytokine, 3*, 165–183.

18. Muller, W. A., Weigl, S. A., Deng, X., & Phillips, D. M. (1993) PECAM-I is required for transendothelial migration of leucocytes, *J. Exp. Med., 179*, 449–460.

19. Giachelli, C. M., Lombardi, D., Johnson, R. J., Murry, C. E., & Almeida, M. (1998) Evidence for a role of osteopontin in macrophage infiltration in response to pathological stimuli in vivo, *Am. J. Pathol., 152*, 353–358.

20. Nagel, T., Resnick, N., Arkinson, W. J., Dewey, C. F. Jr., & Gimbrone, M. A. Jr. (1994) Shear stress selectively upregulates intercellular adhesion molecule-1 expression in cultured human vascular endothelial cells, *J. Clin. Invest., 94*, 885–891.

21. Mondy, J. S., Lindner, V., Miyashimo, J. K., Berk, B. C., Dean, R. H., & Geary, R. L. (1997) Platelet-derived growth factor ligand and receptor expression in response to altered blood flow in vivo, *Circ. Res., 81*, 320–327.

22. Rosenfeld, M., & Ross, R. (1990) Macrophage and smooth muscle cell proliferation in atherosclerotic lesions of WHHL and comparably hypercholesterolemic fed rabbits, *Arteriosclerosis, 10*, 680–687.

23. Hannson, G. K., & Libby, P. (1996) The role of the lymphocytes, in V. Fuster, R. Ross, & E. J. Topol (eds.) *Atherosclerosis and coronary artery disease* (Vol. 1, pp. 557–568), Philadelphia: Lippincott-Raven.

24. Hannson, G. K., Jonasson, L., Siefert, P. S., & Stemme, S. (1989) Immune mechanisms in atherosclerosis, *Arteriosclerosis, 9*, 567–578.

25. Stemme, S., Faber, B., Holm, J., Wiklund, O., Witztum, J. L., & Hannson, G. K. (1995) T-lymphocytes from human atherosclerotic plaques recognized oxidized low density lipoprotein, *Proc. Natl. Acad. Sci. USA, 92*, 3893–3897.

26. Wick, G., Romen, M., Amberger, A., Metzler, B., Mayer, M., Falkensammer, G., & Xu, Q. (1997) Atherosclerosis, autoimmunity and vascular associated lymphoid tissue, *FASEB J. 11*, 1199–1207.

27. Bombeli, T., Schwartz, B. R., & Harlan, J. M. (1998) Adhesion of activated platelets to endothelial cells: evidence for a GP IIbIIIa-dependent bridging mechanism and novel roles for endothelial intercellular adhesion molecule I (ICAM-I), $\alpha_v\beta_3$ integrin, and GP1bα, *J. Exp. Med., 187*, 329–339.

28. Badimon, J. J., Meyer, B., Feigen, L. P., Baron, D. A., Chesebro, J. H., Fuster, V., & Badimon, L. (1997) Thrombosis triggered by severe arterial lesions is inhibited by oral administration of a glycoprotein IIb/IIIa antagonist, *Eur. J. Clin. Invest.*, *27*, 568–574.

29. Sjölund, M., Hedin, U., Sejersen, T., Heldin, C. H., & Thyberg, J. J. (1988) Arterial smooth muscle cell expresses platelet derived growth factor (PDGF), A chain mRNA, secrete a PDGF-like mitogen, and bind exogenous PDGF in a phenotype-and growth state dependent manner, *J. Cell Biol.*, *106*, 403–413.

30. Baird, A., & Böhlen, P. (1990) Fibroblast growth factors, in M. B. Sporn & A. B. Roberts (Eds.), *Peptide growth factors and their receptors* (pp. 369–418), Berlin: Springer.

31. Smith, R. E., Hogaboam, C. M., Stricter, R. M., Lukacs, N. W., & Kinkrel, S. L. (1997) Cell-to-cell and cell-to-matrix interactions mediate chemokine expression: an important component of the inflammatory lesion, *J. Leukoc. Biol.*, *62*, 612–619.

32. Stary, H. C. (1996) The histological classification of atherosclerotic lesions in human coronary arteries, in V. Fuster, R. Ross, & E. J. Topol (Eds.), *Atherosclerosis and coronary artery disease* (Vol. I, pp. 463–474), Philadelphia: Lippincott-Raven.

33. Schwenke, D. C., & Carew, T. E. (1989) The initiation of atherosclerotic lesions in cholesterol-fed rabbits I. Focal increase in arterial LDL concentrations precede development of fatty streak lesions, *Arteriosclerosis*, *9*, 895–907.

34. Yin, J., & Stary, H. C. (1994) Differences in thrombosis and composition of advanced atherosclerotic lesions between natives and non-natives of Alaska, *FASEB J.*, *8*, A268.

35. Rader, D. J. (2000) Inflammatory markers of coronary risk (Editorial), *N. Engl. J. Med.*, *343*, 1179–1182.

36. Ernst, E., & Resch, K. L. (1993) Fibrinogen as a cardiovascular risk factor, *Ann. Intern. Med.*, *118*, 956–963.

37. Danesh, J., Colins, R., Appleby, P., & Peto, R. (1998) Association of fibrinogen, C-reactive protein, albumin or leucocyte count with coronary heart disease: meta analysis of prospective studies, *JAMA*, *279*, 1477–1482.

38. Thompson, W. D., Stirk, C. M., & Smith, E. B. (1992) Fibrin degradation products as the pathological growth stimulus to atherosclerotic plaque formation, in E. Ernest, W. Koenig, G. D. O. Lowe, & T. W. Meade (Eds.), *Fibrinogen: a "new" cardiovascular risk factor* (pp. 35–40), Vienna: Blackwell-MZW.

39. Simzinger, H., & Pirich C. (1992) Platelet function and fibrinogen, in E. Ernst, W. Koenig, G. D. O. Lowe, & T. W. Meade (Eds.), *Fibrinogen: a "new" cardiovascular risk factor* (pp. 46–50), Vienna: Blackwell-MZW.

40. Chambers, R. E., Hutton, C. W., Dieppe, P. A., & Whicher, J. T. (1991) Comparative study of C-reactive protein and serum amyloid A protein in experimental inflammation, *Ann. Rhem. Dis.*, *150*, 677–679.

41. Luizzo, G., Biasucci, L. M., Gallimore, J. R., Grillo, R. L., Rebuzzi, A. G., Pepys, M. B., & Maseri, A. (1994) The prognostic value of C-reactive protein and serum amyloid A protein in severe unstable angina, *N. Engl. J. Med.*, *331*, 417–424.

42. Oltrona, L., Merlini, P. A., & Pezzano, A. (1995) C-reactive protein and serum amyloid A protein in unstable angina, *N. Engl. J. Med.*, *332*, 399.
43. Pietila, K. O., Harmoinen, A. P., Jokincity, J., & Pasternack, A. I. (1996) Serum C-reactive protein concentration in acute myocardial infarction and its relationship to mortality during 24 months of follow up in patients with thrombolytic therapy, *Eur. Heart J.*, *17*, 1345–1349.
44. Mach, F., Lovis, C., Gaspoz, J. M., Unger, P. F., Bouillie, M., Urban, P., & Rutishauser, W. (1997) C-reactive protein as a marker for acute coronary syndromes, *Eur. Heart J.*, *18*, 1897–1902.
45. Ridker, P. M., Hennekens, C. H., Buring, J. E., & Rifali, N. (2000) C-reactive protein and other markers of inflammation in the prediction of cardiovascular disease in women, *N. Engl. J. Med.*, *342*, 836–842.
46. Cermak, J. C., Key, N. S., Bach, R. R., Balla, J., Jacob, H. S., & Vercelloth, G. M. (1993) C-reactive protein induces peripheral blood monocytes to synthesize tissue factor, *Blood*, *82*, 513–520.
47. Pepys, M. B., Rowe, I. F., & Baltz, M. L. (1985) C-reactive protein: binding to lipids and lipoproteins, *Int. Rev. Exp. Pathol.*, *27*, 83–111.
48. Lagrand, W. K., Niessen, H. W. M., Wolbink, G. J., Jaspars, L. H., Visser, C. A., Verheugt, F. W., Meijers, C. J., & Hack, C. E. (1997) C-reactive protein colocalizes with complement in human hearts during acute myocardial infarction, *Circulation*, *95*, 97–103.
49. Maseri, A. (1997) Inflammation, atherosclerosis and ischaemic events—exploring the hidden side of the moon, *N. Engl. J. Med.*, *336*, 1014–1016.
50. Kanel, W. B., Anderson, K., & Wilson, P. W. F. (1992) White blood count and cardiovascular disease, *JAMA*, *267*, 1253–1256.
51. Gillum, R. F., Ingram, D. D., & Makuc, D. M. (1993) White blood cell count, coronary artery disease and death: the NHANES I—Epidemiological follow up study, *Am. Heart J.*, *125*, 855–863.
52. Wiejenberg, M. P., Feskens, E. J. M., & Kromhout, D. (1996) White blood cell count and the risk of coronary heart disease and all-cause mortality in elderly men, *Arterioscler. Thromb. Vasc. Biol.*, *16*, 499–503.
53. Gillum, R. F., & Makuc, D. M. (1992) Serum albumin, coronary heart disease and death, *Am. Heart J.*, *123*, 507–513.
54. Kuller, L. H., Eichner, J. E., Orchard, J. T., Grandits, G. A., & Tracy, R. P. (1991) The reaction between serum albumin levels and risk of coronary disease in the Multiple Risk Factor Intervention Trial, *Am. J. Epidemiol.*, *134*, 1266–1277.
55. Xu, L., Badolato, R., Murphy, W. J., Longo, D. L., Anver, M., Hale, S., Oppenheim, J. J., & Wang, J. M. (1995) A novel biological function of serum amyloid A-induction of T-lymphocyte migration and adhesion, *J. Immunol.*, *155*, 1184–1190.
56. Kisilevsky, R., & Subrahmanyan, L. (1992) Serum amyloid A changes high density lipoproteins cellular affinity, *Lab. Invest.*, *66*, 778–785.
57. Berliner, J. A., Navab, M., Fogelman, A. M., Frank, J. S., Demer, L. L., Edwards, P. A., Watson, A. D., & Lusis, A. J. (1995) Atherosclerosis basic mechanisms—oxidation, inflammation and genetics, *Circulation*, *91*, 2488–2496.

58. Meek, R. L., Urieli-Shoval, S., & Benditt, E. P. (1994) Expression of apolipo-protein serum amyloid A mRNA in human atherosclerotic lesions and cultured vascular cells: implications for serum amyloid A, *Proc. Acad. Sci. USA*, *91*, 3186–3190.

59. Liao, F., Lusis, A. J., Berliner, J. A., Fogelman, A. M., Kindy, M., de Beer, M. C., & de Beer, F. C. (1994) Serum amyloid A, protein family: differential induction by oxidized lipids in mouse strains, *Arterioscler. Thromb.*, *14*, 1475–1479.

60. Fyfe, A. I., Rottenberg, L. S., de Beer, F. C., Cantor, R. M., Rotter, J. I., & Lusis, A. J. (1997) Association between serum amyloid A, proteins and coronary artery disease: evidence from two distinct atherosclerotic process, *Circulation*, *96*, 2914–2919.

61. Luizzo, G., Biasucci, L. M., Gallimore, J. R., Grillo, R. L, Rebuzzi, A. G., Pepys, M. B., & Maseri, A. (1994) Prognostic value of C-reactive protein and serum amyloid A protein in severe unstable angina, *N. Engl. J. Med.*, *331*, 417–424.

62. Danesh, J., Muir, J., Wong, Y. K., Ward, M., Gallimore, J. R., & Pepys, M. B. (1999) Risk factors for coronary heart disease and acute phase proteins. A population-based study, *Eur. Heart J.*, *20*, 954–959.

63. Stafforini, D. M., McIntyre, T. M., Zimmerman, G. A., & Prescott, S. M. (1997). Platelet activation factor acetylhydrolases, *J. Biol. Chem.*, *272*, 17895–17898.

64. Tjoelker, L. W., Wilder, C., Eberhardt, C., Stafforini, D. M., Dietsch, G., Schimpf, B., Hooper, S., Le Trong, H., Cousens, L. S., & Zimmerman, G. A. (1995) Anti-inflammatory properties of a platelet-activating factor acetylhydrolase, *Nature*, *374*, 549–553.

65. Berliner, J. A., Leitinger, N., Watson, A., Huber, J., Fogelman, A., & Navab, M. (1997) Oxidized lipids in atherogenesis: formation, destruction and action, *Thromb. Haemost.*, *78*, 195–199.

66. Kugiyama, K., Ota, Y., Takazoe, K., Moriyama, Y., Kawano, H., Sakamoto, T., Soejima, H., Ogawa, H., Doi, H., Sugiyama, S., & Yasue, H. (1999) Circulating levels of secretory type II phospholipase A (2) predict coronary events in patients with coronary artery disease, *Circulation*, *100*, 1280–1284.

67. Leitinger, N., Watson, A. D., Hama, S. Y., Ivandic, B., Qiao, J. H., Huber, J., Faull, K. F., Grass, D. S., Fogelman, A. M., de Beer, F. C., Lusis, A. J., & Berliner, A. J. (1999) Role of group II secretory phospholipase A2 in atherosclerosis 2. Potential involvement of biologically active oxidized phospholipids, *Arterioscler. Thromb. Vasc. Biol.*, *19*, 1291–1298.

68. Ivanchi, B., Castellani, L. W., Wang, X. P., Qiao, J. H., Mehrabian, M., Navab, M., Fogelman, A. M., Grass, D. S., Swanson, M. E., de Beer, M. C., de Beer, F., & Lusis, A. J. (1999) Role of Group II phospholipase A2 in atherosclerosis. 1. Increased atherogenosis an altered lipoproteins in transgenic mice expressing group II phospholipase A2, *Arterioscler. Thromb. Vasc. Biol.*, *19*, 1284–1290.

69. Cao, Y., Stafforini, D. M., Zimmerman, G. A., McIntyre, T. M., & Prescott, S. M. (1998) Expression of plasma platelet-activating factor acetylhydrolase is transcriptionally regulated by mediators of inflammation, *J. Biol. Chem.*, *273*, 4012–4020.

70. Caslake, M. J., Packard, C. J., Suckling, K. E., Holmes, S. D., Chamberlain, P., & MacPhee, C. H. (2000) Lipoprotein-associated phospholipase A2, platelet-activating

factor acetylhydrolase: a potential new risk factor for coronary artery disease. *Atherosclerosis*, *150*, 413–419.

71. Packard, C. J., O'Reilly, D. S. J., Caslake, M. J., McMahon, A. D., Ford, I., Cooney, J., MacPhee, C. H., Suckling, K. E., Krishna, M., Wilkinson, F. E., Rumley, A., Lowe, G. D. O., for the West of Scotland Coronary Prevention Study Group (2000) Lipoprotein-associated phospholipase A2, as an independent predictor of coronary heart disease, *N. Engl. J. Med.*, *343*, 1148–1155.

72. Biasucci, L. M., Batelli, A., Luizzo, G., Altamura, S., Caligiuri, G., Monaco, C., Rebuzzi, A. G., Ciliberto, G., & Maseri, A. (1996) Elevated levels of interleukin-6 in unstable angina, *Circulation*, *94*, 874–877.

73. Mendall, M. A., Patel, A., Asante, M., Ballam, L., Morris, J., Strachan, D. P., Camm, A. J., & Northfield, T. C. (1997) Relation of serum cytokine concentrations to cardiovascular risk factors and coronary heart disease, *Heart*, *78*, 273–277.

74. Harris, T. B., Fenrucci, L., Tracy, R. P., Corti, M. C., Wacholder, S., Ettinger, W. H., Jr., Heimovitz, H., Cohen, H. J., & Wallace, R. (1999) Association of elevated interleukin-6 and C reactive protein levels with mortality in the elderly. *Am. J. Med.*, *106*, 502–512.

75. Ridker, P. M., Rifai, N., Stampfer, M. J., & Hennekens, C. H. (2000) Plasma concentrations of interleukin-6 and the risk of future myocardial infarction among apparently healthy men, *Circulation*, *101*, 1767–1772.

76. Bataille, R., & Klein, B. (1992) C-reactive protein levels as a direct indicator of interleukin-6 levels in human in vivo, *Arthritis Rheum.*, *35*, 982–984.

77. Van Snick, J. (1990) Interleukin-6: an overview, *Annu. Rev. Immunol.*, *8*, 253–278.

78. Papanicolaou, D. A., Wilder, R. L., Manolagas, S. C., & Chrousos, G. P. (1998) The pathophysiologic roles of interluekin-6 in human disease, *Ann. Intern. Med.*, *128*, 127–137.

79. Seino, Y., Dkeda, U., Ikeda, M., Yamamoto, K., Misawa, Y., Hasegawa, T., Kano, S., & Shimada, K. (1994) Interleukin-6 gene transcripts are expressed in human atherosclerotic lesions, *Cytokine*, *6*, 87–91.

80. Hojo, Y., Ikeda, U., Katsuki, T., Mizumo, O., Fukazawa, H., Kurosaki, K., Fujikawa, H., & Shimada, K. I. (2000) Interleukin-6 expression in coronary circulation after coronary agionplasty as a risk factor for restenosis, *Heart*, *84*, 83–87.

81. Biasucci, L. M., Luizzo, G., Fortuzzi, G., Caligiuri, G., Rebuzzi, A. G., Ginetti, F., Dinarello, C. A., & Maseri, A. (1999) Increasing levels of interleukin (IL) – IRa and IL-6 during the first 2 days of hospitalization in unstable angina are associated with increased risk of in hospital coronary events, *Circulation*, *99*, 2079–2084.

82. Francis, S. E., Camp, N. J., Dewberry, R. M., Gunn, J., Syrris, P., Carter, N. D., Jeffrey, S., Kaski, J. C., Cumberland, D. C., Duff, G. W., & Crossman, D. C. (1999) Interleukin-1 receptor antagonist gene polymorphism and coronary artery disease, *Circulation*, *99*, 861–866.

83. Hasdai, D., Scheinowitz, M., Liebowitz, E., Sclarovsky, S., Eldar, M., & Barak, V. (1996) Increased serum concentrations of interleukin 1- beta in patients with coronary artery disease, *Heart*, *76*, 24–28.

84. Ridker, P. M., Rifai, N., Pfeffer, M., Sacks, F., Lepage, S., & Braunwald, E. (2000) Elevation of tumour necrosis factor-alpha and increased risk of recurrent coronary events after myocardial infarction, *Circulation*, *101*, 2149–2153.

85. Bevilacqua, M. P., Nelson, R. M., Mannori, G., & Cecconi, O. (1994) Endothelial-leucocyte adhesion molecules in human disease, *Annu. Rev. Med.*, *45*, 361–378.

86. Ridker, P. M., Hennekens, E. H., Roitman-Johnson, B., Stampfer, M. J., & Allen, J. (1998) Plasma concentrations of soluble intercellular adhesion molecule I and risks of future myocardial infarction in apparently healthy mean, *Lancet*, *351*, 88–92.

87. Haught, W. H., Mansour, M., Rothlein, R., Kishmoto, T. K., Mainolfi, E. A., Hendricks, C., & Mehta J. L. (1996) Alterations in circulating adhesion molecule-1 and L-selectin: further evidence for chronic inflammation in ischaemic heart disease, *Am. Heart J.*, *132*, 1–8.

88. Ogawa, H., Yasue, H., Miyao, Y., Sakamoto, T., Soljima, H., Nishiyama, K., Kaikita, K., Suefuji, H., Misumi, K., Takazoe, K., Kugiyama, K., & Yoshimura, M. (1999) Plasma soluble intercellular adhesion molecule-1 levels in coronary circulation in patients with unstable angina, *Am. J. Cardiol.*, *83*, 38–42.

89. Rifai, N., Jourbran, R., Yu, H., Asami, M., & Joumu, M. (1999) Inflammatory markers in men with angiographically documented coronary heart disease, *Clin. Chem.*, *45*, 1967–1973.

90. Porsch-Oezcueruemez, M., Kurz, D., Kloer, H. U., & Luley, C. (1999) Evaluation of serum levels of solubilized adhesion molecules and cytokine receptors in coronary heart disease, *J. Am. Coll. Cardiol.*, *34*, 1995–2001.

91. Paiker, J. E., Raal, F. J., Veller, M., von Arb, M., Chetty, N., & Naram, N. H. (2000) Cell adhesion molecules—can they be used to predict coronary artery disease in patients with hypercholesterolaemia? *Clin. Chim. Acta.*, *293*, 105–113.

92. Sinisalo, J., Paronen, J., Mattila, K. J., Syrjala, M., Alfthan, G., Palonio, T., Merrinen, M. S., & Vaarala, O. (2000) Relation of inflammation to vascular function in patients with coronary heart disease, *Atherosclerosis*, *149*, 403–411.

93. John, S., Jacobi, J., Delles, C., Schlaich, M. P., Alter, O., & Schmieder, R. E. (2000) Plasma soluble adhesion molecules and endothelium dependent vasodilation in early human atherosclerosis, *Clin. Sci.*, *98*, 521–529.

94. Semaan, H. B., Gurbel, P. A., Anderson, J. L., Muhlestein, J. B., Carlquist, J. F., Horne, B. D., & Serebruany, V. L. (2000) Soluble VCAM-I and E-selectin but not ICAM-I discriminate endothelial injury in patients with documented coronary artery disease, *Cardiology*, *93*, 7–10.

95. Ghaisas, N. K., Shahi, C. N., Foley, B., Goggins, M., Crean, P., Kelly, A., Kelleher, D., & Walsh, M. (1997) Elevated levels of soluble adhesion molecules in peripheral blood of patients with unstable angina, *Am. J. Cardiol.*, *80*, 617–619.

96. Caulin-Glaser, T., Farrell, W. J., Pfau, S. E., Zaret, B., Bunger, K., Setaro, J. F., Brennam, J. J., Bender, J. R., Cleman, M. W., Cabin, H. S., & Remetz, M. S. (1998) Modulation of circulating cellular adhesion molecules in postmenopausal women with coronary artery disease, *J. Am. Coll. Cardiol*, *31*, 1555–1560.

97. Sburouni, E., Kroupsis, C., Kyriakides, Z. S., Koniavitou, K., & Kremastinos, D. T. (2000) Cell adhesion molecules in relation to simvastatin and hormone replacement therapy in coronary artery disease, *Eur. Heart J.*, *21*, 963–964.
98. McCarty, M. F. (1998) Interleukin-6 as a central mediator of cardiovascular risk associated with chronic inflammation, smoking, diabetes and visceral obesity: down-regulation with essential fatty acids, ethanol and pentoxiphylline. *Med. Hypotheses*, *52*, 465–477.
99. Yudkin, J. S., Kumari, M., Humphries, S. E., & Mohamed-Ali, V. (2000) Inflammation, obesity, stress and coronary heart disease: is interleukin-6 the link? [Review], *Atherosclerosis*, *148*, 209–214.

3

Traditional Risk Factors and Newly Recognized Emerging Risk Factors for Cardiovascular Disease

3.1. INTRODUCTION

Hypercholesterolemia has been considered the main factor leading to atherosclerosis and coronary heart disease (CHD) since 1913, when Anitschkow[1] showed that cholesterol could induce changes of atherosclerosis of the aorta in rabbits, resembling disease in human. However, it was not until 1961 with the Framingham Heart Study report[2] that hypercholesterolemia and hypertension were clearly established as major contributors to cardiovascular disease in humans. It was about this time or soon after that cigarette smoking was recognized as the third important risk factor for CHD, and was listed in the Surgeon General (United States) report in 1964. Since that time numerous studies have confirmed that causal link with traditional risk factors and atherosclerotic CHD. Moreover, many new risk factors have been added to the list over the past several decades and even at the present time new risk factors are continually being recognized.

3.2. HYPERCHOLESTEROLEMIA

The role of elevated concentrations of serum cholesterol and low-density lipoprotein (LDL) in the pathogenesis of atherosclerosis is well established.

Evidence supporting the atherogenic effects of LDL includes studies of diet-induced atherosclerosis in animals; clinical studies in humans with genetic disorders, such as familial hypercholesterolemia, that are associated with a high risk of premature atherosclerosis; and pathological studies, demonstrating that cholesterol derived from LDL is present in atherosclerotic plaques. Epidemiological studies have consistently shown higher rates of CHD in populations with higher mean concentrations of total and LDL cholesterol. The Multiple Risk Factor Intervention Trial (MRFIT) involving 356,222 men followed for 6 years demonstrated a curvilinear relationship between increasing plasma concentrations of total cholesterol and risk of CHD[3]. The risk increased slightly as total cholesterol values rose from 150 to 200 mg/dL but was approximately two- to fourfold higher when cholesterol values were increased to 250 and 300 mg/dL compared with values at 200 mg/dL.

There are overwhelming data that reduction in total and LDL cholesterol reduces the risk of atherosclerosis in patients with or without preexistent cardiovascular disease. Results from early clinical trials demonstrated that reduction of 8–14% in total cholesterol reduced the incidence of coronary events by 19–34%[4]. These trials led to the conclusion that for every 1% decrease in total cholesterol, 5 years of treatment would result in a 2% decrease in the incidence of CHD. In the past decade results of five major trials with potent hypolipidemic agents (hydroxy-methylglutaryl coenzyme A reductase inhibitors [statins]) have provided unequivocal evidence of the benefits of cholesterol or LDL reductions[5–9]. Significant decreases in cardiovascular endpoints and mortality were seen in patients treated for about 5 years. Similar reduction in relative risk of coronary events occurred in patients with and without clinically evident CHD and in patients with mild or severe dyslipidemia. Although treatment was aimed primarily at reducing LDL cholesterol levels, there were concurrent increased high-density lipoprotein (HDL) by 5–8% and reduced triglycerides by 12–15%.

There is convincing evidence that for any given lipoprotein concentration in the plasma, LDL is found in higher concentration in the arterial wall than in the plasma[10,11]. Oxidative modification of the trapped lipoprotein then occurs in two stages[12]. The first stage occurs before monocytes are recruited and results in the oxidization of lipids in LDL with little change in apolipoprotein B, the major protein of LDL. The second stage begins when monocytes are recruited to the lesion, convert into macrophages and LDL lipids are further oxidized with the protein portion as well. There is a shift in receptor recognition from LDL receptor to scavenger receptors and/or oxidized LDL receptor, which leads to uptake of LDL that is not regulated by the cholesterol content of the cell. Massive accumulation of cholesterol in the cytoplasm gives rise to the foam cells.

Oxidized LDL is a potent inducer of inflammatory molecules such as P-selectin, monocyte chemoattractant protein-1 (MCP-1), monocyte colony stimulating factor (M-CSF), and GRO (a C-X-C chemokine). These factors lead to further monocyte adherence, migration and conversion into macrophages in the intima of the artery[12]. Oxidized LDL is believed to induce these inflammatory molecules both by inducing increased rates of gene transcription and by stabilizing the mRNA for these genes[13].

HDL may protect by inhibiting LDL oxidation through two enzyme systems associated with normal HDL. Platelet activating factors acetylhydrolase and paraoxonase have been found to protect against LDL modification in the coculture system[14,15]. The inverse relationships between HDL levels and the risk for atherosclerotic events may be partly related to these enzymes associated with HDL that protect against LDL oxidation, and the putative role of HDL in reverse cholesterol transport[16].

It has been postulated that genetic factors may influence lipid oxidation and inflammation; that oxidized lipids may be responsible for the induction of a set of genes that induce chronic inflammatory response characteristic of the fatty streak. Experiments in mice suggest that a major gene contributing to aortic lesion development, termed Ath-1, may control either the accumulation of lipid peroxides in tissues or the cellular responses to such lipid peroxides[17]. High levels of oxidized lipids activate the NF_kB-like transcription factor and the expression of genes that contain NF_kB binding sites (the inflammatory genes) result in upregulation of MCP-1, colony stimulating factors, serum amyloid A (SAA), and hemeoxygenase in the fatty streak-susceptible mice[18,19].

3.3. DYSLIPIDEMIAS

Hypertriglyceridemia, low HDL cholesterol, and lipoprotein(a). Reduction of plasma LDL cholesterol reduces cardiovascular events and total mortality; however, many mature patients with premature CHD do not have elevated LDL cholesterol but instead have elevated triglycerides or low HDL cholesterol or both, and recent data suggest that interventions to modulate these lipoprotein fractions may reduce cardiovascular risk.

The association between triglycerides levels and cardiovascular disease has been controversial but it is now recognized as an independent risk factor for atherosclerotic vascular disease[20-22]. Triglycerides are transported in a number of different lipoprotein fractions, which have atherogenic propensity[23]. Also, a number of proatherogenic metabolic and physiologic changes are associated with elevated triglyceride levels, such as increased small dense LDL particles, low HDL cholesterol levels, and increased levels of procoagulant molecules[24]. Hypertriglyceridemia can be the result of elevated chylomicrons (Type I or V hyperlipoproteinemia), very low-density lipoproteins

(VLDL) (Type IV or IIb hyperlipoproteinemia), or lipoprotein remnants (Type III hyperlipoproteinemia). The type of lipoprotein that is elevated is an important determinant of the degree of cardiovascular risk. Premature atherosclerosis is not a feature of familial chylomicronemia syndromes (Type I hyperlipoproteinemia) and large chylomicrons are not atherogenic but can cause pancreatitis and eruptive exanthomas. Conditions associated with elevated VLDL are often associated with increased risk of premature cardiovascular disease such as obesity, Type II diabetes, excessive alcohol consumption, Type III and Type IV patterns of hyperlipoproteinemia[25].

There is epidemiological evidence that HDL cholesterol is associated inversely with CHD[26,27], low levels being associated with increased cardiovascular risk[28]. Rare genetic disorders of high HDL, as a result of increased production of apoA-1 (the major HDL protein), are associated with decreased incidence of CHD[29,30]. Low HDL cholesterol levels are frequently associated with elevated triglyceride levels, and reduction of triglycerides usually results in some increase of HDL cholesterol concentration. Many persons with low HDL cholesterol have normal triglycerides, isolated low HDL cholesterol or primary hypoalphalipoproteinemia. Premature CHD is common in families with primary hypoalphalipoproteinemia but the development of premature atherosclerosis may depend on the specific gene defect or metabolic cause of the low HDL cholesterol. Evidence in animals indicates that interventions to increase plasma HDL cholesterol or apoA-1 is associated with reduced atherosclerosis[31-33]. Studies in humans are more limited and show similar reduction in cardiovascular events with increased HDL cholesterol levels but with concomitant decrease in triglyceride levels[34-36].

Lipoprotein(a) [Lp(a)] is similar in structure to LDL with an additional protein called apolipoprotein(a) [apo(a)], which is linked by a disulfide bond to apoB. A number of epidemiological studies indicate an independent association between elevated plasma levels of Lp(a) and atherosclerotic vascular disease[37-39], but not all have found this association[40]. It has been estimated that a normolipidemic patient with Lp(a) concentration greater than 30 mg/L has a 1.75 fold elevated risk of CHD and that a combined elevation with increased LDL cholesterol levels raises the relative risk to 6.0[41]. However, in studies of African Americans, elevated levels of Lp(a) were not associated with increased risk for cardiovascular disease[25]. It is postulated that Lp(a) inhibits the activation of plasminogen to plasmin at the vessel wall leading to inadequate fibrinolysis and increasing the likelihood of atherosclerotic plaque development and thrombosis[42,43]. The gene for apo(a) is the major genetic factor controlling the plasma level of Lp(a) and this is inherited as an autosomal codominant trait with expression in childhood[44]. However, the plasma levels of Lp(a) are determined primarily by the rate of production and the catabolism. Lp(a) levels increased in postmenopausal women, nephrotic syndrome, end stage renal disease and were reduced by estrogen therapy[25].

Although elevated Lp(a) is an independent risk factor for atherosclerosis and cardiovascular disease, measurement of Lp(a) is not currently recommended in routine screening for CHD risk assessment.

3.4. SMOKING

Cigarette smoking is a major risk factor for CHD, stroke, and peripheral vascular disease. Large body of data from cohort and prospective studies has firmly established the strong relationships between smoking and atherosclerotic vascular disease[45,46]. It has been estimated that smoking cause 17–30% of all deaths attributed to cardiovascular disease[47]. The risk for CHD in smokers is dose-related and as few as four cigarettes per day can increase the risk. Smoking may be additive or synergistic with other risk factors for cardiovascular disease, such as hypertension, hypercholesterolemia, etc.

Smoking may play a role at different stages of the development of CHD, including promotion of atherosclerosis, triggering of acute coronary thrombosis, coronary artery spasm, cardiac arrhythmia, and reduction of the capacity of blood to deliver oxygen[46]. Its role in the pathogenesis of atherosclerosis has been attributed to several mechanisms: direct endothelial damage, increased proliferation of smooth muscle in atheromatous lesions, decreased endothelium-dependent coronary vasodilation, and reduced levels of HDL[46,48]. Smoking-induced endothelial injury may result from oxidation caused by lipid peroxidation and the production of free radicals[49]. Smooth-muscle proliferation appears to be stimulated by smoking-induced increases in the adherence of platelets to arterial endothelium[48]. Lipid infiltration of the arterial wall may be increased in smoking by reducing the levels of HDL cholesterol.

Besides promoting atherosclerosis, smoking may precipitate acute coronary artery thrombosis by increasing platelet aggregation, fibrinogen levels, plasma viscosity, and decreasing red cell deformity[48]. It may also increase the risk of plaque rupture and acute ischemic events by the short-term increases in arterial wall stiffness[50].

Cessation of smoking greatly reduces the risk of CHD and the mortality from cardiovascular disease in patients with symptomatic CHD. Smoking cessation by the age of 65 reduced the risk of recurrent serious coronary events by 50% compared to those who continued smoking[51]. In survivors of out-of-hospital cardiac arrest followed for 3 years, smoking cessation decreased the risk of recurrent cardiac arrest by 30%[52]. Smoking cessation may also decrease the rate of restenosis after percutaneous transluminal coronary angioplasty[53] and decreases recurrence of disease after coronary artery bypass surgery[54].

3.5. HYPERTENSION

Hypertension is one of the three major risk factors for the initial development of CHD and it also increased the risk of mortality and reinfarction in post-myocardial infarction patients. Mechanical stress on blood vessels, such as coronary arteries, resulting from high blood pressure is an important factor in endothelial cell dysfunction, the progression of atherosclerosis, and plaque rupture[55]. Transient surges in the blood pressure can trigger rupture of soft and vulnerable lipid-rich plaques to cause acute ischemic events[56]. Hypertension decreases coronary artery blood flow reserve and myocardial oxygen supply is limited during exercise[57]. Moreover, increased systolic blood pressure increases the left ventricular afterload that leads to ventricular hypertrophy and increased oxygen demand. Thus, there is an imbalance between myocardial oxygen supply and demand and is prone to develop myocardial ischemia.

It is clearly established that lowering the blood pressure with anti-hypertensive therapy reduces coronary events, and in post-myocardial infarction patients, the prognosis is affected by previous history of hypertension and the post-infarction blood pressure levels[58,59]. In hypertensive patients with acute myocardial infarction, the overall 5 year mortality rate was 58% versus 49% among non-hypertensive patients ($p < 0.05$); and reinfarction occurred in 43% of hypertensives versus 31% of non-hypertensives ($p < 0.01$)[59]. Treatment with an antihypertensive, ACE inhibitor trandolapril, as compared with placebo was associated with a reduction in the relative risk of death to 0.59 in the hypertensive patients[60]. After control of various confounders, the benefit from ACE inhibition increased with higher blood pressure at randomization. Thus, treatment with ACE inhibitors is important in acute myocardial infarction with a history of hypertension.

Excessive diastolic blood pressure reduction below a certain limit may result in a paradoxic increase in cardiac events[61,62]. This J-curve phenomenon was originally demonstrated for hypertensive patients for events related to myocardial ischemia but not for strokes. In hypertensive patients with myocardial ischemia, coronary deaths decreased with the blood pressure reduction until the diastolic pressure of 85–90 mmHg was reached, and further reduction below 85 mmHg was associated with increased coronary deaths[61]. Most coronary blood flow occurs during diastole and so blood flow is greatly influenced by the diastolic blood pressure level. However, in a large randomized trial of 18,790 patients with hypertension, there was no evidence of a J-curve phenomenon for the relationship of cardiovascular mortality[63]. For systolic blood pressure, the benefits of lowering blood pressure levels were observed to 140 mmHg, but further reduction down to 120 mmHg did not provide further benefit. The lowest incidence of major cardiovascular events occurred at a mean diastolic blood pressure of 83 mmHg but further reduction to 70 mmHg was not harmful.

3.6. DIABETES MELLITUS

Diabetic patients have a two- to threefold increased risk for cardiovascular disease compared with non-diabetic subjects[64,65]. This excess risk is present in both Type I and II diabetes, and may affect women to a greater degree than men, and is influenced by ethnic background. Cardiovascular disease is responsible for 75–85% of hospital admissions and deaths in diabetes, and more than 50% of diabetic patients have CHD at diagnosis[65].

There are several mechanisms by which diabetes may increase the risk of atherosclerotic cardiovascular disease. Hyperglycemia itself may be harmful by directly causing tissue damage through processes such as glyco-oxidation, protein kinase C activation, and cellular myoinosital depletion[66]. Clinical evidence also demonstrates that the degree of hyperglycemia in diabetic patients correlates with the risk and severity of microvascular complications, and improving hyperglycemia reduces the risk incrementally[67]. However, observational and intervention trials have produced mixed results and the data do not suggest a dominant effect of hyperglycemia on the excess risk for cardiovascular disease in diabetes[68]. Aggressive treatment of hyperglycemia is beneficial to future health in diabetic subjects particularly to prevention and amelioration of microangiopathy, but is unlikely to lower the excess risk of CHD substantially.

Insulin resistance or hyperinsulinemia may increase the risk for atherosclerosis, as there is a strong association between fasting insulin levels and CHD mortality in population studies[69,70]. Fasting insulin levels in normoglycemia subjects reflect the degree of insulin resistance. The notion that hyperinsulinemia may be atherogenic is supported by in vitro studies demonstrating that pharmacologic range of insulin has a mitogenic action in smooth-muscle cells, is lipogenic, and stimulates plasminogen activator inhibitor (PAI-1) production[71]. In non-diabetic men followed prospectively, insulin levels and resistance had independent predictive values for CHD, beyond an association with other risk factors[72]. There is also a direct relationship between insulin resistance and carotid wall intimal medial thickness (IMT) as assessed by β-mode ultrasound[73]. However, it is not known whether reduction of insulin resistance protect against CHD. Recent evidence that the insulin sensitizer troglitazone was shown to reduce carotid wall IMT in Type II diabetic patients[74] is encouraging. Weight reduction and exercise and metformin, which reduce insulin resistance[75] may have beneficial effects on cardiovascular events partly through this mechanism among others.

Dyslipidemia may be a major factor contributing to increase risk for cardiovascular disease in diabetes. Although total and LDL cholesterol levels are not significantly elevated over non-diabetics, the triglyceride values are higher and their HDL cholesterol levels are lower[76,77]. Although the prevalence hypercholesterolemia is not increased, its impact on CHD in diabetic subjects is much greater than that in the general population. In the MRFIT following 6,000 men with diabetes, there was a fourfold greater risk for CHD than in men without diabetes for parallel levels of total cholesterol[78]. Several cross-sectional and prospective studies, however, have demonstrated that triglyceride and HDL cholesterol have significantly greater predictive power for cardiovascular disease in diabetic subjects than does the total or LDL cholesterol[68]. Epidemiological observations have demonstrated that hypertriglyceridemia is an independent cardiovascular risk factor in the general population. In addition, triglyceride-rich particles are frequently associated with the atherogenic small dense forms of LDL (phenotype β), and reduced HDL cholesterol, which is a powerful risk factor by itself. Whether the risk associated with hypertriglyceridemia and low HDL cholesterol in diabetes is a result of insulin deficiency or resistance or associated with some other diabetic specific factor is not known.

Renal disease and hypertension is more prevalent in diabetic patients and contribute to the accelerated vascular disease. Hypertension is not only more frequent in diabetic patients, but also has a greater impact on CHD than in non-diabetic subjects. Multiple abnormalities in platelet function, coagulation, and fibrinolysis have been described in diabetic patients as well in experimental induced diabetics. There is increased platelet stickiness and aggregability, an increase in fibrinogen and Factor VII levels, and an increase in the concentration of PAI-1[79].

3.7. OBESITY

Obesity is emerging as one of the most important contributors to increase morbidity and mortality, especially from cardiovascular diseases[80]. Obesity is associated with an increased risk for Type II diabetes, dyslipidemia, hypertension, left ventricular hypertrophy, congestive heart failure, and CHD. The greater the degree of adiposity, greater is the level of risk factors. The American Heart Association (AHA) reclassified obesity as a major, modifiable risk factor for CHD in 1998, and this has been sanctioned by the World Health Organization. It is recently estimated that approximately one of every two US adults is considered overweight or obese (Body Mass Index (BMI) 25.0 kg/m^2 or greater).

The direct causal relationship between obesity and cardiovascular disease is complex and likely multifactorial in nature. CHD in obesity may be related to development of hyperlipidemia, diabetes or hypertension or inactivity. Furthermore, increased body weight is associated with adaptive cardiovascular changes for the increased hemodynamic demands. One of the most important clinical effects of obesity is increased blood pressure. Cross-sectional and longitudinal studies have consistently shown a higher prevalence of hypertension in obese subjects, and there is a strong correlation with weight gain or loss with increased or decreased blood pressure. Obesity and hypertension are more marked in younger adults, which then gradually decreased with age. The relationships between hypertension and obesity is not fully understood, but may result from hemodynamic alterations, renal dysfunction, increase in sympathetic nervous activity, and possibly related to insulin resistance[81].

The association between obesity and CHD is well established. Long-term epidemiologic studies have shown that CHD mortality increases on average 4–6% for every one BMI starting at about a BMI of 20–24 kg/m[82]. Besides the increased risk of atherosclerotic cardiovascular disease related to hypertension, diabetes, and hypercholesterolemia in obesity, other related comorbidities include hypertriglyceridemia, low HDL cholesterol, increased PAI-1, tissue type plasminogen activator and Factor VII. Clustering of these metabolic abnormalities in obese patients with increased abdominal girth has been labeled the "insulin resistance syndrome"[83]. An enlarged waist circumference (40 in. for men and 35 in. for women) is independently associated with increased risk for CHD[84].

Weight loss has shown to reverse many of pathologic and coexisting cardiovascular risk factors associated with obesity. Most of the metabolic abnormalities can be improved with modest reduction of 5–10 kg, although gender differences have been seen[85]. The mechanisms underlying the improvement may be multifactorial, however, from reduction in calories, total and saturated fat, alcohol, and increased physical activity. However, no prospective studies to date have demonstrated that intentional weight loss reduces the cardiovascular risk, probably because of the difficulties in sustaining long-term weight loss.

3.8. GENETICS

A family history of premature CHD has been demonstrated to be a major risk factor for cardiovascular disease[86–88]. The risk of ischemia as evidenced by electrocardiogram is about 40% higher and the risk of death from cardiac events is about 2.5–7 times higher in persons with a parenteral history of premature CHD (before age of 60 years), than in persons without such a family history[89,90]. Moreover, recent studies have found greater arterial abnormalities in the young, asymptomatic offspring of patients with premature myocardial infarction compared to controls. In the Bogalusa Heart Study, children and adolescents had an increased pressure-strain modulus of elasticity of the common carotid artery, an index of arterial stiffness[91]. Impaired flow-mediated, endothelium-dependent vasodilation in first degree relatives (young healthy subjects) of patients with angiographic or clinical evidence of premature CHD has also been reported[92]. In a very recent study comparing 40 healthy young people (mean age 19 ± 5.2 years) whose parents had premature myocardial infarction and 40 control, age, sex-matched subjects, the offspring of patients with premature CHD had lower flow-mediated reactivity of the brachial arterial ($p = 0.01$), and greater mean intima-media thickness of the common carotid artery ($p = 0.0004$)[93]. Flow-mediated brachial artery reactivity is impaired in persons with overt atherosclerosis and in asymptomatic persons with risk factors for CHD[94], whilst increased thickness of the intima-media of the carotid artery is a powerful predictor of CHD and clinical sequelae[95,96]. The presence of any disease in a family, however, may not necessary be by genetic inheritance, but could represent environment factors or lifestyle influence.

Several reports from longitudinal epidemiological studies have shown higher serum concentration of lipoproteins, homocysteine, and higher blood pressure in children and young adults with a parenteral history of premature CHD than in those without such a background[97-99]. Gaeta et al. (2000)[93] had also confirmed that offspring of patients with premature CHD had higher concentrations of Lp(a) lipoprotein and apolipoprotein B (lipid profiles associated with atherosclerotic vascular disease) than controls. It has been suggested that 30% of the variation in the thickness of the common carotid intima and media may be explained by genetic factors[100]. Furthermore, there is a link between different mutations of the gene that code for endothelial nitric oxide synthase either with smoking-related risk of coronary artery disease or with coronary vasospasm[101,102].

A number of monogenic disorders have been shown to cause hypertension[103]. It appears that in the majority of cases hypertension results from the interaction between multiple genes and the environment (or dietary influences such as increased sodium intake and body weight). Mutations responsible for several monogenic cardiovascular disorders have also been identified. The association between familial hypercholesterolemia and premature CHD was first noted in families and subsequently in populations. A number of genetic abnormalities are associated with reduction or abnormalities in the expression of the LDL receptor, which leads to elevation of LDL cholesterol[104]. However, these mutations by a single gene appear to be responsible for only a minority of the cases of hypercholesterolemia. Instead, like hypertension most cases of hypercholesterolemia result from interaction between multiple genes and environmental and dietary influences. Obviously genetic factors may predisclose to premature atherosclerosis by different mechanisms or risk factors. For instance, the racial differences in the prevalence of coronary risk factors, such as the incidences of diabetes mellitus in Puma Indians and South Pacific Islanders, as well as in the differing contributions that these risk factors make to the prevalence of CHD in the populations at large. Other examples include mutation in the MTHFR gene, that cause elevations in homocysteine, may increase the risk for CHD; or genetic abnormalities that may lead to a procoagulant state.

3.9. NEW RISK FACTORS FOR ATHEROSCLEROTIC CARDIOVASCULAR DISEASE

A number of new risk factors for CHD have been emerging over the past two decades (see Table 3.1). Inflammatory markers which are listed as risk

Table 3.1
New Risk Factors for Atherosclerotic Cardiovascular Disease

Traditional cardiovascular risk factors

- Hypercholesterolemia
- Hypertension
- Smoking
- Diabetes mellitus
- Obesity
- Dyslipidemia
- Genetics.

New emerging risk factors

- Estrogen deficiency
- Left ventricular hypertrophy
- C-reactive protein
- Fibrinogen
- Homocysteine
- Lipoprotein(a)
- Factor VII
- Endogenous tissue plasminogen activator
- Plasminogen-activator inhibitor Type I
- Serum amyloid A
- Lipoprotein-associated phospholipase A
- Cytokines and adhesion molecules
- Renal insufficiency
- Certain infections, i.e., *Chlamydia pneumoniae.*

factors were dealt with in Chapter 2 and will not be discussed in this section. The best known of these new risk factors is estrogen deficiency, which appears to be responsible for the higher prevalence of CHD in post-menopausal women. The incidence of CHD is low among premenopausal women compared to men in all populations that have been studied[105]. Estrogen therapy results in an increase in HDL cholesterol, that may be related to reduction in cardiovascular disease, and improves the function of the vascular endothelium, including that of the coronary arteries[105,106]. The benefits of the use of estrogen (hormone replacement therapy) for prevention of clinical CHD among post menopausal women have been documented for most, but not all, observational studies but the issue is contentious and not all settled[107]. Ongoing clinical trials comparing the benefits of estrogen in women with hysterectomy only and estrogen–progesterone and placebo in postmenopausal women may provide a more definitive answer about the risks and benefits of hormone replacement therapy. In a recent meta-analysis of observational studies it is estimated that estrogen alone was associated with a 35–50% reduction and estrogen–progesterone with about 33% reduction in the risk of CHD comparing users versus non-users[108].

3.9.1. Homocysteine

Homocysteine is a sulfur-containing amino acid formed during the metabolism of methionine. The metabolism of homocysteine is influenced by folic acid, vitamin B_{12}, and vitamin B_6. Severe hyperhomocysteinemia, a rare inherited disorder, is associated with premature atherosclerosis and arterial thrombosis even in children[109]. However, homocysteinemia occurs in approximately 5–7% of the general population and may be associated with pre-mature CHD in the third or fourth decade of life[110,111]. Abundant epidemiological evidence has demonstrated that the presence of mild hyperhomocysteinemia is an independent risk factor for atherosclerosis in the coronary, cerebral, and peripheral arteries[112,113]. Normal total plasma homocysteine range from 5 to 15 μmol/L, moderate concentration is considered 15 to 30 μg/ml, intermediate > 30 to 100 μmol/L and severe elevation >100 μmol/L during fasting[112]. Many epidemiological, cross-sectional, case study, nested case-control, and cohort studies by and large indicate an independent association between moderate elevated plasma homocysteine levels and cardiovascular disease[113]. However, although the association between homocysteine levels and CHD is generally strong and biologically plausible, the data from the prospective studies are less consistent and weaker. It has been suggested that elevated plasma homocysteine level merely indicates lower socioeconomic status and poor nutrition, or that it may be a result of cardiovascular disease rather than the cause. Although the association between genetic hyperhomocysteinemia and vascular disease indicates that the elevated homocysteine levels precede the disease, these issues are not completely resolved.

Plasma homocysteine is a sensitive marker of folate and vitamin B_{12} status, and the plasma levels of homocysteine are inversely related to plasma concentrations of these vitamins. However, an increase in homocysteine levels occurs long before the usual manifestation of folate or vitamin B_{12} deficiency. A number of other factors can influence homocysteine metabolism and blood levels including chronic renal failure, hypothyroidism, several types of carcinomas (breast, ovarian, and pancreatic), acute lymphoblastic leukemia, drugs (methotrexate, phenytoin, theophyline), and cigarette smoking[114].

Experimental evidence suggests that hyperhomocysteinemia may predispose to atherosclerosis by endothelial dysfunction and injury followed by platelet activation and thrombus formation. It has been proposed that homocysteine-induced endothelial injury exposes the subendothelial matrix, leading to platelet activation, as homocysteine-induced atherosclerosis is characterized by substantial platelet accumulation and platelet thrombus[115,116]. In primates hyperhomocysteinemia leads to impaired vasomotor regulation and endothelial antithrombotic function[117] and similar findings are presenting in young patients with hyperhomocysteinemia and peripheral vascular disease[118]. Although the exact mechanism of endothelial dysfunction is unknown, there is evidence that homocysteine exerts its effects by oxidative damage.

Auto-oxidation of homocysteine to homocystine produces potent oxygen species, including superoxide anion radical, hydroxyl radical, and hydrogen peroxide. There is evidence that homocysteine-induced endothelial cell injury in vitro is largely due to the generation of hydrogen peroxide[119], but several mechanisms may be involved as homocysteine can inhibit expression of thrombomodulin, induce the expression of tissue factors, suppress activation of protein C, and enhance activities of Factor XII and Factor V to create a procoagulation environment[114]. Auto-oxidation of homocysteine also initiates lipid peroxidation or supports the oxidation of LDL through the generation of superoxide formation or hydroxyl radical and anion radical[120,121]. Homocysteine may also affect nitric oxide availability at the endothelium, increase smooth-muscle cell proliferation, damage vascular matrix, activate elastase, and increase calcium deposition[114].

Observational and interventional studies have provided a rationale for the use of folic acid in the secondary prevention of vascular disease. In a recent uncontrolled study, a combination of folic acid with vitamins B_6 or B_{12} decreased the progression of carotid plaque when assessed by ultrasound[122].

There are now several large, controlled, intervention trials in patients with vascular disease in progress.

3.9.2. Left Ventricular Hypertrophy

Left ventricular hypertrophy is the response of the heart to chronic pressure or volume overload. It is defined as left ventricular mass exceeding 131 g/m^2 of body surface area in men and 100 g/m^2 in women[123]. Echocardiogram appears to be the best method for assessing left ventricular mass. Age, blood pressure, obesity, valve disease, and myocardial infarction are associated with left ventricular hypertrophy. Sodium intake, hereditary factors, and neurohumoral factors may also play a role in development of increased left ventricular mass[124].

Left ventricular hypertrophy is independently associated with increased incidence of cardiovascular disease and mortality and stroke[125]. Although multiple studies have shown increased cardiovascular mortality associated with left ventricular hypertrophy compared to those without, adjusted odds ratio 1.4–5.4[126], these effects are difficult to separate from just the effect of severe hypertension. Diminished coronary vasodilator reserve, increased myocardial oxygen demand, subendocardial ischemia, arrhythmia and left ventricular failure may explain the increased mortality risk associated with left ventricular hypertrophy. Interventional trials will always have difficulty showing improved clinical outcome of reversing left ventricular hypertrophy over and above that achievable with blood pressure control alone.

3.9.3. Coagulation Factors

Thrombosis is involved in two critical points in CHD, initially in atherogenesis and later in the conversion of chronic CHD to acute ischemic syndromes. Coagulation factors now emerging as cardiovascular risk factors include fibrinogen (previously discussed), Factor VII, PAI-1, tissue plasminogen activator, and D-dimer.

Several large-scale studies have shown that the fibrinolytic markers tissue-type plasminogen activator and PAI are consistent markers of risk for cardiovascular disease[127–130]. The fibrinolytic markers predict future cardiovascular disease in univariate analysis, but the predictive value in multivariate analysis appears marginal[131].

Advanced atheromatous lesions are the substrates for arterial thrombosis, leading to acute ischemic events. The lipid core of Type IV and V lesions

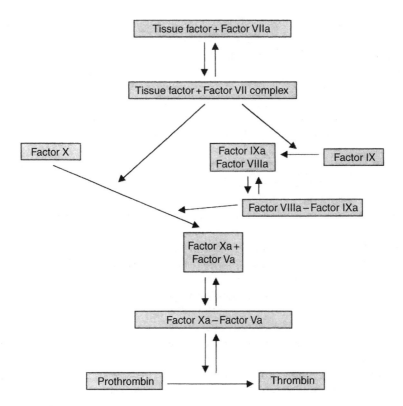

Figure 3.1.   An outline of the tissue factor pathway activation of coagulation. Adapted from Rauch et al.[132] with the permission of the publishers.

is rich in tissue factor, upon plaque rupture, initiates the coagulation cascade and thrombin generation. Tissue factor interacts with Factor VII and subsequently activates Factor X, which leads to the conversion of prothrombin to thrombin in the prothrombinase complex (see Figure 3.1)[132]. Recent studies showed increased levels of circulating tissue factor antigen with cardiovascular disease and increased blood thrombogenicity in patients with acute and chronic coronary syndromes[133,134].

3.9.4. Renal Impairment

Patients with renal disease have elevated risk for cardiovascular disease, even in the absence of classic risk factors[135,136]. This association is well established in patients with advanced renal insufficiency[136]. However, this association may largely be due to secondary hypertension and dyslipidemia. Lipid abnormalities begin to develop when the glomerular filtration rate falls below 40–50 ml/min and becomes more pronounced with progression of renal insufficiency[137]. Chronic renal insufficiency is usually accompanied by hypertriglyceridemia without hypercholesterolemia. VLDL cholesterol is often moderately elevated, whereas LDL cholesterol is not. Plasma concentrations of apoB are moderately increased, in addition HDL cholesterol and apoA-1 levels are usually decreased, factors that are associated with increased premature atherosclerosis.

The cardiovascular risk associated with early or mild renal insufficiency is now an emerging or more controversial issue. It has been reported in patients with hypertension that a serum creatinine concentration greater than 133 μmol/L (1.5 mg/dL) was a strong predictor of cardiovascular disease[138,139]. In contrast, mild renal insufficiency failed to predict cardiovascular disease in 6,233 adult participants who were followed for 15 years in the Framingham Heart Study[140]. However, in a more recent trial, not confined to hypertensive patients, with 980 subjects with mild renal insufficiency and 8,307 without renal impairment but all with preexisting vascular disease, renal insufficiency significantly increased cardiovascular events[141]. The cumulative incidence of primary outcome and cardiovascular death, independent of known cardiovascular risks, were higher in patients with renal insufficiency than those without. In another study, mild renal insufficiency was associated with increased risk of stroke[142]. Micro-albuminuria is a more sensitive marker of renal damage than serum creatinine and is more firmly associated with cardiovascular disease. However, the same risk factors that lead to cardiovascular disease could contribute to intra-renal vascular disease, and mild renal impairment may be a result of atherosclerotic damage—nephrosclerosis. Mild to moderate decrease in renal function is known to correlate with several vascular risk factors—insulin resistance, hypertriglyceridemia, reduced HDL cholesterol, elevated LDL, hyperuricemia, and hyperhomocysteinemia[143].

3.10. UNRESOLVED ISSUES

It is clear that atherosclerosis and cardiovascular disease are multifactorial in pathogenesis and that there are many risk factors. However, it appears that there need to be some consensus or further investigations to distinguish between true risk factors (that predispose to the disease) from markers of early or latent disease. For instance, true risk factors for atherosclerosis appear to be hypercholesterolemia, smoking, dyslipidemia, hypertension, diabetes, and obesity, whereas, CRP, SAA, fibrinogen, cytokines, and adhesion factors etc., appears more likely to be early markers of atherosclerosis. However, investigators and reports in the literature have lumped all these risk factors and "markers" together. A parallel example would be to consider a high erythrocyte sedimentation rate (ESR) above 60 mm/hr as a risk factor for multiple myeloma or giant cell arteries when clearly this is a laboratory marker or sign of the disease.

Furthermore, epidemiological studies are likely to underestimate certain groups of "true risk factors" by adjusting for confounding "markers" of early, latent, disease which may also happen to be nonspecific markers of inflammation. For instance, if a "true risk factor" is always associated with laboratory evidence of inflammation (CRP, SAA, etc.), then adjusting for those confounding variables will dampen or mask the association with that risk factor. At present, epidemiologists and statisticians have not addressed this issue to find ways to overcome the hurdles.

REFERENCES

1. Finging, G., & Hanke, H. (1997) Nicolai Nikolajewitsch Anitschkow (1883–1964) established the cholesterol fed rabbit as a model for atherosclerosis research, *Atherosclerosis, 135*, 1–7.
2. Kannel, W. B., Dawber, T. R., Kagan, A., Revotskie, N., & Stokes, J., III (1961) Factors of risk in the development of coronary heart disease—six year follow up experience: the Framingham Study, *Ann. Intern. Med., 55*, 33–50.
3. Stamler, M., Wentworth, D., & Neaton, J. D., for the MRFIT Research Group (1986) Is the relationship between serum cholesterol and the risk of premature death from coronary heart disease continuous or graded? Findings in 356,222 primary screenees of the multiple risk factor intervention trial (MRFIT), *JAMA, 256*, 2823–2828.
4. Kwiterovitch, P. O. (1998) State of the art update and review; clinical trials of lipid-lowering agent, *Am. J. Cardiol., 82*, 3U–17U.
5. Downs, J. R., Clearfield, M., Weis, S., Whitney, E., Shapiro, D. R., Beere, P. A., Langendorfer, A., Stein, E. A., Kruyer, W., & Gotto, A. M. (1998) Primary prevention of acute coronary events with lovastatin in men and women with average cholesterol levels; results of AFCAPS/Tex CAPS. Air Force/Texas Coronary Atherosclerosis Prevention Study, *JAMA, 279*, 1615–1622.
6. Long Term Intervention with Pravastatin in Ischaemic Disease (LIPID) Study Group (1998) Prevention of cardiovascular events and death with pravastatin in patients with coronary heart disease and a broad range of initial cholesterol levels, *N. Engl. J. Med., 339*, 1349–1357.
7. Sacks, F. M., Pfeffer, M. A., Moye, L. A., Rouleau, J. L., Rutherford, J. D., Cole, T. G., Brown, L., Warnica, J. W., Arnold, J. M., Wun, C. C., Davis, B. R., &

Braunwald, E. (1996) The effects of pravastatin on coronary events after myocardial infarction in patients with average cholesterol levels, *N. Engl. J. Med., 335,* 1001–1009.

8. Scandinavian Simvastatin Survival Group (1994) Randomized trial of cholesterol lowering in 4444 patients with coronary heart disease: the Scandinavian Simvastatin Survival Study, *Lancet, 344,* 1383–1389.

9. Shepherd, J., Cobbe, S. M., Ford, I., Isles, C. G., Lorimer, A. R., MacFarlane, P. W., McKillop, J. H., & Packard, C. J. (1995) Prevention of coronary heart disease with pravastatin in men with hypercholesterolemia, *N. Engl. J. Med., 333,* 1301–1307.

10. Smith, E. B. (1974) The relationship between plasma and tissue lipids in human atherosclerosis, *Adv. Lipid Res., 12,* 1–49.

11. Hoff, H. F., Heideman, C. L., Gotto, A. M. Jr., & Gaubatz, J. W. (1977) Apolipoprotein B retention in the grossly normal and atherosclerotic human aorta, *Circ. Res., 40,* 56–64.

12. Berliner, J. A., Navab, M., Fogelman, A. M., Frank, J. S., Demer, L. L., Edwards, P. A., Watson, A. O., & Lusis, A. J. (1995) Atherosclerosis: basic mechanisms—oxidation, inflammation and genetics, *Circulation,* 91, 2488–2496.

13. Bork, R. W., Svenson, K. L., Melrabian, M., Lusis, A. J., Fogelman, A. M., & Edwards, P. A. (1992) Mechanisms controlling competence gene expression in murine fibroblasts stimulated with minimally modified LDL, *Arterioscler. Thromb., 12,* 800–806.

14. Watson, A. D., Navab, M., Hama, S. Y., Sevanian, A., Prescott, S. M., Stafforini, D. M., McIntyre, T. M., La Du, B. N., Fogelman, A. M., & Berliner, J. A. (1995) Effect of platelet-activating factor acetylhydrolase on the formation and action of minimally oxidized-low density lipoprotein, *J. Clin. Invest, 95,* 774–782.

15. Watson, A. D., Navab, M., Hough, G. P., Hama, S. Y., La Du, B. N., Young, L., Laks, H., Hermut, L. C., Fogelman, A. M., & Berliner, J. A. (1994) Biologically active phospholipids in MM-LDL are transferred to HDL and are hydrolyzed by HDL-associated esterases, *Circulation, 90,* I-353 [Abstract].

16. Gordon, D. J., Probstfield, J. L., Garrison, R. J., Neaton, J. D., Castelli, W. P., Jacobs, J. D. Jr., Bangdiwala, S., & Tyroler, H. A. (1989) High-density lipoprotein cholesterol and cardiovascular disease, *Circulation, 79,* 8–15.

17. Lao, F., And alibi, A., Ciao, J.-H., Allayed, H., Foeman, A. M., & Luis, A. J. (1993) Genetic evidence for a common pathway mediating oxidative stress, inflammatory gene induction, and aortic fatty streak formation in mice, *J. Clin. Invest., 94,* 877–884.

18. Lao, F., And alibi, A., de Boer, F. C., Foeman, A. M., & Luis, A. J. (1993) Genetic control of inflammatory gene induction and NF_kB-like transcription factor activation in response to an atherogenic diet in mice, *J. Clin. Invest., 91,* 2572–2579.

19. Ciao, J.-H., Welch, C. L., Xie, P.-Z., Fishbein, M. C., & Luis, A. J. (1993) Involvement of the tyrosine gene in the deposition of cardiac lipofuscin in mice: association with aortic fatty streak development, *J. Clin. Invest., 92,* 2386–2393.

20. Austin, M. A. (1991) Plasma triglyceride and coronary heart disease, *Arterioscler. Thromb., 11,* 2–14.

21. Castelli, W. P. (1992) Epidemiology of triglycerides: a view from Framingham [see comments], *Am. J. Cardiol., 70,* 3H–9H.
22. Jeppensen, J., Hein, H. O., Saudicani, P., & Gyntelberg, F. (1998) Triglyceride concentration and ischaemic heart disease: an eight-year follow-up in the Copenhagen Male Study [published erratum appears in *Circulation* (1998) *97,* 1995] [see comments], *Circulation, 97,* 1029–1036.
23. Bradley, W. A., & Gianturco, S. H. (1994) Triglyceride-rich lipoprotein and atherosclerosis: pathophysiological considerations, *J. Intern. Med. Suppl., 736,* 33–39.
24. Akmal, M., Kasim, S. E., Soliman, A. R., & Massry, S. G. (1990) Excess parathyroid hormone adversely affects lipid metabolism in chronic renal failure, *Kidney Int., 37,* 854–858.
25. Rader, D. J., & Rosas, S. (2000) Management of selected lipid abnormalities: hypertriglyceridemia, low HDL cholesterol, lipoprotein(a) in thyroid and renal diseases, and post-transplantation, *Med. Clin. North Am., 84,* 43–61.
26. Goldbourt, U., Yaari, S., & Medulie, J. H. (1997) Isolated low HDL cholesterol as a risk factor for coronary heart disease mortality: a 21 year follow-up of 8000 men, *Arterioscler. Thromb. Vasc. Biol., 17,* 107–113.
27. Gordon, D. J., & Rifkind, B. M. (1989) High density lipoproteins—the clinical implications of recent studies, *N. Engl. J. Med., 321,* 1311–1316.
28. Vega, G. L., & Grundy, S. M. (1996) Hypoalphalipoproteinemia (low high density lipoprotein) as a risk factor for coronary heart disease, *Curr. Opin. Lipidol., 7,* 209–216.
29. Glueck, C. J., Fallat, R. W., Millett, F., Gartside, P., Elston, R. C., & Go, R. C. (1975) Familial hyper-alpha—lipoproteinemia: studies in eighteen kindreds, *Metabolism, 24,* 1243–1265.
30. Rader, D. J., Shaefer, J. R., Lohse, P., Ikewaki, K., Thomas, F., Harris, W. A., Zech, L. A., Dujovne, C. A., & Brewer, H. B. (1993) Increased production of apolipoprotein A-1 associated with elevated plasma levels of high-density lipoproteins, apolipoprotein A-1, and lipoprotein A-1 in a patient with familial hyperalphalipoproteinemia, *Metab. Clin. Exp., 42,* 1429–1434.
31. Badimon, J. J., Badimon, L., & Fuster, V. (1990) Regression of atherosclerotic lesions by high density lipoprotein plasma fraction in the cholesterol-fed rabbit, *J. Clin. Invest., 85,* 1234–1243.
32. Miyazaki, A., Sakuma, S., Morikawa, W., Takine, T., Miake, F., Terano, T., Sakai, M., Hakamata, H., Sakamoto, Y., & Natio, M. (1995) Intravenous injection of rabbit apolipoprotein A-1 inhibits the progression of atherosclerosis in cholesterol-fed rabbits, *Arterioscler. Thromb. Vasc. Biol., 15,* 1882–1885.
33. Plump, A., Scott, C., & Breslow, J. (1994) Human apolipoprotein A-1 gene expression increases high density lipoprotein and suppresses atherosclerosis in the apolipoprotein-E-deficient mouse, *Proc. Natl. Acad. Sci. USA, 91,* 9607–9611.
34. Golbourt, U., Behar, S., Reicher-Riess, H., Agmon, J., Kaplinsky, E., Graff, E., Kishon, Y., Caspi, A., Weisbort, J., & Mandelzweig, L. (1993) Rationale and design of a secondary prevention trial of increasing serum high-density lipoprotein cholesterol and reducing triglycerides in patients with clinically manifest

atherosclerotic heart disease (the Bezafibrate Infarction Prevention Trial), *Am. J. Cardiol., 71*, 909–915.

35. Rubins, H. B., Robins, S. J., Iwane, M. K., Boden, W. E., Elam, M. B., Fye, C. L., Gordon, D. J., Schaefer, E. J., Schectman, G., & Wittes, J. T. (1993) Rationale and design of the Department of Veterans Affairs High Density Lipoprotein Cholesterol Intervention Trial (CHIT) for secondary prevention of coronary artery disease in men with low/high-density lipoprotein cholesterol and desirable low-density lipoprotein cholesterol, *Am. J. Cardiol., 71*, 45–52.

36. Tenkanen, L., Pietila, K., Manninen, V., & Manttari, M. (1994) The triglyceride issue revisited: findings from the Helsinki Heart Study, *Arch. Intern. Med., 154*, 2714–2720.

37. Boston, A. G., Cupples, L. A., Jenner, J. L., Ordovas, J. M., Seman, L. J., Wilson, P. W., Schaefer, E. J., & Castelli, W. P. (1996) Elevated plasma lipoprotein(a) and coronary heart disease in men 55 years and younger, *JAMA, 276*, 544–548.

38. Rosengren, A., Wilhelmsen, L., Ericksson, E., Risberg, B., & Wedel, H. (1990) Lipoprotein (a) and coronary heart disease: a prospective case-control study in general population sample of middle aged men, *BMJ, 301*, 1248–1251.

39. Schaefer, E. J., Lamon-Fava, S., Jenner, J. L., McNamara, I. R., Ordovas, J. M., Davis, C. E., Abolafia, J. M., Lippel, K., & Levy, R. I. (1994) Lipoprotein(a) levels and increased risk of coronary heart disease in men. The Lipid Research Clinics Coronary Primary Prevention Trial [see comments], *JAMA, 271*, 999–1003.

40. Ridker, P. M., Hennekens, C. H., & Stampfer, M. J. (1993) A prospective study of lipoprotein(a) and the risk of myocardial infarction [see comments], *JAMA, 270*, 2195–2199.

41. Sandholzer, C., Saha, N., Kark, J. D., Rees, A., Jaross, W., Dieplinger, H., Hoppichler, F., Boerwinkle, E., & Utermann, G. (1992) Apo(a) isoforms predict risk for coronary heart disease: a study in six populations, *Arterioscler. Thromb., 12*, 1214–1226.

42. Miles, L. A., Fless, G. M., Levin, E. G., Scanu, A. M., & Plow, E. F. (1989) A potential basis for the thrombotic risks associated with lipoprotein(a), *Nature, 339*, 301–303.

43. Scanu, A. M. (1988) Lipoprotein(a): a potential bridge between the fields of atherosclerosis and thrombosis, *Arch. Pathol. Lab. Med., 112*, 1045–1047.

44. Utermann, G. (1995) Lipoprotein(a), in C. R. Scriver, A. L. Beaudet, & W. S. Sly (Eds.), *Metabolic and molecular basis of inherited disease* (pp. 1887–1912), New York: McGraw Hill.

45. Fielding, J. (1985) Smoking: health effects and control (first of two parts), *N. Engl. J. Med., 313*, 491–498.

46. Goldstein, M. J., & Niaura, R. (1998) Smoking, in E. J. Topol, R. M. Calif, J. M. Isner, E. N. Prystowsky, P. W. Serrauys, J. D., E. J. Swain, Thomas, & P. D. Thompson (Eds.), *Textbook of cardiovascular medicine* (pp. 145–169), Philadelphia: Lippincott-Raven.

47. McGinnis, J., & Foege, W. (1993) Actual causes of death in the United States, *JAMA, 270*, 2207–2212.

48. US Department of Health and Human Services (1990) The health benefits of smoking cessation. A report of the Surgeon General, DHHS Publication No. (CDC) 90-8416, US Department of Health and Human Services, Public Health Service, Centers for Disease Control, Rockville, MD.

49. Morrow, J. D., Frei, B., Longmire, A. W., Gaziano, J. M., Lynch, S. M., Shyr, Y., Strauss, W. E., Oates, J. A., & Roberta, L. J. (1995) Increase in circulating products of lipid peroxidation (F2-isoprostanes) in smokers: smoking as a cause of oxidative damage, *N. Engl. J. Med., 332*, 1198–1203.

50. Kool, M. J., Hoeks, A. P., Struijker Boudier, H. A., Reneman, R. S., & Von Bortel, L. M. (1993) Short and long-term effects of smoking on arterial wall properties in habitual smokers, *J. Am. Coll. Cardiol., 22*, 1881–1886.

51. Kannell, W., McGee, D., & Castelli, W. (1984) Latest perspectives on cigarette smoking and cardiovascular disease: the Framingham study, *J. Cardiac Rehabil., 4*, 267–277.

52. Hallstrom, A., Cobb, L., & Ray, R. (1986) Smoking as a risk for recurrence of sudden cardiac arrest, *N. Engl. J. Med., 314*, 271–275.

53. Galan, K., Deligonul, U., Kern, M., Chaitman, B. R., & Vandormael, M. G. (1988) Increased frequency of restenosis in patients continuing to smoke cigarettes after percutaneous transluminal coronary angioplasty, *Am. J. Cardiol., 61*, 260–263.

54. Solymoss, B., Nadeau, P., Millette, D., & Campeau, L. (1988) Late thrombosis of saphenous vein coronary bypass grafts related to risk factors, *Circulation, 78*(Suppl I), I-140–143.

55. Kario, K., & Pickering, T. G. (2000) Modification of high blood pressure after myocardial infarction, *Med. Clin. North Am., 84*, 1–21.

56. Neutel, J. M., & Smith, D. H. (1997) The circadian pattern of blood pressure: cardiovascular risk and therapeutic opportunities, *Curr. Opin. Nephrol. Hypertens., 6*, 250–256.

57. Brush, J. E., Cannon, R. O. III., Schenke, W. H., Bonow, R. O., Leon, M. B., Maron, B. J., & Epstein, S. E. (1988) Angina due to coronary microvascular disease in hypertensive patients without left ventricular hypertrophy, *N. Engl. J. Med., 319*, 1302–1307.

58. Flack, J. M., Neaton, J., Grimm, R. J., Shih, J., Cutler, J., Ensrud, K., & MacMahon, S. (1995) Blood pressure and mortality among men with prior myocardial infarction, Multiple Risk Factor Intervention Trial Research Group, *Circulation, 92*, 2437–2445.

59. Herlitz, J., Bang, A., & Karlson, B. W. (1996) Five-year prognosis after acute myocardial infarction in relation to a history of hypertension, *Am. J. Hypertens., 9*, 70–76.

60. Gustafsson, F., Kober, L., Torp-Pedersen, C., & Hildebrandt, P. (1998) Influence of a history of arterial hypertension and pre-treatment blood pressure on the effect of angiotensin converting enzyme inhibition after acute myocardial infarction. Trandolapril Cardiac Evaluation Study, *J. Hypertens., 16*(Suppl), S65–S70.

61. Cruickshank, J. M., Thorp, J. M., & Zacharias, F. J. (1987) Benefits and potential harm of lowering high blood pressure, *Lancet, 1*, 581–584.

62. Farnett, L., Mulrow, C. D., Linn, W. D., Lucey, C. R., & Tuley, M. R. (1991) The J-curve phenomenon and the treatment of hypertension: is there a point beyond which pressure reduction is dangerous? *JAMA, 265,* 489–495.

63. Hansson, L., Zanchetti, A., Carruthers, S. G., Dahlof, B., Elmfeldt, D., Julius, S., Menard, J., Rahn, K. H., Wedel, H., & Westerling, S. (1998) Effects of intensive blood pressure lowering and low dose aspirin in patients with hypertension: principal results of the Hypertension Optimal Treatment (HOT), randomized trial. HOT Study Group, *Lancet, 351,* 1755–1762.

64. Kannel, W. B., & McGee, D. L. (1979) Diabetes and cardiovascular disease. The Framingham study, *JAMA, 241,* 2035–2038.

65. Wingard, D. L., & Barrett-Connor, E. (1995) Heart disease and diabetes, in National Diabetes Data Group (Ed.), *Diabetes in America* (2nd ed., pp. 428–448), National Institutes of Health, Bethesda, MD: National Institute of Diabetes and Digestive Disease and Kidney Diseases.

66. Ruderman, N., Williamson, J., & Brownlee, J. (Eds.) (1992) *Hyperglycemia, diabetes, and vascular disease,* New York: Oxford University Press.

67. Diabetes Control and Complications Trials Research Group (DCCT) (1993) The effects of intensive treatment of diabetes on the development and progression of long-term complications in insulin-dependent diabetes mellitus, *N. Engl. J. Med., 329,* 977–986.

68. Goldberg, R. B. (2000) Cardiovascular disease in diabetic patients, *Med. Clin. North Am., 84,* 81–93.

69. Pyörälä, K. (1979) Relationship of glucose intolerance and plasma insulin to the incidence of coronary heart disease: results from two population studies in Finland, *Diabetes Care, 20,* 614–620.

70. Welborn, T. A. & Wearne, K. (1979) Coronary heart disease incidence and cardiovascular mortality in Busselton with reference to glucose and insulin concentrations, *Diabetes Care, 2,* 154–160.

71. Stout, R. W. (1990) Insulin and atheroma, *Diabetes Care, 13,* 631–634.

72. Lamarche, B., Tchernof, A., Mauriege, P., Cantin, B., Dagenais, G. R., Lupien, P. J., & Despres, J. P. (1998) Fasting insulin and apolipoprotein B levels and low-density lipoprotein particle size as risk factors for ischaemic heart disease, *JAMA, 279,* 1955–1961.

73. Howard, G., O'Leary, D. H., Zaccaro, D., Haffner, S., Rewers, M., Hamman, R., Selby, J. V., Saad, M. F., Savage, P., & Bergman, R. (1996) Insulin sensitivity and atherosclerosis, *Circulation, 93,* 1809–1817.

74. Minamikawa, J., Tanaka, S., Yamauchi, M., Inoue, & Koshiyama, J. (1998) Potent inhibiting effect of troglitazone on carotid arterial wall thickness in type 2 diabetes, *J. Clin. Endocrinol. Metab., 83,* 1818–1820.

75. DeFronzo, R. A., & Goodman, A. M., for the Multicenter Metformin Study Group (1995) Efficacy of metformin in patients with non-insulin dependent diabetes mellitus, *N. Engl. J. Med., 333,* 541–549.

76. National Center for Health Statistics (1981) Plan and operation of the Second National Health Interview Survey, 1976–1980, in *Viral and Health Statistics,* Ser. 1, No. 15, DHHS, pub. no. PHS81-1317, US Government Printing Office, Washington, DC.

77. Wilson, P. W., Kannell, W. B., & Anderson, K. M. (1985) Lipids, glucose tolerance and vascular disease: the Framingham study, *Manogr. Atheroscler, 13*, 1–11.
78. Stamler, J., Vaccaro, O., Neaton, J. D. & Wentworth, D. (1993) Diabetes, other risk factors and 12 year cardiovascular mortality for men screened in the Multiple Risk Factor Intervention Trial, *Diabetes Care, 16*, 434–444.
79. Coldwell, J. A. (1997) Aspirin therapy in diabetes, *Diabetes Care, 20*, 1767–1771.
80. Eckel, R. H. (1997) Obesity and heart disease: a statement for health care professionals from the Nutrition Committee, America Heart Association, *Circulation, 96*, 3248–3250.
81. Hall, J. E. (1997) Mechanisms of abnormal renal sodium handling in obesity hypertension, *Am. J. Hypertens.*, (SPT-2) *10*, 495–555.
82. Jousilahti, P., Toumilehto, J., Vartianen, E., Pekkanen, J., & Puska, P. (1996) Body weight, cardiovascular risk factors and coronary mortality: 15 year follow up of middle aged men and women in eastern Finland, *Circulation, 93*, 1372–1379.
83. Defronzo, R. A. (1997) Insulin resistance: a multifaceted syndrome responsible for NIDDM, obesity, hypertension, dyslipidaemia and atherosclerosis, *Neth. J. Med., 50*, 191–197.
84. Lean, M. E. J., Han, T. S., & Seidell, J. C. (1998) Impairment of health and quality of life in people with large waist circumference, *Lancet, 351*, 853–856.
85. Van Gall, L. F., Wanters, M. A., & De Leeuw, I. H. (1997) The beneficial effects of modest weight loss on cardiovascular risk factors, *Int. J. Obes. Rehab. Metab. Disord., 21* (Suppl), S5–S9.
86. Barrett-Connor, E., & Khaw, K. (1984) Family history of heart attack as an independent predictor of death due to cardiovascular disease, *Circulation, 69*, 1065–1069.
87. Jousilahti, P., Puska, P., Vartianen, E., Pekhanen, J., & Toumilehto, J. (1996) Parenteral history of premature coronary heart disease: an independent risk factor of myocardial infarction, *J. Clin. Epidemiol., 49*, 497–503.
88. Friedlander, Y., Siscovick, D. S., Weinmann, S., Austin, M. A., Psaty, B. M., Lemaitre, R. N., Arbogast, P., Raghunathan, T. E., & Cobb, L. A. (1998) Family history as a risk factor for primary cardiac arrest, *Circulation, 97*, 155–160.
89. De Bacqner, D., De Backer, G., Kornitzer, M., & Blackburn, H. (1999) Parenteral history of premature coronary heart disease mortality and signs of ischaemia on the resting electrocardiogram, *J. Am. Coll. Cardiol., 33*, 1491–1498.
90. Slack, J., & Evans, K. A. (1966) The increased risk of death from ischaemia heart disease in the first degree relatives of 121 men and 96 women with ischaemic heart disease, *J. Med. Genet., 3*, 239–257.
91. Riley, W. A., Freedman, D. S., Higgs, N. A,. Barnes, R. W., Zinkgraf, S. A., & Berenson, G. S. (1986) Decreased arterial elasticity associated with cardiovascular disease risk factors in the young: Bogalusa Heart Study, *Arteriosclerosis, 6*, 378–386.
92. Clarkson, P., Celermajer, D. S., Powe, A. J., Donald, A. E., Henry, R. M. A., & Deanfield, J. E. (1997) Endothelium-dependent dilatation is impaired in young healthy subjects with a family history of premature coronary disease, *Circulation, 96*, 3378–3383.

93. Gaeta, G., De Michelle, M., Cuomo, S., Guarini, P., Foglia, M. C., Bond, G., & Trevisan, M. (2000) Arterial abnormalities in the offspring of patients with premature myocardial infarction, *N. Engl. J. Med., 343*, 840–846.

94. Celermajer, D. S, Sorensen, K. E., Bull, C., Robinson, J., & Deanfield, J. E. (1994) Endothelium-dependent dilatation in the systemic arteries of asymptomatic subjects relates to coronary risk factors and their interaction, *J. Am. Coll. Cardiol., 24*, 1468–1474.

95. Bots, M. L., Hoes, A. W., Koudstaal, P. J., Hofman, A., & Grobbee, D. E. (1997) Common carotid intima-media thickness and risk of stroke and myocardial infarction: the Rotterdam study, *Circulation, 96*, 1432–1437.

96. O'Leary, D. H., Polak, J. F., Kronmal, R. A., Manolio, T. A., Burke, G. L., & Wolfson, S. K. Jr. (1999) Carotid-artery intima and media thickness as a risk factor for myocardial infarction and stroke in older adults, *N. Engl. J. Med., 340*, 14–22.

97. Freedman, D. S., Srinivasan, S. R., Shear, C. L., Franklin, F. A., Webber, L. S., & Berenson, G. S. (1986) The relation of apolipoproteins A-1 and B in children to parenteral myocardial infarction, *N. Engl. J. Med., 315*, 721–726.

98. Bao, W., Srinivasan, S. R., Wattigney, W. A., & Berenson, G. S. (1995) The relation of parenteral cardiovascular disease to risk factors in children and young adults: the Bogalusa heart study, *Circulation, 91*, 365–371.

99. Greenlund, K. J., Srinivasan, S. R., Xu, J. H., Dalzers, E., Myers, L., Pickoff, A., & Borenson, G. S. (1999) Plasma homocysteine distribution and its association with parenteral history of coronary artery disease in black and white children: the Bogalusa heart study, *Circulation, 99*, 2144–2149.

100. Zannad, F., Visvikis, S., Gueguen, R., Sass, C., Chapet, O., Herbeth B., & Siest, G. (1998) Genetics strongly determines the wall thickness of the left and right carotid arteries, *Hum. Genet., 103*, 183–188.

101. Wang, X. L., Sim, A. S., Badenhop, R. F., McCredie, R. M., & Wilcken, D. E. (1996) A smoking-dependent risk of coronary artery disease associated with a polymorphism of the endothelial nitric oxide synthase gene, *Nat. Med., 2*, 41–45.

102. Nakayama, M., Yasue, H., Yoshimura, M., Shimasaki, Y., Kugiyama, K., Ogawa, H., Motoyama, T., Saito, Y., Miyamoto, Y., Ogawa, Y., & Nakao, K. (1999) T-786→C mutation in the 5′-flanking region of the endothelial nitric oxide synthase gene is associated with coronary spasm, *Circulation, 99*, 2864–2870.

103. Lifton, R. P. (1996) Molecular genetics of human blood pressure variation, *Science, 272*, 676–680.

104. Brown, M. S., & Goldstein, J. L. (1986) A receptor-mediated pathway for cholesterol homeostasis, *Science, 232*, 34–47.

105. Meilahan, E. (1999) Sex steroid hormonal influences on coronary artery disease, in R. B. Ness, & L. H. Kuller (Eds.), *Health and disease among women, biological and environmental influences* (p. 155), New York: Oxford University Press.

106. Lieberman, E. H., Gerhard, M. D., Uehata, A., Walsh, B. W., Selwyn, A. P., Ganz, P., Yeung, A. C., & Creager, M. A. (1994) Estrogen improves endothelium-dependent, flow-mediated vasodilation in post-menopausal women, *Ann. Intern. Med., 121*, 936–941.

107. Kuller, L. H. (2000) Hormone replacement therapy and coronary heart disease: a new debate, *Med. Clin. North Am., 84*, 181–198.
108. Barrett-Connor, E., & Grady, D. (1998) Hormone replacement therapy, heart disease and other considerations, *Annu. Rev. Public Health, 19*, 55–72.
109. McCully, K. S. (1969) Vascular pathology of homocysteinemia: implications for the pathogenesis of arteriosclerosis, *Am. J. Pathol., 56*, 111–128.
110. Ueland, P. M., & Refsum, H. (1989) Plasma homocysteine, a risk factor for vascular disease: plasma levels in health, disease, and drug therapy, *J. Lab. Clin. Med., 114*, 473–501.
111. McCully, K. S. (1996) Homocysteine and vascular disease, *Nat. Med., 2*, 386–389.
112. Kang, S. S., Wong, P. W., & Malinow, M. R. (1992) Hyperhomocysteinemia as a risk factor for occlusive vascular disease, *Ann. Rev. Nutr., 12*, 279–298.
113. Eikelboom, J. W., Lonn, E., Genest, J. Jr., Hankey, G., & Yusuf, S. (1999) Homocysteine and cardiovascular disease: a critical review of epidemiological evidence, *Ann. Intern. Med., 131*, 363–375.
114. Welch, G. N., & Loscalzo, J. (1998) Homocysteine and atherosclerosis: mechanism of disease [Review article], *N. Engl. J. Med., 338*, 1042–1050.
115. Harker, L. A., Slicheter, S. J., Scott, C. R., & Ross, R. (1974) Homocysteinemia: vascular injury and arterial thrombosis, *N. Engl. J. Med., 291*, 537–543.
116. Harker, L. A., Ross, R., Slichter, S. J., & Scott, C. R. (1976) Homocysteine-induced arteriosclerosis: the role of endothelial cell injury and platelet response in its genesis, *J. Clin. Invest., 58*, 731–741.
117. Lentz, S. R., Sobey, C. G., Piegors, D. J., Bhopatkar, M. Y., Faraci, F. M., Malinow, M. R., & Heistad, D. D. (1996) Vascular dysfunction in monkeys with diet-induced hyperhomocyst(e)inemia, *J. Clin. Invest., 98*, 24–29.
118. Van den Berg, M., Boers, G. H., Franken, D. G., Blom, H. J., Van Kamp, G. J., Jakobs, C., Rauwerda, J. A., Kluft, C., & Stehouwert, C. D. (1995) Hyperhomocysteinemia and endothelial dysfunction in young patients with peripheral arterial occlusive disease, *Eur. J. Clin. Invest., 25*, 176–181.
119. Starkebaum, G., & Harlan, J. M. (1986) Endothelial cell injury due to copper-catalysed hydrogen peroxide generation from homocysteine, *J. Clin. Invest., 77*, 1370–1376.
120. Rowley, D. A., & Halliwell, B. (1982) Superoxide-dependent formation of hydroxyl radicals in the presence of thiol compounds, *FEBS Lett., 138*, 33–36.
121. Loscalzo, J. (1996) The oxidant stress of hyperhomocyst(e)inemia, *J. Clin. Invest., 98*, 5–7.
122. Peterson, J. C., & Spence, J. D. (1998) Vitamins and progression of atherosclerosis in hyperhomocyst(e)inaemia [Letter], *Lancet, 351*, 263.
123. Savage, D. D., Garrison, R. J., Kannell, W. B., Levy, D., Anderson, S. J., Stokes, J. 3rd, Feinlieb, M., & Castelli, W. P. (1987) The spectrum of left ventricular hypertrophy in a general population sample: the Framingham study, *Circulation, 75*(1 PT2,) I26–I33.
124. Harjai, K. J. (1999) Potential new cardiovascular risk factors: left ventricular hypertrophy, homocysteine, lipoprotein(a) triglycerides, oxidative stress, and fibrinogen, *Ann. Intern. Med., 131*, 376–386.

125. Levy, D., Garrison, R. J., Savage, D. D., Kannel, W. B., & Castelli, W. P. (1990) Prognostic implications of echocardiographically demonstrated left ventricular mass in the Framingham heart study, *N. Engl. J. Med., 322*, 1561–1566.
126. Devereux, R. B., Agabiti-Rosei, E., Dahlof, B., Gosse, P., Hahn, R. T., Okin, P. M., & Roman, M. J. (1996) Regression of left ventricular hypertrophy as a surrogate end-point for morbid events in hypertension trials, *J. Hypertens., 14*(Suppl), S95–S101.
127. Thompson, S. G., Kienast, J., Pyke, S. D., Haverkate, F., & van de Loo, J. C. (1995) Hemostatic factors and the risk of myocardial infarction or sudden death in patients with angina pectoris. European Concerted Action on Thrombosis and Disabilities Angina Pectoris Study Group, *N. Engl. J. Med., 332*, 635–641.
128. Jansson, J. H., Olofsson, B. O., & Nilsson, T. K. (1993) Predictive value of tissue plasminogen activator mass concentration on long term mortality in patients with coronary artery disease. A 7 year follow-up, *Circulation, 88*(5 PT.1), 2030–2034.
129. Ridker, P. M., Vaughan, D. E., Stampfer, M. J., Manson, J. E., & Hennekens, C. H. (1993) Endogenous tissue-type plasminogen activator and risk of myocardial infarction, *Lancet, 341*, 1165–1168.
130. Ridker, P. M., Hennekens, C. H., Stampfer, M. J., Manson, J. E., & Vaughan, D. E. (1994) Prospective study of endogenous tissue plasminogen activator and risk of stroke, *Lancet, 343*, 940–943.
131. Ridker, P. M. (1997), Fibrinolytic and inflammatory markers for arterial occlusion: the evolving epidemiology of thrombosis and hemostasis, *Thromb. Haemost., 78*, 53–59.
132. Rauch, U., Osende, J. I., Fuster, V., Badimon, J. J., Fayad, Z., & Chesebro, J. H. (2001) Thrombus formation on atherosclerotic plaques: pathogenesis and clinical consequences, *Ann. Intern. Med., 134*, 224–238.
133. Soejima, H., Ogawa, H., Yasue, H., Kaikita, K., Nishiyama, K., Misumi, K., Takazoe, K., Miyao, Y., Yoshimura, M., Kugiyama, K., Nakamura, S., Tsuji, I., & Kumeda, K. (1999) Heightened tissue factors associated with tissue factor pathway inhibitor and prognosis in patients with unstable angina, *Circulation, 99*, 2908–2913.
134. Saito, Y., Wada, H., Yamamuro, M., Inoue, A., Shimura, M., Hiyoyama, K., Gabazza, E. C., Isaka, N., Shiku, H., Takeya, H., Suzuki, K., Kumeda, K., Kato, H., & Nakano, T. (1999) Changes of plasma hemostatic markers during percutaneous transluminal coronary angioplasty in patients with chronic coronary artery disease, *Am. J. Hematol., 61*, 238–242.
135. Hall, W. D. (1999) Abnormalities of kidney function as a cause and a consequence of cardiovascular disease, *Am. J. Med. Sci., 317*, 176–182.
136. Parfrey, P. S., & Foley, R. N. (1999) The clinical epidemiology of cardiac disease in chronic renal failure, *J. Am. Soc. Nephrol., 10*, 1606–1615.
137. Mittman, N., & Auram, M. M. (1996) Dyslipidemia in renal disease, *Semin. Nephrol., 16*, 202–213.
138. Shulman, N. B., Ford, C. E., Hall, W. D., Blaufox, M. D., Simon, D., Lanford, H. G., & Schneider, K. A. (1989) Prognostic value of serum creatinine and effect

of treatment of hypertension on renal function. Results from the hypertension detection and follow-up program. The Hypertension Detection and Follow-up Program Cooperative Group, *Hypertension, 13*, 180–193.

139. Flack, J., Neaton, J., Daniels, B., & Esunge, P. (1993) Ethnicity and renal disease: lessons from the Multiple Risk Factor Intervention Trial and the Treatment of Mild Hypertension Study, *Am. J. Kidney Dis., 21*, 31–40.

140. Culleton, B., Larson, M., Wilson, P., Evans, J., Parfrey, P., & Levy, D. (1999) Cardiovascular disease and mortality in a community-based cohort with mild renal insufficiency, *Kidney Int., 56*, 2214–2219.

141. Mann, J. F. E., Hertzel, C. G., Pogue, J., Bosch, J., & Yusuf, S. for the Hope Investigators (2001) Renal insufficiency as a predictor of cardiovascular outcomes and the impact of ramipril: the Hope randomized trial, *Ann. Intern. Med., 134*, 629–636.

142. Wannamettree, S., Sharper, A., & Perry, I. (1997) Serum creatinine concentration and risk of cardiovascular disease: a possible marker for increased risk of stroke, *Stroke, 28*, 557–563.

143. Kasiske, B. L. (2001) The kidney in cardiovascular disease [Editorial], *Ann. Intern. Med. 134*, 707–709.

4

Effect of Infection on Lipoproteins and the Coagulation System

4.1. INTRODUCTION

The link or association between various infections and complications of atherosclerosis (myocardial infarction and stroke) could potentially be related to changes in lipoprotein patterns. Infection and inflammation can produce a wide range of changes in the metabolism that could produce a proatherogenic environment. Infections normally result in the stimulation of the proinflammatory cytokines, as a defense mechanism against invading microbes, which are potent inducers of acute phase reactants, C-reactive protein (CRP), fibrinogen, serum amyloid A (SAA), which are early markers of atherosclerosis and cardiovascular disease.

4.2. LIPOPROTEIN AND ATHEROSCLEROSIS

As discussed in Chapter 3, lipids and lipoproteins are well-established as playing a major role in atherogenesis. Hypercholesterolemia, especially elevated levels of low-density lipoprotein (LDL) cholesterol, is a major risk factor for coronary heart disease (CHD), and therapeutic reductions in total cholesterol and LDL result in decrease in cardiovascular mortality and morbidity[1-3]. Hypertriglyceridemia and elevated levels of triglyceride-rich lipoproteins (very low-density lipoprotein (VLDL) and remnants) are now considered established risk factors for CHD[4,5]. However, blood levels of high-density lipoprotein (HDL) cholesterol are inversely correlated with the risk for atherosclerotic complications[6]. Therapies that raise HDL and reduce triglyceride concentrations have resulted in reduced cardiovascular events and mortality[7,8].

4.2.1. Acute Phase Response

When the host defense is breached by an invader, there is a generalized, coordinated, but non-specific reaction termed the "acute phase response," which helps protect the host from further injury and facilitates the repair process. This response augments (positive acute phase proteins), or depresses (negative acute phase proteins) the concentration and function of humoral defense components. The acute phase proteins include CRP, SAA, lipopolysaccharide-binding protein (LBP), haptoglobulin, fibrinogen, ceruloplasminα, acid glycoprotein, complement components (C3 and C4), transferrin, calcitonin, pre-albumen, natural anticoagulants such as protein C, protein S, antithrombin plasminogen, tissue plasminogen activator, urokinase, vitronectin, plasminogen activator inhibitor-I (PAI-1), α_1-protease inhibitor, α-antichymotrypsin, pancreatic secretory trypsin inhibitor, ferritin, angiotensinogen, α-fetoprotein, thyroxine-binding globulin, Factor XII, fibronectin, granulocyte colony stimulating factor (GCSF), and interleukin (IL)-1 receptor antagonist[9]. Classical positive phase response proteins include fibrinogen, CRP and SAA, ferritin, etc., whereas, negative acute phase response proteins include albumin, transthyretin, α_2-HS glycoprotein, and transferrin. These important proteins increase the number and function of phagocytic cells, facilitate delivery of humoral and cellular components to sites of inflammation, and direct the pattern of antigen-specific immune responses. The acute phase response is mediated by gamma-delta T-cells[10], reactions of humoral defenses, and by de novo production of regulatory molecules (i.e., cytokines, chemokines, prostaglandins, hormones) by phagocytes, lymphocytes, and endothelial cells. Cytokines, such as tumor necrosis factor (TNF) or IL-1, are prime mediators of these metabolic changes during infection and inflammation. It has been postulated that prolonged exposure to these metabolic changes may be harmful to the host, for example, development of secondary amyloidosis after chronic infection or inflammation, and possibly atherosclerosis.

Many acute-phase proteins are thought to be anti-infective. CRP binds to phosphocholine on the surfaces of invading microbes to enhance killing by complement and phagocytes, and secretory phospholipase A_2 is a potent anti-staphylococcal and antistreptococcal enzyme. Acute phase proteins can also be anti-inflammatory, neutralizing proinflammatory cytokines, proteases and oxidants released into the blood from areas of inflammation[11].

The acute phase response may also lead to a procoagulant environment. This is a defense mechanism to localize invading microbes, as clotting is required to wall off microorganisms in an abscess. The main procoagulant cytokine is IL-6 and through mediators such as fibrinogen, PAI-1 and CRP stimulate tissue factor on monocytes, which initiates the clotting cascade.

The acute phase responses may also alter the use and metabolism of endogenous nutrients. Increases in fatty acid and triglycerides in the blood can result from cytokine mediated increased lipolysis within adipocytes and hepatic synthesis[12]. Thus, metabolic changes resulting from infection or inflammation can lead to alterations in cholesterol and lipoprotein or other proteins that produce a favorable environment for development of atherosclerosis (see Table 4.1, adapted from Khovidhunkit et al.[12]).

Table 4.1
Potential Proatherogenic Changes and Effects of Lipoproteins During Infection and Inflammation

Changes	Effects
VLDL	
Increased VLDL levels	Provides lipid substrates for macrophage uptake
Decreased LPL and HL	Decreases clearance of triglyceride-rich lipoproteins
Increased sphingolipid content	Decreases clearance of triglyceride-rich lipoproteins
Decreased tissue apoE expression	Decreases lipoprotein clearance
LDL	
Increased small dense LDL	Increases susceptibility to oxidation; increases LDL penetration through endothelium; increases interaction with arterial wall proteoglycans and LDL retention in arterial wall
Increased PAF-AH activity	Increases LPC production
Increased sPLA$_2$	Releases polyunsaturated fatty acids from phospholipids that can become oxidized fatty acids
Increased sphingolipid content	Facilitates LDL aggregation and uptake into macrophages
Increased ceruloplasmin	Increases LDL oxidation
HDL	
Decreased HDL and apoA-1	Impairs apolipoprotein-mediated cholesterol removal from cells
Decreased LCAT	Impairs cholesterol removal from cells by diffusion mechanism
Decreased CETP	Impairs cholesterol transfer to triglyceride-rich lipoproteins
Decreased HL	Reduces pre-β HDL generation
Decreased PLTP	Reduces pre-β HDL generation; decreases HDL phospholipid content and impairs cholesterol removal by increasing cholesterol flux from HDL into cells
Increased SAA	Decreases availability of cholesterol in HDL to be metabolized by hepatocytes; increases cholesterol uptake into macrophages

Table 4.1

(*continued*)

Changes	Effects
Increased sPLA$_2$	Decreases HDL phospholipid content and impairs cholesterol removal by increasing cholesterol flux from HDL into cells
Increased PAF-AH activity	Increases LPC production
Decreased PON	Decreases ability of HDL to protect against LDL oxidation
Decreased transferrin	Impairs the ability of HDL to prevent LDL oxidation
Increased apoJ	Induces smooth-muscle cell differentiation in arterial wall

Note. apo, apolipoprotein; CETP, cholesterol ester transfer protein; HDL, high-density lipoprotein; HL, hepatic lipase; LCAT, lecithin: cholesterol acyltransferase; LDL, low-density lipoprotein; LPC, lysophosphatidylcholine; LPL, lipoprotein lipase; PAF-AH, platelet-activating factor acetylhydrolase; sPLA$_2$, secretory phospholipase A$_2$; PLTP, phospholipid transfer protein; PON, paraoxanase; VLDL, very low-density lipoprotein; SAA, serum amyloid A. Adapted from Khovidhunkit et al.[12] with permission of the publishers.

4.2.2. Alterations of Triglyceride and VLDL Metabolism

The main effect of infection and inflammation on the metabolism and lipoprotein is hypertriglyceridemia[13]. This is mainly due to an increase in VLDL, as a result of an increased production and decreased clearance. Interferon-α appears to be the primary cytokine responsible for the increased hepatic lipogenesis and decreased triglyceride clearance[12,14]. Lipopolysaccharide (LPS) from gram-negative bacteria in low doses increases hepatic fatty acid synthesis, decreases hepatic fatty acid oxidation, and increases adipose tissue lypolysis— all resulting in increased fatty acid for esterification into triglycerides and assembly into VLDL in the liver[15,16] in rodents. High-dose LPS decreases lipoprotein lipase activity, thus decreasing the clearance of triglyceride-rich lipoprotein[17] but does not increase hepatic VLDL synthesis. Lipoteichoic acid (LTA) from gram-positive bacteria is also capable of raising triglyceride levels in rodents by increasing hepatic VLDL triglyceride production[18]. Infection can also impair the clearance of VLDL particles by reduction of apolipoprotein (apo)E expression in tissues, since uptake of VLDL particles by the LDL receptor and LDL-receptor-related protein is enhanced by apoE[19].

The proinflammatory cytokines such as TNF-α, IL-1, IL-6, and interferon-α are the mediators of LPS and LTA effect on triglyceride metabolism, as they can increase hepatic fatty acid synthesis with increased VLDL and triglycerides in animal models[15,20]. Although the cytokine profiles stimulated with bacterial infections (primarily TNF-α and IL-1), viral infections (IFN-α), and noninfectious inflammation (mainly IL-1) are somewhat different, the effect on triglyceride metabolism is similar[12].

Besides an increase in VLDL and triglycerides, infection and inflammation result in a more sphingolipid-enriched VLDL which have potentially greater proatherogenic properties. Sphingomyelin impairs the clearance of triglyceride-rich lipoproteins resulting in accumulation of proatherogenic remnant particles[21].

4.2.3. Cholesterol and LDL Alterations

Infection and inflammation can affect cholesterol and LDL metabolism by several mechanisms, reviewed recently by Khovidhunkit et al.[12], see Table 4.1. Oxidative modification of lipoproteins plays a major role in atherosclerosis and infection or inflammatory mediators can induce LDL oxidation in vivo. In a recent study by Memon et al.[22], bacterial LPS to mimic acute infection, zymosan to induce acute systemic inflammation, and turpentine to produce acute local inflammation were found to increase oxidized lipids in serum and induce LDL oxidation in vivo in hamsters. Furthermore, in response to infection and inflammation, the component of LDL may change from the predominantly large buoyant LDL to the small dense LDL (subclass B) that appears to be more proatherogenic, due to greater susceptibility to oxidation and can penetrate the endothelium and bind more effectively to the intima proteoglycans than the larger LDL particle[23,24]. Besides a greater tendency to retention in the arterial wall there is also decreased clearance of small dense LDL due to poor binding affinity to LDL receptor[25]. In humans with chronic infections such as in patients with the acquired immunodeficiency syndrome (AIDS), a decrease in LDL cholesterol is associated with an increase in small dense LDL[26].

In animals LPS increases the triglyceride and cholesterol content in LDL, resulting in triglyceride and cholesterol-rich particles[27]. This LDL is also enriched with sphingolipids, such as sphingomyelin and ceramide[28]. Infection through cytokines may also increase ceramide generation by upregulation of secretion of sphingomyelinase by endothelial cells and macrophages[29]. Lipoproteins rich in sphingolipid is proposed to increase the atherogenicity of LDL. Ceramide-rich lipoproteins enhance LDL uptake by macrophages to form foam cells[30], and LDL from atheromas are enriched with ceramide with increased tendency to aggregate[29].

Besides an increase in sphingomyelin and ceramide, LPS increases the glucosylceramide content of lipoproteins[28], through TNF-α and IL-1 upregulation of liver synthesis and activity of glucosylceramide synthase[31], and this glycosylated sphingolipid has increased atherogenic potential[32].

Activation of leukocytes, platelets, and endothelial cells by infection or inflammation increases the proinflammatory phospholipid, platelet-activating factor (PAF), and the catalyzing enzyme PAF acetylhydrolase (PAF-AH) that hydrolyzes oxidized fatty acids from phospholipids[33]. Most plasma PAF-AH activity (60–70%) is found in LDL and the rest in HDL in humans. PAF-AH hydrolyzes phosphatidylcholine to lysophosphatidylcholine that may be responsible for many of the biologic effects of LDL, such as chemotaxis of monocytes, stimulation of adhesion molecules and impairment of blood vessel relaxation[34,35], proatherogenic properties. Conversely, PAF-AH may protect LDL against further oxidation as it removes oxidized fatty acids from the phospholipids in LDL.

Another acute phase protein that is induced in infection and inflammation, secretory non-pancreatic phospholipase A_2 (sPLA$_2$), hydrolyzes phospholipids, mainly phosphatidylethanolamine, liberating polyunsaturated fatty acids. Thus, more fatty acid substrate for oxidation with increased oxidized fatty acids are provided, resulting in modification of LDL to oxidized LDL[36]. Transgenic mice over expressing human sPLA$_2$ can develop atherosclerosis even on a low-fat diet[37].

4.2.4. Alteration of HDL Metabolism

Probably one of the major proatherogenic lipid effects of infection or inflammation is a reduction in serum levels of HDL. Clinical and epidemiological studies have established that low HDL is a risk factor for cardiovascular disease. The mechanism for a low HDL in infection and inflammation is not well understood. Besides, a low HDL chronic infection may affect the composition and function of HDL, through the effect of apolipoproteins, enzymes, and transfer proteins that regulate the metabolism and function of HDL. The antiatherogenic properties of HDL putatively include protection against LDL oxidation and the removal of cholesterol from cells to the liver for elimination (reverse cholesterol transport).

Acute phase HDL (produced during infection or inflammation) are low in cholesterol ester but enriched with free cholesterol, triglyceride, and sphingolipids[27,38,39]. Other plasma proteins that may play a role in HDL metabolism and function such as lecithin: cholesterol acyltransferase (LCAT), cholesterol ester transfer protein, hepatic lipase, and phospholipid transfer protein (PLTP) are also reduced during infection[40–42].

HDL may protect against LDL oxidation through several HDL-associated proteins with antioxidant properties, including PAF-AH, paraoxonase, ceruloplasmin, and transferin[43,44]. The response of PAF-AH to inflammation or infection may vary with the animal species. In humans infected with HIV, an increase in PAF-AH activity is found in LDL but not in HDL[43]. Although PAF-AH increase may protect against LDL oxidation, a prolonged increase can result in the production of lysophosphatidylcholine which has proathero-genic effects. Serum paraoxonase activity decreases in humans and rodents with infection or inflammation[44]. Since paraoxonase hydrolyzes oxidized phospholipids, the acute phase HDL is unable to protect against LDL oxida-tion and may promote the oxidation process and migration of monocytes[45], thus, being pro-oxidant and proatherogenic. The role of paraoxonase is sup-ported by the demonstration that paraoxonase deficient mice have increased susceptibility of atherosclerosis, and increasing paraoxonase content of HDL particles improves the protective function of HDL[46].

Two metal binding acute-phase proteins associated with HDL (transfer-rin and ceruloplasmin) are affected during infection or inflammation and may also influence the protective function of HDL. Transferrin is an antioxidant which improves the ability of HDL to protect against LDL oxidation[47], and reduction in concentration during infection or inflammation result in less transferrin in HDL and reduced antioxidant properties. Ceruloplasmin (which binds copper) plasma concentration is increased with infection and inflam-mation. Although ceruloplasmin is considered an antioxidant, there is evi-dence that increase in intact ceruloplasmin can enhance LDL oxidation[48], and is considered a cardiovascular risk factor[49].

HDL plays an important role in the removal of cholesterol from periph-eral cells, such as foam cells in atheromas—the reverse cholesterol transport. This allows cholesterol to be transported to the liver for metabolism and excretion. The initial process of cholesterol removal appears to involve an energy-dependent active step with apolipoprotein-mediated mechanism and a diffusion mechanism[50,51.] In the former mechanism cholesterol is removed from peripheral cells by apoA-1 on small, lipid-poor pre-β HDL through the assistance of ATP-binding cassette transporter I on the cell surface[52]. Diffusion of free cholesterol across plasma membrane to HDL also can occur by maintaining a free cholesterol gradient, by converting free cholesterol into cholesterol ester catalyzed by LCAT. The generated cholesterol ester then binds to the core of HDL particles, resulting in a larger α-HDL. Cholesterol ester in HDL is transported to the liver for elimination by several routes. Cholesterol ester in HDL is transferred to triglyceride-rich lipoprotein in exchange for triglyceride in the presence of cholesterol ester transfer protein.

Infection and inflammation can result in reduction of HDL concentrations, apoA-1 levels and LTP activity. This results in impaired apolipoprotein-mediated cholesterol removal from cells, and PLTP-reduced activity results in lower HDL levels and further decrease in cellular cholesterol removal[53]. Plasma LCAT activ-ity is also reduced during infection and inflammation[40], with resulting decrease in free cholesterol gradient and removal of cellular cholesterol by diffusion. Reduction of LCAT also impairs esterification of free cholesterol and the amount of cholesterol ester in HDL core. Other changes with infection include reduction of hepatic lipase and cholesterol ester transfer protein activity, which could impair the transfer of cholesterol to triglyceride-rich lipoproteins and delivery to the liver. A decrease in hepatic lipase could reduce the generation of pre-β HDL and impair the transfer of cellular cholesterol to HDL.

Secretory non-pancreatic phospholipase A_2 (sPLA$_2$), an acute phase protein, that is induced in infection hydrolyzes phospholipids in HDL, leads to decreased phospholipid content, and could increase cholesterol efflux from HDL into cells[54]. Another acute phase protein SAA is increased with inflammation and associated with HDL. SAA-rich HDL preferentially binds to macrophages than hepatocytes[55], thus less cholesterol in HDL is available to be metabolized and excreted by the liver. Furthermore, more cholesterol directed to macrophage could lead to more foam cells and increased atherosclerosis.

Infection and inflammation may also increase apoJ (clusterin), a glycoprotein associated with HDL in plasma. ApoJ is found in atherosclerotic lesions and regulates vascular smooth-muscle cell differentiation in vitro[56]. Thus, an increase in apoJ during infection could enhance the progression of atherosclerotic lesions through its effects on vascular smooth-muscle cells.

4.3. COAGULATION AND ATHEROSCLEROSIS

It has been postulated that the coagulation system plays a critical role in the development of atherosclerosis based on a variety of observations, including the expression of procoagulants and fibrinolytic factors within atherosclerotic vessels, the presence of substantial amounts of fibrinogen and fibrin degradation products within intimal lesions, assimilation of mural thrombi into developing plaques, and the identification of high plasma levels of fibrinogen as an independent risk factor for cardiovascular disease. Rokitansky proposed in the 19th century that fibrin formation promoted early atherosclerosis by the covering of microthrombi by vessel wall endothelium and Duguid[57] refined this theory, on the evidence that thrombus formation occurred under the endothelium during progression of atherosclerosis.

The role of fibrin in atherosclerosis requires an understanding of the coagulation system and the mechanism controlling the entry of macromolecules in vessel wall. Fibrin formation from the inactivated circulating fibrinogen results from a cascade of events that is initiated by tissue factor, a transmembrane protein present on non-vascular cells and on stimulated monocytes and endothelial cells[58,59] (see Figure 4.1). Studies show that fibrinogen permeates into and accumulates within the plaque[60,61] and studies using monoclonal antibodies show that fibrin is commonly detected in atherosclerotic advances lesions, while fibrinogen is detected in early lesions or non-atherosclerotic intima of the aorta and peripheral arteries[62,63].

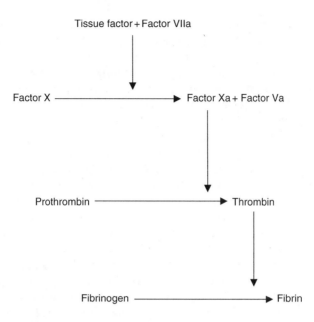

Figure 4.1.   A schematic diagram of the coagulation cascade.

The mechanisms leading to deposition of fibrin in plaque are not well understood. It has been asserted that plaque rupture or intramural hemorrhage releases fibrinogen into the vessel wall where tissue factor initiates coagulation[64]. Although 93% of carotid specimens with advanced atheroma had intramural hemorrhage and plaque rupture or fissuring[65], plaques are very permeable and unruptured plaques may contain the full complement of clotting factors[60]. Fibrin has also been found in non-atherosclerotic regions of intima in the carotid artery, although the amount of fibrin is much greater with the progression of atherosclerosis[66]. Fibrin is often colocalized with tissue factor and macrophages in non-atherosclerotic diffuse intimal thickening and may be deposited episodically with a period of transient inflammation[66]. It has also been shown that passive accumulation of fibrinogen without transforming to fibrin can occur in the aortic intima[67].

4.3.1. The Role of Plaque Rupture

The current paradigm of sudden death or acute myocardial infarction, from atherosclerosis is rupture of the fibrous cap from an atheroma, exposing thrombogenic and procoagulant material, initiating platelet aggregation at the disrupted endothelial surface by the interaction of platelets and active thrombogenic matrix and activation of the clotting cascade by tissue factors and phospholipid[68,69]. Coagulation of the infiltrating and overlying blood with extrusion of the thrombogenic plaque contents results in sudden occlusion of the arterial lumen[70]. Evidence of plaque rupture associated with thrombosis and sudden death have been reported in up to 73% of cases, while 8% consists of plaque fissure with intraplaque hemorrhage, and 19% show no evidence of thrombi[71]. Limitations of these data include selective bias by autopsy studies, limited ability of clinical imaging methods to accurately delineate atheromas of vessel wall, and lack of advanced lesions in animal models with vulnerable plaques.

The main hypothesis of this paradigm to explain plaque rupture involves inflammatory cytokine-mediated expression of proteins, especially metalloproteases directed at collagen and the matrix proteins necessary to maintain integrity of the fibrous cap. It is unclear why the inflammatory process becomes critical to create a vulnerable plaque. A protease able to digest proteolytic inhibitors, stromelysin 3, or accumulation of oxidative products that inactivate protease serpins, could tip the proteolytic balance[72-74], as these products are found in advanced human lesions as opposed to earlier lesions. The proteolytic digestion of the fibrous cap (capsule) with inability to generate new smooth-muscle cells through apoptosis and senescence may account for atrophy and eventual rupture of the plaque. There is extensive apoptosis of smooth-muscle cells within the cap of advanced atherosclerosis and from those cultured from the plaques[75-76].

Cell death may be controlled by interaction of the death receptor Fas with its ligand FasL (death signaling pathway). It has recently been found that the normal intima expresses C-FLIP, an anti-apoptotic gene, but this gene is lost in areas of apotosis of the fibrous cap[66]. Macrophages and endothelial cells express FasL in vivo in atherosclerotic plaques and in vitro these cells can enhance vascular smooth-muscle cell apoptosis by a Fas/FasL-dependent mechanism[66]. FasL is released from macrophages soon after stimulation and soluble FasL can kill vascular smooth-muscle cells[77]. In human coronary plaque, FasL is upregulated in endothelial cells and macrophages, which is correlated with apoptosis of plaque cells, and, thus, suggests that FasL may be the cause of cell death in the plaque.

Recent autopsy studies have questioned the necessity of plaque rupture preceding thrombotic occlusion of arterial lumen. There is evidence to suggest that advanced plaques may undergo many non-fatal ruptures without causing death or clinical acute ischemic syndrome. People dying of non-cardiovascular causes may exhibit plaque rupture of 10% as an incidental finding[78]. Thrombotic coronary artery death can also occur without rupture.

In one study of 20 cases of sudden cardiac death, plaque rupture was found in only 60% of lesions with thrombi and the remaining 40% showed superficial erosion[79]. Other studies have also found similar results in larger numbers of sudden coronary death and one third of the lesions can be described as plaque rupture and 40% of lesions with thrombi failed to show rupture[79-81]. It is not clear how simple denudation of the endothelium can initiate the coagulation process leading to thrombosis, as many of these lesion did not show significant inflammation or stainable tissue factor in the eroded intima[79]. However, activation of stealth tissue factor derived from monocytes/ macrophages may explain the thrombosis[79], or from vascular smooth-muscle cells or endothelial cells undergoing apoptosis[82,83].

4.3.2. Pathophysiology of Thrombus Formation on Atheroma

It has been more than 100 years since Virchow described the main factors determining arterial thrombosis, Virchow's Triad: the arterial wall substrates, the local rheologic characteristics of blood flow, and systemic factors in the circulating blood, Table 4.2 (adapted from Rauch et al.[84]). Advanced atheromatous lesions are the substrates for arterial thrombosis. The lipid core of advanced atheroma is rich in tissue factors, which initiates the coagulation cascade and thrombus generation, on exposure to the circulating blood by rupture or erosion of the plaque. The degree of plaque disruption (rupture, erosion, fissure, or ulceration) and the amount of stenosis caused by the disrupted plaque, and the overlying mural thrombus are the main factors determining clinical manifestation of ischemia. Tissue factor activates Factor VII and subsequently Factor X, which lead to conversion of prothrombin to thrombin in the prothrombinase complex (Figure 4.1). Release of highly procoagulant lipid core into the blood stream triggers formation of thrombi up to six times larger than thrombi generated by other components of the arterial wall[85]. The vulnerability of plaques to rupture or disruption is related to the size of the lipid core, thickness of the fibrous cap, content and metabolic activity of lipids, activity, and density of macrophages and matrix metalloproteinases, and the shear stress of blood flow[86-88].

Vasoconstriction, plaque disruption, and thrombus formation induce changes in shear rate of flowing blood, and increasing shear force increases thrombus formation[88]. Shear force is directly related to flow velocity and inversely to the lumen diameter. Platelet deposition may depend on arterial size, geometric changes, and degree of narrowing after plaque disruption. Most platelets are deposited at the apex of a stenosis, which is the site of maximal shear force[89]. This may cause further growth of thrombus at the injury

Table 4.2

Virchow Triad on Arterial Thrombosis

Local vessel wall substrates

Atherosclerosis
- Degree of plaque disruption, components of plaque (e.g., lipid core and tissue factor content), generation of microparticles through apoptosis

Vessel wall inflammation
- Plaque infiltrates, macrophages (source of tissue factor)

Interventional vessel wall injury
- Endothelial denudation; injury of smooth-muscle cells (rich in prothrombin); plaque disruption after coronary angioplasty

Rheology

High shear stress
- Severely stenotic arteries, dysfunction of endothelium, vasoconstriction

Oscillatory shear stress
- Bifurcation of arteries, plaque irregularities

Slow blood flow/local stasis
- Dissection of intima, aneurysms

Systemic factors of circulating blood

Metabolic or hormonal factors
- Hyperproteinemia or dyslipoproteinemia, diabetes mellitus (glycosylation), catecholamines (e.g., stress, smoking, cocaine use), high-renin hypertension

Plasma variables of hemostasis
- Tissue factor, Factor VII, Factor VIII, fibrinogen, thrombin generation (fragments 1 and 2), thrombin activity (fibrinopeptide A), plasminogen activator inhibitor-1, tissue plasminogen activator

Cellular blood elements
- Cell count (leukocytosis, erythrocytosis), blood viscosity, activation of blood particles, cell aggregation (platelet–platelet, platelet–leukocyte), platelet volume

Note. Adapted from Rauch et al.[84] with permission of the publishers.

site and create further severe stenosis and thrombotic occlusion. Thrombin generation causes vasoconstriction when the endothelium is dysfunctional or denuded, which leads to increase in shear force. Traditional risk factors for atherosclerosis such as smoking, hypertension, or diabetes mellitus may cause endothelial dysfunction, promote vasoconstriction and increase shear force and platelet deposition.

Systemic factors that are associated with blood hypercoagulable state include changes in lipid and hormonal metabolism, hyperglycemia, hemostasis, fibrinolysis, platelet and leukocyte function[86]. Patients with coronary thrombosis or plaque erosion frequently have systemic risk factors associated with a hypercoagulable state[81].

Lipoprotein(a) has a similar structure to that of plasminogen and reduces plasmin formation and impairs thrombolysis, thus predisposing to thrombosis[90]. LDL cholesterol elevation also increases thrombogenicity of blood and thrombus growth under defined conditions[91,92]. Furthermore, reduction of LDL cholesterol levels by statins decreases thrombus growth by 20%[92].

Other cardiovascular risk factors such as smoking and diabetes mellitus can increase blood thrombogenicity; smoking, increase catecholamine release, causes endothelial dysfunction and is associated with increased fibrinogen[93]. High plasma levels of catecholamines potentiate platelet activation and enhance vasospasm and high fibrinogen (precursor of fibrin) all of which produce a procoagulant environment. Poorly controlled diabetes predispose to increased blood thrombogenicity by several mechanisms. There is increased plasma fibrinogen and PAI-1, glycosylation of collagen and proteins, increased platelet reactivity and hyperaggregability, more leukocyte–platelet aggregates in the blood of patients with diabetic vasculopathy, increased expression of monocyte procoagulant activity, partly through tissue factor pathway activation[94–99]—all contribute to high blood thrombogenicity in diabetic patients.

4.3.3. Infection and the Coagulation System

Hemostasis and control of intravascular thrombosis is regulated by a balance of prothrombotic and antithrombotic mechanisms on the vessel wall and in the circulation. Sepsis and severe infection has been well-established and recognized to cause disseminated intravascular coagulation and vascular thrombosis and compromise[100,101]. When gram-negative bacteria release endotoxin into the blood stream, LPS can change the endothelial lining of blood vessels from an anticoagulant, profibrinolytic surface into a procoagulant one. Bacteria endotoxin potently stimulates expression of the gene encoding tissue factor, a procoagulant molecule that greatly increases the activity of coagulation factors VIIa and Xa[102]. LPS can also stimulate endothelial cell production of fibrinolytic inhibitor, PAI-1. These alterations in endothelial function and dysfunction of the protein C activation pathway[101,103] are important in the development of disseminated intravascular coagulation in gram-negative sepsis and purpura fulminans in meningococcemia.

The three most important regulators of coagulation are (1) the tissue factor pathway inhibitor, which directly inhibits activated Factor X (Factor Xa) and complexed to Factor Xa, inhibits tissue factor and activated Factor VII (Factor VIIa); (2) antithrombin, which mainly inhibits thrombin and Factor Xa; (3) the protein C pathway (Figure 4.2). Protein C becomes activated by

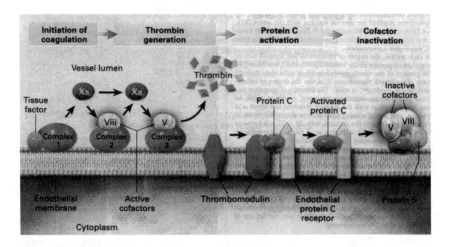

Figure 4.2. Activation of coagulation and the protein C pathway, adapted from Faust et al. with permission of the publishers. Faust, S. N., Levin, M., Harrison, O. B., Yoedin, R. D., Lockhart, M. S., Kondaveeti, S., Laszik, Z., Esmon, C. T., Heyderman, R. S. (2001) Dysfunction of endothelial protein C activation in severe meningococcal sepsis, *N. Engl. J. Med.*, *345*, 408–416.

thrombin bound to vascular thrombomodulin and can degrade activated Factor VIII (Factor VIIIa), and activated Factor V (Factor Va), co-factors of the coagulation complexes that activate Factor X and prothrombin. Thrombomodulin acts as a molecular switch for thrombin, as thrombin bound to thrombomodulin activates an important anticoagulant pathway and no longer functions as a procoagulant. The protein C pathway is designed to block efficiently the procoagulant activity of thrombin, to inhibit the amplification of the coagulation response brought about by co-factors Factor Va and Factor VIIIa, and to stimulate endogenous fibrinolysis[104].

4.3.4. Links between Inflammation and Coagulation

Infection and microbial products such as LPS interact with a variety of lipophilic proteins and inflammatory mediators, including PAF and an array of proinflammatory cytokines to produce a systemic inflammatory response. LPS binds avidly to the LPS receptor, CD14, which is found on monocytes, macrophages, and neutrophils[105], and activates complement generating the membrane attack complex C569[106]. Challenge of healthy volunteers with LPS and TNF-α indicates that the extrinsic pathway is the predominant mechanism by which the coagulation system is activated in sepsis[107,108].

LPS and TNF-α both can induce synthesis and expression of tissue factor on monocytes and endothelium in vitro[109,110]. Platelet activation and assembly of platelet prothrombinase complex can be brought about by the membrane attack complex C569[111]. These mechanisms provide a trigger to initiate and amplify the coagulation response. Also, there is evidence that circulating microparticles play a major role in disseminated coagulopathy[112]. Activation of the contact activation system, Factor XII, prekallikrein and kinnogen, potentiates LPS-induced activation of the complement system.

In addition, the inflammatory response inhibits the anticoagulation system. Antithrombin becomes complexed with thrombin and other proteases, and activated protein C becomes complexed with protein C inhibitor and α1-antitrypsin, and both are consumed[104]. Furthermore, antithrombin acts as a negative acute-phase protein and its synthesis is diminished[100,113]. LPS and TNF-α can interact with the endothelium to downregulate thrombomodulin[110,114], activated neutrophils can also release elastase which can cleave thrombomodulin[115] and decreases its function by releasing reactive oxygen species, through oxidation of methionine on thrombomodulin[116]. These mechanisms lead to decreased thrombin inactivation and decreased generation of activated protein C. With complement activation and cytokine secretion, the serum level of C4b-binding increases and diminishes free protein S for supporting activated protein C[117]. In addition, α1-antitrypsin (acute phase reactant) level increases with infection and inflammation and, thus, is one on the major inhibitors of activated protein C[118]. Furthermore, the concentration of PAI-1 increases with the inflammatory response and this decreases fibrinolytic activity[119]. Thus, infection and systemic inflammation disrupt the balance between procoagulant, anticoagulant, and fibrinolytic systems, leading to activation of intravascular coagulation, resulting in microthrombi and depletion of coagulation factors.

These events are likely protective host mechanisms against invading microbes. For instance, thrombin appears to be directly chemotactic for neutrophils[120] and promotes synthesis by endothelial cells of PAF, a potent neutrophil agonist, and of IL-8, the most potent neutrophil chemotactic molecule of neutrophils in vivo[121]. Thrombin is also chemotactic for monocytes[122] and may induce the synthesis of IL-6 and IL-8[123] and causes expression of P-selectin and E-selectin for tethering and activation of phagocytes on the endothelial surface[124]. Activated platelets stimulate increase in the synthesis of IL-1 and TNF-α by monocytes[125] and induce IL-8 production by endothelial cells[126]. Furthermore, Factor Xa may function as a mediator of acute inflammation in vivo[127]. Thus, several factors important in the coagulation cascade mediate cellular proliferation and inflammation as the propagation of a procoagulant state appears to amplify the inflammatory response.

Conversely, the natural anticoagulant response due to formation of activated protein C through thrombin–thrombomodulin complex has an anti-inflammatory role in the host response to infection. Activated protein C may be protective against endotoxin-induced septic shock[128,129], and in addition to its anticoagulant function it is an important modulator of the inflammatory response in sepsis. This effect of activated protein C on the inflammatory response is related to a direct effect on monocytes. Activated protein C, in conjunction with protein S is capable of suppressing endotoxin-induced cytokine synthesis by >90% by monocytes in vitro[130].

4.3.5. Links between Inflammation, Thrombosis, and Atherosclerosis

Although it is well-established that severe infection and sepsis can stimulate the clotting cascade and cause widespread thrombosis, there is little or no data on mild, low grade infection or inflammation on coagulation. However, it is postulated that chronic low grade infection or inflammation may cause more limited endothelial activation that could contribute to local thrombosis in atherosclerotic vessels. Several inflammatory mediators present in atherosclerotic plaque can stimulate or augment tissue factor gene expression by endothelial cells. TNF-α and IL-1 can augment tissue factor expression and PAI-1 production by human endothelial cells. Bacterial endotoxin (LPS) within atheroma possibly derived from *Chlamydia pneumoniae* or other bacteria, could induce expression of tissue factor and PAI-1 by the endothelium that promotes or lead to thrombotic complications in plaque[102].

Bacterial LPS potently stimulates tissue factor gene expression in human macrophages[131] and foamy macrophages in atheroma expresses tissue factor[132]. When plaques rupture, exposure and blood contact with these tissue factor-bearing macrophages can lead to thrombosis. Blood monocytes and resting macrophages do not express tissue factor, and unlike endothelial cells do not express tissue factor gene expression significantly in response to IL-1 or TNF-α. A cell surface based signaling system, CD154 (CD40 ligand), binding to CD40 receptor on leukocytes can induce tissue factor expression[133]. Several cell types in atheroma carry CD154 and contribute to macrophage tissue factor expression in human atheroma[134]. Local inflammation or bacterial LPS could also stimulate smooth-muscle cells in the artery wall leading to amplification of the inflammatory response (augmentation of IL-6), and procoagulation activation through tissue factor expression via CD154, or systemically from increased fibrinogen and PAI-1 levels as part of the acute phase response.

The interaction of platelets and leukocytes in the inflammatory response also plays a role in thrombosis and platelets can both produce and respond to chemoattractant cytokines[135]. The chemokine stromal cell-derived factor-1 potently stimulates platelet aggregation, and platelet Factor IV produced by platelets is a CXC chemokine family of inflammatory mediators. Moreover, platelets can express CD154 that regulates tissue factor expression in the macrophage and smooth-muscle cell[136].

Platelets and their products (P-selectin) play a role in leukocytes adhesion and transmigration, and accumulation of platelet at sites curvature within the vasculature. Also, binding of platelets to neutrophils influences cellular effector responses by inducing leukocyte activation; augmenting cell molecule expression; and promotes integrin activation, chemokine synthesis, and the respiratory burst. Moreover, neutrophil-platelet and monocyte-platelet aggregates circulate in the peripheral blood of patients with coronary artery disease and may correlate with disease activity[137].

REFERENCES

1. Stamler, M., Wentworth, D., & Neaton, J. D. for the MRFIT Research Group (1986) Is the relationship between serum cholesterol and the risk of premature death from coronary heart disease continuous or graded? Findings in 356,222 primary screenees of the Multiple Risk Factor Intervention Trial (MRFIT), *JAMA*, *256*, 2823–2828.
2. Kwiterovitch, P. O. (1998) State of the art update and review: clinical trials of lipid-lowering agents, *Am. J. Cardiol.*, *82*, 3u–17u.
3. Long Term Intervention with Pravastatin in Ischaemic Disease (LIPID) Study Group (1998) Prevention of cardiovascular events and death with pravastatin in patients with coronary heart disease and a broad range of initial cholesterol levels, *N. Engl. J. Med.*, *339*, 1349–1357.
4. Bradley, W. A., & Gianturco, S. H. (1994) Triglyceride-rich lipoprotein and atherosclerosis: pathophysiological considerations, *J. Intern. Med. Suppl.*, *736*, 33–39.
5. Rader, D. J., & Rosas, S. (2000) Management of selected lipid abnormalities: hypertriglyceridemia, low HDL cholesterol, lipoprotein (a), in thyroid and renal diseases, and post-transplantation, *Med. Clin. North Am.*, *84*, 43–61.
6. Goldbourt, U., Yeari, S., & Medalie, J. H. (1997) Isolated low HDL cholesterol as a risk factor for coronary heart disease mortality: a 21 year follow-up of 8000 men, *Arterioscler. Thromb. Vasc. Biol.*, *17*, 107–113.
7. Goldbourt, U., Behar, S., Reicher-Reiss, H., Agmon, J., Kaplinsky, E., Graff, E., Kishon,Y., Caspi, A., Weisbort, J., & Mandezulig, L. (1993) Rationale and design of a secondary prevention trial of increasing serum high-density lipoprotein cholesterol and reducing triglycerides in patients with clinically manifest atherosclerotic heart disease (The Bezafibrate Infarction Prevention Trial), *Am. J. Cardiol.*, *71*, 909–915.

8. Rubins, H. B., Robins, S. J., Iwane, M. K., Boden, W. E., Elam, M. B., Fye, L. L., Gorden, D. J., Schaefer, E. J., Schectman, G., & Wittes, J. T. (1993) Rationale and design of the Department of Veterans Affairs High-Density Lipoprotein Cholesterol Intervention Trial (HIT) for secondary prevention of coronary artery disease in men with low high-density lipoprotein cholesterol and desirable low-density lipoprotein cholesterol, *Am. J. Cardiol.*, *71*, 45–52.

9. Gabay, C., & Kushner, I. (1999) Acute-phase proteins and other systemic response to inflammation, *N. Engl. J. Med.*, *340*, 448–454.

10. Mak, T. W., & Ferrick, D. A. (1998) The γ δT-cell bridge: linking innate and acquired immunity. *Nat. Med.*, *4*, 764–765.

11. Tilg, H., Dinarello, G. A., & Mier, J. W. (1997) IL-6 and APPS: anti-inflammatory and immunosuppressive mediators, *Immunol. Today*, *18*, 428–432.

12. Khovidhunkit, W., Memon, R. A., Feingold, K. R., & Grunfeld, C. (2000) Infection and inflammation-induced proatherogenic changes of lipoproteins, *J. Infect. Dis.*, *181*(Suppl. 3), S462–472.

13. Gallin, J. I., Kaye, D., & O'Leary, W. M. (1969) Serum lipids in infection, *N. Engl. J. Med.*, *281*, 1081–1086.

14. Grunfield, C., Pang, M., Doerrler, W., Shingenaga, J. K., Jensen, P., & Feingold, K. R. (1992) Lipids, lipoproteins, triglyceride clearance and cytokines in human immunodeficiency virus infection and the acquired immunodeficiency syndrome, *J. Clin. Endocrinol. Metab.*, *74*, 1045–1052.

15. Memon, R. A., Grunfeld, C., Moser, A. H., & Feingold, K. R. (1993) Tumor necrosis factor mediates the effects of endotoxin in cholesterol and triglyceride metabolism in mice, *Endocrinology*, *132*, 2246–2253.

16. Memon, R. A., Feingold, K. R., Moser, A. H., Doerrler, W., Adi, S., Dinarello, C. A., & Grunfeld, C. (1992) Differential effects of interleukin-I and tumour necrosis factor on ketogenesis, *Am. J. Physiol.*, *262*, E301–E309.

17. Feingold, K. R., Staprans, I., Memon, R. A., Moser, A. H., Shigenaga, J. K., Doerrler, W., & Dinarello, C. A. (1992) Endotoxin rapidly induces changes in lipid metabolism that produce hypertriglyceridemia: low doses stimulate hepatic triglyceride production while high doses inhibit clearance, *Lipid Res.*, *33*, 1765–1776.

18. Nonogaki, K., Moser, A. H., Pan, X. M., Staprans, I., Grunfeld, C., & Feingold, K. R. (1995) Lipoteichoic acid stimulates lipolysis and hepatic triglyceride secretion in rats in vivo, *J. Lipid Res.*, *36*, 1987–1995.

19. Hardardóttir, I., Sipe, J., Moser, A. H., Fielding, C. J., Feingold, K. R., & Grünfeld, C. (1997) LPS and cytokines regulate extra hepatic mRNA levels of apolipoproteins during the acute phase response in Syrian hamsters, *Biochem. Biophys. Acta*, *1344*, 210–222.

20. Feingold, K. R., Soued, M., Serio, M. K., Moser, A. H., Dinarello, C. A., & Grünfeld, C. (1989) Multiple cytokines stimulate hepatic lipid synthesis in vivo, *Endocrinology*, *125*, 267–274.

21. Redgrave, T. G., Rakic, V., Mortimer, B. C., & Mamo, J. C. (1992) Effects of sphingomyelin and phosphatidylcholine acyl chains on the clearance of triacylglycerol-rich lipoproteins from plasma. Studies with lipid emulsions in rats, *Biochem. Biophys. Acta*, *1126*, 65–72.

22. Memon, R. A., Staprans, I., Noor, M., Holleran, W. M., Uchida, Y., Moser, A. H., Feingold, K. R., & Grunfeld, C. (2000) Infection and inflammation induce LDL oxidation in vivo, *Arterioscler. Thromb. Vasc. Biol.*, *20*, 1536–1542.
23. Chait, A., Bragg, R. L., Tribble, D. L., & Krauss, R. M. (1993) Susceptibility of small, dense, low-density lipoproteins to oxidative modification in subjects with the atherogenic lipoprotein phenotype, pattern B, *Am. J. Med.*, *94*, 350–356.
24. Hurt-Cumejo, E., Camejo, G., Rosengren, B., Lopez, F., Wiklund, O., & Bondjers, G. (1990) Differential uptake of proteoglycan-selected subfractions of low density lipoprotein by human macrophages, *J. Lipid Res.*, *31*, 1387–1398.
25. Nigon, F., Lesnik, P., Rouis, M., & Chapman, M. J. (1991) Discrete subspecies of human low density lipoproteins are heterogenous in their interaction with the cellular LDL receptor, *J. Lipid Res.*, *32*, 1741–1753.
26. Feingold, K. R., Krauss, R. M., Pang, M., Doerrler, W., Jensen, P., & Grunfeld, C. (1993) The hypertriglyceridemia of acquired immunodeficiency syndrome is associated with an increased prevalence of low density lipoprotein subclass pattern B, *J. Clin. Endocrinol. Metab.*, *76*, 1423–1427.
27. Feingold, K. R., Hardardottir, I., Memon, R., Krul, E. J., Moser, A. H., Taylor, J. M., & Grunfeld, C. (1993) Effect of endotoxin on cholesterol biosynthesis and distribution in serum lipoproteins in Syrian hamsters, *J. Lipid Res.*, *34*, 2147–2158.
28. Memon, R. A., Holleran, W. M., Moser, A. H., Seki, T., Uchida, Y., Fuller, J., Shingenaga, J. K., Grunfeld, C., & Feingold, K. R. (1998) Endotoxin and cytokines increase hepatic sphingolipid biosynthesis and produce lipoproteins enriched in ceramides and sphingomyelin, *Arterioscler. Thromb. Vasc. Biol.*, *18*, 1257–1265.
29. Schissel, S. L., Tweedie-Hardman, J., Rapp, J. H., Graham, G., Williams, K. J., & Tabas, I. (1996) Rabbit aorta and human atherosclerotic lesions hydrolyze the sphingomyelin of retained low-density lipoprotein. Proposed role for arterial wall sphingomyelinase in subendothelial retention and aggregation of atherogenic lipoproteins, *J. Clin. Invest.*, *98*, 1455–1464.
30. Xu, X. X., & Tabas, I. (1991) Sphingomyelinase enhances low density lipoprotein uptake and ability to induce cholesteryl ester accumulation in macrophages, *J. Biol. Chem.*, *266*, 24849–24858.
31. Memon, R. A., Holleran, W. M., Uchida, Y., Moser, A. H., Ichikawa, S., Hirabayashi, Y., Grunfeld, C., & Feingold, K. R. (1999) Regulation of glycosphingolipid metabolism in liver during the acute phase response, *J. Biol. Chem.*, *274*, 19707–19713.
32. Mukhin, D. N., Chao, F. F., & Kruth, H. S. (1995) Glycosphingolipid accumulation in the aortic wall is another feature of human atherosclerosis, *Arterioscler. Thromb. Vasc. Biol.*, *15*, 1607–1615.
33. Imaizumi, T. A., Stafforini, D. M., Yamada, Y., McIntyre, T. M., Prescott, S. M., & Zimmerman, G. A. (1995) Platelet-activating factor: a mediator for clinicians, *J. Intern. Med.*, *238*, 5–20.
34. Quinn, M. T., Parthasarathy, S., & Steinberg, D. (1988) Lipophosphatidylcholine: a chemotactic factor for human monocytes and its potential role in atherogenesis, *Proc. Natl. Acad. Sci. USA.*, *85*, 2805–2809.

35. Kugiyama, K., Kerns, S. A., Morrisett, J. D., Roberts, R., & Henry, P. D. (1990) Impairment of endothelium-dependent arterial relaxation by lysolecithin in modified low-density lipoprotein, *Nature*, *344*, 160–162.

36. Leitinger, N., Watson, A. D., Hama, S. Y., Ivandic, B., Qiao, J. H., Huber, J., Faull, F. K., Grass, D. S., Navab, M., Fogelman, A. M., de Beer, F. C., Lusis, A. J., & Berlinger, J. A. (1999) Role of Group II secretory phospholipase A2 in atherosclerosis. 2. Potential involvement of biologically active oxidized phospholipids, *Arterioscler. Thromb. Vasc. Biol.*, *19*, 1291–1298.

37. Ivandic, B., Castellani, L. W., Wang, X., P., Qiao, J. H., Mehrabian, M., Navab, M., Fogelman, A. M., Grass, D. S., Swanson, M. E., de Beer, M. C., de Beer, F., & Lusis, A. J. (1999) Role of Group II secretory phospholipase A2 in atherosclerosis. 1. Increased atherogenesis and altered lipoproteins in transgenic mice expressing Group IIa phospholipase A2, *Arterioscler. Thromb. Vasc. Biol.*, *19*, 1284–1290.

38. Auerbach, B. J., & Parks, J. S. (1989) Lipoprotein abnormalities associated with lipopolysaccharide-induced lecithin: cholesterol acyltransferase and lipase deficiency, *J. Biol. Chem.*, *264*, 10264–10270.

39. Ettinger, W. H., Miller, L. D., Albers, J. J., Smith, T. K., & Parks, J. S. (1990) Lipopolysaccharide and tumour necrosis factor cause a fall in plasma concentration of lecithin: cholesterol acyltransferase in cynomologus monkeys, *J. Lipid Res.*, *31*, 1099–1107.

40. Ly, H., Francone, O. L., Fielding, C. J., Shigenaga, J. K., Moser, A. H., Grunfeld, C., & Feingold, K. R. (1995) Endotoxin and TNF lead to reduced plasma LCAT activity and decreases hepatic LCAT mRNA levels in Syrian hamsters, *J. Lipid. Res.*, *36*, 1254–1263.

41. Hardardottir, I., Moser, A. H., Fullerr, J., Fielding, C., Feingold, K., & Grunfeld, C. (1996) Endotoxin and cytokines decreases serum levels and extra hepatic protein and mRNA levels of cholesteryl ester transfer protein in Syrian hamsters, *J. Clin. Invest.*, *97*, 2585–2592.

42. Feingold, K. R., Memon, R. A., Moser, A. H., Shigenga, J. K., & Grunfeld, C. (1999) Endotoxin and interleukin-1 decrease hepatic lipase mRNA, *Atherosclerosis*, *142*, 379–387.

43. Khovidhunkit, W., Memon, R. A., Shigenaga, J. K., Pang, M., Schambelan, M., Mulligan, K., Feingold, K. R., & Grunfeld, C. (1999) Plasma platelet-activating factor acetylhydrolase activity in human immunodeficiency virus infection and the acquired immunodeficiency syndrome, *Metab. Clin. Exp.*, *48*, 1524–1531.

44. Feingold, K. R., Memon, R. A., Moser, A. H., & Grunfeld, C. (1998) Paraoxanase activity in the serum and hepatic mRNA levels decrease during the acute phase response, *Atherosclerosis*, *139*, 307–315.

45. Van Lenten, B. J., Hama, S. Y., de Beer, F. C., Stafforini, D. M., McIntyre, T. M., Prescott, S. M., La Du, B. N., Fogelman, A. M., & Navab, M. (1995) Anti-inflammatory HDL becomes pro-inflammatory during the acute phase response. Loss of protective effect of HDL against LDL oxidation in aortic wall cell co-cultures, *J. Clin. Invest.*, *96*, 2758–2767.

46. Shih, D. M., Gu, L., Xia, Y. R., Navab, M., Li, W. F., Hama, S., Castellani, L. W., Furlong, C. E., Costa, L. G., Fogelman, A. M., & Lusis, A. J. (1998) Mice

lacking paraoxanase are susceptible to organophosphate toxicity and atherosclerosis, *Nature*, *394*, 284–287.

47. Kunitake, S. T., Jarvis, M. F., Hamilton, R. L., Kane, J. P. (1992) Binding of transition metals by apolipoprotein A-1-containing plasma lipoproteins: inhibition of oxidation of low density lipoproteins, *Proc. Natl. Acad. Sci. USA*, *89*, 6993–6997.

48. Ehrenwald, E., Chisolm, G. M., & Fox, P. L. (1994) Intact human ceruloplasmin oxidatively modifies low density lipoprotein, *J. Clin. Invest.*, *93*, 14493–14501.

49. Manttari, M., Manninen, V., Huttunen, J. K., Palosuo, T., Ehnholm, C., Heinonen, O. P., & Frick, M. H. (1994) Serum ferritin and ceruloplasmin as coronary risk factors, *Eur. Heart J.*, *15*, 1599–1603.

50. Oram, J. F., & Yokoyama, S. (1996) Apolipoprotein-mediated removal of cellular cholesterol and phospholipids, *J. Lipid Res.*, *37*, 2473–2491.

51. Rothblat, G. H., de la Llera-Moya, M., Atger, V., Kellner-Weiber, G., Williams, D. L., & Phillips, M. C. (1999) Cells cholesterol efflux: integration of old and new observations provides new insights, *J. Lipids Res.*, *40*, 781–796.

52. Lawn, R. M., Wade, D. P., Garvin, M. R., Wang, X., Schwartz, K., Porter, J. G., Seilhamer, J. J., Vaughan, A. M., & Oram, J. F. (1999) The Tangier disease gene product ABC1 controls the cellular apolipoprotein-mediated lipid removal pathway, *J. Clin. Invest.*, *104*, R25–31.

53. Jiang, X. C., Bruce, C., Mar, J., Lin, M., Yi, Y., Francome, O. L., & Tall, A. R. (1999) Targeted mutation of plasma phospholipid transfer protein gene markedly reduces high-density lipoprotein levels, *J. Clin. Invest.*, *103*, 907–914.

54. Johnson, W. J., Bamberger, M. J., Latta, R. A., Rapp, P. E., Phillips, M. C., & Rothblat, G. H. (1986) The bidirectional flux of cholesterol between cells and lipoproteins. Effect of phospholipid depletion of high density lipoprotein, *J. Biol. Chem.*, *261*, 5766–5776.

55. Kisilevsky, R., & Subrahmanyan, L. (1992) Serum amyloid A changes high density lipoproteins cellular affinity: a clue to serum amyloid A's principal function, *Lab. Invest.*, *66*, 778–785; [Erratum] *1992*, *67*, 151.

56. Moulson, C. L., & Millis, A. J. (1999) Clusterin (apoJ) regulates vascular smooth muscle cell differentiation in vitro, *J. Cell Physiol.*, *180*, 355–364.

57. Mannusic, P. M. (1981) The Rokitanski–Duguid project [Letter], *Thromb. Haemost.*, *45*, 300.

58. Neimetz, J. (1972) Coagulant activity of leucocytes. Tissue factor activity, *J. Clin. Invest.*, *51*, 307–313.

59. Colucci, M., Balconi, G., Lorenzet, R., Pietra, A., Locati, D., Donati, M. B., & Semeraro, N. (1983) Cultured human endothelial cells generate tissue factor in response to endotoxin, *J. Clin. Invest.*, *71*, 1893–1896.

60. Smith, E. B. (1994) Fibrin deposition and fibrin degradation products in atherosclerotic plaques, *Thromb. Res.*, *74*, 329–335.

61. Penn, M. S., Chisolm, G. M., & Schwartz, S. M. (1990) Visualization and quantification of transmural concentration profiles of macromolecules across the arterial wall, *Circ. Res.*, *67*, 11–22.

62. Bini, A., Fenoglio, J. J. Jr., Mesa-Tejada, R., Kudryk, R., & Kaplan, K. L. (1989) Identification and distribution of fibrinogen, fibrin and fibrin(ogen) degradation

products in atherosclerosis. Use of monoclonal antibodies, *Arteriosclerosis*, *9*, 109–121.

63. Shekhonin, B. V., Tararak, E. M., Samokhin, G. P., Mitkevich, O. V., Mazurov, A. V., Vinogradov, D. V., Vlasik, T. N., Kalantarov, G. F., & Koteliansky, V. E. (1990) Visualization of apo B, fibrinogen/fibrin and fibronectin in the intima of normal human aorta and large arteries during atherosclerosis, *Atherosclerosis*, *82*, 213–226.

64. Taubman, M. B., Fallon, J. T., Schecter, A. D., Giesen, P., Mendlowitz, M., Fyfe, B. S., Marmur, J. D., & Nemerson, Y. (1997) Tissue factor in the pathogenesis of atherosclerosis, *Thromb. Haemost.*, *78*, 200–204.

65. Fisher, M., Sacoolidge, J. C., & Taylor, C. R. (1987) Patterns of fibrin deposits in carotid artery plaques, *Angiology*, *38*, 393–399.

66. Yee, K.O., Ikari, Y., & Schwartz, S. M. (2001) An update of the Grützbalg hypothesis: the role of thrombosis and coagulation in atherosclerotic progression, *Thromb. Haemost.*, *85*, 207–217.

67. Valenzuela, R., Shianoff, J. R., DiBello, P. M., Urbanic, D. A., Anderson, J. M., Matsueda, G. R., & Kudryk, B. J. (1992) Immunoelectrophorectic and immunohistochemical characterization of fibrinogen derivatives in atherosclerotic aortic intimas and vascular prosthesis pseudointimas, *Am. J. Pathol.*, *141*, 861–880.

68. Fuster, V. (1996) Elucidation of the role of plaque instability and rupture in acute coronary events, *Am. J. Cardiol.*, *76*, 24C–33C.

69. Giesen, P. L., Rauch, U., Bohrmann, B., Kling, D., Roque, M., Fallon, J. T., Badimon, J. J., Himber, J., Riederer, M. A., & Nemerson, Y. (1999) Blood borne tissue factor: another view of thrombosis, *Proc. Natl. Acad. Sci. USA*, *96*, 2311–2315.

70. Falk, E., Shah, P. K., & Fuster, V. (1995) Coronary plaque disruption, *Circulation*, *92*, 657–671.

71. Davies, M. J. (1992) Anatomic features in victims of sudden death. Coronary artery pathology, *Circulation*, *85*(Suppl. 1), 119–124.

72. Schonbeck, U., Mach, F., Sukhova, G. R., Atkinson, E., Levesque, E., Herman, M., Graber, P., Bassett, P., & Libby, P. (1999) Expression of stromelysin-3 in atherosclerotic lesions: regulation via CD40-CD40 ligand signaling in vitro and in vivo, *J. Exp. Med.*, *189*, 843–853.

73. Hazen, S. L., Hsu, F. F., Gaut, J. P., Crowley, J. R., & Heinecke, J. W. (1999) Modification of proteins and lipids by myeloperoxidase, *Methods Enzymol.*, *300*, 88–105.

74. Desrochers, P. E., Mookhtiar, K., Van Wort, H. E., Hasty, K. A., & Weiss, S. J. (1992) Proteolytic inactivation of alpha 1-proteinase inhibitor and alpha-1 antichymotrypsin by oxidatively activated human neutrophil metalloproteinase-S, *J. Biol. Chem.*, *267*, 5005–5012.

75. Bennett, M. R., Evan, G. I., & Schwartz, S. M. (1995) Apoptosis of human vascular smooth muscle cells derived from normal vessels and coronary atherosclerotic plaques, *J. Clin. Invest.*, *95*, 2266–2274.

76. Geng, Y. J., Henderson, L. E., Levesque, E. B., Muszynski, M., & Libby, P. (1997) Fas is expressed in human atherosclerotic intima and promotes apoptosis of

cytokine-primed human vascular smooth muscle cells, *Arterioscler. Thromb. Vasc. Biol.*, *17*, 2200–2208.

77. Kiener, P. A., Davis, P. M., Starling, G. C., Mehlin, C., Klebanoff, S. J., Ledbetter, J. A., & Lilies, W. C. (1997) Differential induction of apoptosis by Fas-Fas ligand interactions in human monocytes and macrophages, *J. Exp. Med.*, *185*, 1511–1516.

78. Arbustini, E., Grasso, M., Diegoli, M., Morbini, P., Aguzzi, A., Fasani, R., & Specchia, G. (1993) Coronary thrombosis in non-cardiac death, *Coron. Artery. Dis.*, *4*, 751–759.

79. Farb, A., Burke, A. P., Tang, A. L., Liang, Y. H., Mannan, P., Smialek, J., & Virmani, R. (1996) Coronary plaque erosion without rupture into a lipid core: a frequent cause of coronary thrombosis in sudden coronary death, *Circulation*, *93*, 1354–1363.

80. Farb, A., Tang, A. L., Burke, A. P., Sessums, L., Liang, Y., & Virmani, R. (1995) Sudden coronary death. Frequency of active coronary lesions, inactive coronary lesions, and myocardial infarction, *Circulation*, *92*, 1701–1709.

81. Burke, A. P., Farb, A., Malcom, G. T., Liang, Y. H., Smialek, J., & Virmani, R. (1997) Coronary risk factors and plaque morphology in men with coronary disease who died suddenly [see comments], *N. Engl. J. Med.*, *336*, 1276–1282.

82. Flynn, P. D., Byrne, C. D., Baglin, T. P., Weissberg, P. L., & Bennett, M. R. (1997) Thrombin generation by apoptotic vascular smooth muscle cells, *Blood*, *89*, 4378–4384.

83. Bombeli, T., Karsan, A., Tait, J. F., & Harlan, J. M. (1997) Apoptotic vascular endothelial cells become procoagulant, *Blood*, *89*, 2429–2442.

84. Rauch, U., Osende, J. I., Fuster, V., Badimon, J. J., Fayad, Z., & Cheseboro, J. H. (2001) Thrombus formation on atherosclerotic plaques: pathogenesis and clinical consequences, *Ann. Intern. Med.*, *134*, 224–238.

85. Fernandez-Ortiz, A., Badimon, J. J., Falk, E., Fuster, V., Meyer, B., Mailhac, A., Weng, D., Shah, P. K., & Badimon, L. (1994) Characterization of the relative thrombogenicity of atherosclerotic plaque components: Implications for consequences of plaque rupture, *J. Am. Coll. Cardiol.*, *23*, 1562–1569.

86. Felton, C. V., Crook, D., Davies, M. J., & Oliver, M. F. (1997) Relation of plaque lipid composition and morphology to the stability of human aortic plaques, *Arterioscler. Thromb. Vasc. Biol.*, *17*, 1337–1345.

87. Moreno, P. R., Falk, E., Palacios, I. F., Newell, J. B., Fuster, V., & Fallon, J. T. (1994) Macrophage infiltration in acute coronary syndromes. Implications for plaque rupture, *Circulation*, *90*, 775–778.

88. Turritto, V. T., & Hall, C. L. (1998) Mechanical factors affecting hemostasis and thrombosis, *Thromb. Res.*, *92*, S25–S31.

89. Badimon, L., & Badimon, J. J. (1989) Mechanisms of arterial thrombosis in non-parallel streamlines. Platelet thrombi grow on the apex of stenotic severely injured vessel wall. Experimental study in the pig model, *J. Clin. Invest.*, *84*, 1134–1144.

90. Loscalzo, J. (1990) Lipoprotein(a). A unique risk factor for atherothrombotic disease, *Arteriosclerosis*, *10*, 672–679.

91. Brook, J. G., & Aviram, M. (1988) Platelet lipoprotein interactions, *Semin. Thromb. Hemostat.*, *14*, 258–265.

92. Rauch, U., Osende, J. I., Chesebro, J. H., Fuster, V., Vorcheimer, D. A., Harris, K., Sandler, D. A., Fallon, J. T., Jayaraman, S., & Badimon, J. J. (2000) Statins and cardiovascular disease: the multiple effects of lipid-lowering therapy by statins, *Atherosclerosis*, *153*, 181–189.

93. Miller, G. J. (1992) Hemostasis and cardiovascular risk. The British and European experience, *Arch. Pathol. Lab. Med.*, *116*, 1318–1321.

94. Meigs, J. B., Mittleman, M. A., Nathan, D. M., Tofler, G. H., Singer, D. E., Murphy-Sheehy, P. M., Lipinska, I., D'Agostino, R. B., & Wilson, P. W. (2000) Hyperinsulinemia, hyperglycemia and impaired hemostasis: The Framingham offspring study, *JAMA*, *283*, 221–228.

95. Matsuda, T., Morishita, E., Jokaji, H., Asakura, H., Saito, M., Yoshida, T., & Takemoto, K. (1996) Mechanism on disorders of coagulation and fibrinolysis in diabetes, *Diabetes*, *45*(Suppl. 3), S109–S110.

96. Tschoepe, E., Rauch, U., & Schwippert, B. (1997) Platelet-leucocytes cross-talk in diabetes mellitus, *Horm. Metab. Res.*, *29*, 631–635.

97. Rauch, U., Schwippert, B., Schultheiss, H. P., & Tschoepe, D. (1998) Platelet activation in diabetic microangiopathy, *Platelets*, *9*, 237–240.

98. Buzzan, M., Gruden, G., Stella, S., Vaccarino, A., Tamponi, G., Olivetti, C., Giunti, S., & Carvallo-Perin, P. (1998) Microalbuminuria in IDDM is associated with increasing expression of monocyte procoagulant activity, *Diabetologia*, *41*, 767–771.

99. Rao, A. K., Chouhan, V., Chen, X., Sun, L., & Boden, G. (1999) Activation of the tissue factor pathway of blood coagulation during prolonged hyperglycemia in young healthy men, *Diabetes*, *48*, 1156–1161.

100. Levi, M., & ten Cate, H. (1999) Disseminated intravascular coagulation, *N. Engl. J. Med.*, *341*, 586–592.

101. Faust, S. N., Heyderman, R. S., & Levin (2000) Disseminated intravascular coagulation and purpura fulminans secondary to infection. Baillieres Best Pract. *Res. Clin. Haematol.*, *13*, 179–197.

102. Libby, P., & Simon, D. I. (2001) Inflammation and thrombosis. The clot thickens, *Circulation*, *103*, 1718–1720.

103. Esmon, C. T., Ding, W., Yasuhiro, K., Gu, J. M., Ferrell, G., Regan, L. M., Stearns-Kurosawa, D. J., Kurosawa, S., Mather, T., Laszik, Z., & Esmon, N. L. (1997) The protein C pathway: new insights, *Thromb. Haemostat.*, *78*, 70–74.

104. Alberio, L., Lämmle, B., & Esmon, C. T. (2001) Protein C replacement in severe meningococcemia: rationale and clinical experience, *Clin. Infect. Dis.*, *32*, 1338–1346.

105. Ulevitch, R. J., & Tobias, P. S. (1995) Receptor-dependent mechanisms of cell stimulation of bacterial endotoxin, *Annu. Rev. Immunol.*, *13*, 437–457.

106. Brandtzaeg, P., Mollness, T. E., & Kierulf, P. (1989) Complement activation and endotoxin levels in systemic meningococcal disease, *J. Infect. Dis.*, *160*, 58–65.

107. Bauer, K. A., ten Cate, H., Barzegar, S., Spriggs, D. R., Sherman, M. L., & Rosenberg, R. D. (1989) Tumour necrosis factor infusions have a procoagulant effect on the hemostasis mechanisms of humans, *Blood*, *74*, 165–172.

108. Van Deventer, S. J., Buller, H. R., ten Cate, J. W., Aarden, L. A., Hack, C. E., & Sturk, A. (1990) Experimental endotoxemia in humans: analysis of cytokines release and coagulation, fibrinolytic and complement pathways, *Blood*, 76, 2520–2526.

109. Edgington, T. S., Mackman, N., Brand, K., & Ruf, W. (1991) The structural biology of expression and function of tissue factor, *Thromb. Haemost.*, 66, 67–79.

110. Moore, K. L., Andreoli, S. P., Esmon, N. L., Esmon, C. T., & Bang, N. U. (1987) Endotoxin enhances tissue factor and suppresses thrombomodulin expression of human vascular endothelium in vitro, *J. Clin. Invest.*, 79, 124–130.

111. Sims, P. J., Wiedmer, T., Esmon, C. T., Weiss, H. J., & Shattil, S. J. (1989) Assembly of platelet prothrombinase complex is linked to vesiculation of the platelet plasma membrane: studies in Scott syndrome—an isolated defect in platelet procoagulant activity, *J. Biol. Chemo.*, 264, 17049–17057.

112. Nieuwland, R., Berckmans, R. J., McGregor, S., Boing, A. N., Romijn, F. P., Westendorp, R. G., Hack, C. E., & Sturk, A. (2000) Cellular origin and procoagulant properties of microparticles in meningococcal sepsis, *Blood*, 95, 930–935.

113. Neissen, R. W., Lamping, R. J., Jansen, P. M., Prins, M. N., Peters, M., Taylor, F. B., de Vijlder, J. J., ten Cate, J. W., Hack, C. E., & Sturk, A. (1997) Antithrombin acts as a negative acute phase protein as established with studies on Hep G2 cells and in baboons, *Thromb. Haemost.*, 78, 1088–1092.

114. Moore, K. L., Esmon, C. T., & Esmon, N. L. (1998) Tumour necrosis factor leads to internalization and degradation of thrombomodulin from the surface of bovine aortic endothelial cells in culture, *Blood*, 73, 159–165.

115. Boehme, M. W., Deng, Y., Raeth, U., Bierhaus, A., Ziegler, R., Stremmel, W., & Nawroth, P. P. (1996) Release of thrombomodulin from endothelial cells by concerted action of TNF-alpha and neutrophils: in vivo and in vitro studies, *Immunology*, 87, 134–140.

116. Glaser, C. B., Morser, J., Clarke, J. H., Blasko, E., McLean, K., Kuhn, I., Chang, R. J., Lin, J. H., Vilander, L., & Andrews, W. H. (1992) Oxidation of a specific methionine in thrombomodulin by activated neutrophil products blocks cofactor activity: a potential rapid mechanism for modulation of coagulation, *J. Clin. Invest.*, 90, 2565–2573.

117. Dahbäck, B. (1991) Protein S and C4b-binding protein: components involved in the regulation of the protein C anticoagulated system, *Thromb. Haemost.*, 66, 49–61.

118. Heeb, M. J., & Griffin, J. H. (1988) Physiologic inhibition of human activated protein C by alpha 1-antitrypsin, *J. Biol. Chem.*, 263, 11613–11616.

119. Colucci, M., Paramo, J. A., & Collen, D. (1985) Generation in plasma of a fast-acting inhibitor of plasminogen activator in response to endotoxin stimulation, *J. Clin. Invest.*, 75, 818–824.

120. Bizios, R., Lai, L., Fenton, J. W., & Malik, A. B. (1986) Thrombin-induced chemotaxis and aggregation of neutrophils, *J. Cell Physiol.*, 128, 485–490.

121. Prescott, S. M., Zimmerman, G. A., & McIntyre, T. M. (1984) Human endothelial cells in culture produce platelet activating factor (1-alkyl-2-acetyl-sn-glkycero-3-phosphocholine) when stimulated with thrombin, *Proc. Natl. Acad. Sci. USA*, 81, 3534–3538.

122. Bar-Shavit, R., Kahn, A., Wilner, G. D., & Fenton, J. W. D. (1983) Monocyte chemotaxis: stimulation by specific exosite region in thrombin, *Science, 220,* 728–731.
123. Johnson, K., Choi, Y., De Groot, E., Samuels, I., Creasey, A., & Aarden, L. (1998) Potential mechanisms for a proinflammatory vascular cytokine response to coagulation activation, *J. Immunol., 160,* 5130–5135.
124. Kaplanski, G., Fabrigoule, M., Boulay, V., Dinarello, C. A., Bongrand, P., Kaplanski, S., & Farnarier, C. (1997) Thrombin induces endothelial Type II activation in vitro: IL-1 and TNF-alpha-independent IL-8 secretion and E-selectin expression, *J. Immunol., 158,* 5435–5441.
125. Aiura, K., Clark, B. D., Dinarello, C. A., Margolis, N. A., Kaplanski, G., Burke, J. F., Tompkins, R. G., & Gelfand, J. A. (1997) Interaction with autologous platelets multiplies interleukin-1- and tumour necrosis factor production in mononuclear cells, *J. Infect Dis., 175,* 123–129.
126. Kaplanski, G., Porat, R., Aiura, K., Erban, J. K., Gelfand, J. A., & Dinarello, C. A. (1993) Activated platelets induce endothelial secretion of interleukin-8 in vitro via an interleukin-1 mediated event, *Blood, 81,* 2492–2495.
127. Cirino, G., Cicala, C., Bucci, M., Sorrentino, L., Ambrosini, G., De Dominicis, G., & Altier, D. C. (1997) Factor Xa as an interface between coagulation and inflammation: molecular mimicry of factor Xa association with effector cell protease receptor-1 induces acute inflammation in vivo, *J. Clin. Invest., 99,* 2446–2451.
128. Taylor, F. B., Jr., Chang, A., Esmon, C. T., D'Angelo, A., Vigano-D'Angelo, S., & Blick, K. E. (1987) Protein C-prevents the coagulatopathic and lethal effects of *Escherichia coli* infusion in the baboon, *J. Clin. Invest., 79,* 918–925.
129. Roback, M. G., Stack, A. M., Thompson, C., Brugnara, C., Schwarz, H. P., & Salidino, R. A. (1998) Activated protein C concentrate for the treatment of meningococcal endotoxin shock in rabbits, *Shock, 9,* 138–142.
130. Gray, S. T., & Hancock, W. W. (1996) A physiologic anti-inflammatory pathway based on thrombomodulin expression and generation of activated protein C by human mononuclear phagocytes, *J. Immunol., 156,* 2256–2263.
131. Brand, K., Fowler, B. J., Edgington, T. S., & Mackman, N. (1991) Tissue factor mRNA in THP-1 monocytic cells is regulated at both transcriptional and post-transcriptional levels in response to lipopolysaccharide, *Mol. Cell Biol., 11,* 4732–4738.
132. Wilcox, J. N., Smith, K. M., Schwartz, S. M., & Gordon, D. (1989) Localization of tissue factor in the normal vessel wall and in the atherosclerotic plaque, *Proc. Natl. Acad. Sci. USA, 86,* 2839–2843.
133. Mach, F., Schonbeck, U., Bonnefoy, J. Y., Pober, J. S., & Libby, P. (1997) Activation of monocyte/macrophage functions related to acute atheroma complication by ligation of CD40: induction of collagenase stromelysin and tissue factor, *Circulation, 96,* 396–399.
134. Mach, F., Schonbeck, U., Sukhova, G. K., Bourcier, T., Bonnefoy, J. Y., Pober, J. S., & Libby, P. (1997) Functional CD40 ligand is expressed on human vascular endothelial cells, smooth muscle cells and macrophages: implications

for CD40–CD40 ligand signaling in atherosclerosis, *Proc. Natl. Acad. Sci. USA*, *94*, 1931–1936.

135. Abi-Younes, S., Sauty, A., Mach, F., Sukhova, G. K., Libby, P., & Luster, A. D. (2000) The stromal cell-derived factor-1 chemokine is a potent platelet agonist highly expressed in atherosclerotic plaques, *Circ. Res.*, *86*, 131–138.

136. Henn, V., Slupsky, J. R., Grafe, M., Anagnostopoulos, I., Forster, R., Muller-Berghaus, G., & Kroczek, R. A. (1998) CD40 ligand on activated platelets triggers an inflammatory reaction of endothelial cells, *Nature*, *391*, 591–594.

137. Ott, I., Neumann, F. J., Gawaz, M., Schmitt, M., & Schomig, A. (1996) Increased neutrophil-platelet adhesion in patients with unstable angina [see comments], *Circulation*, *94*, 1239–1246.

Section II

Emerging Relationships of Infections and the Cardiovascular System

5

Chlamydia pneumoniae and the Cardiovascular System

5.1. MICROBIOLOGY OF *CHLAMYDIA PNEUMONIAE*

Chlamydia pneumoniae is the most recently discovered human species of the genus *Chlamydia*, which are obligate intracellular bacteria that have a unique biphasic developmental cycle. There are four species of *Chlamydia*: *Chlamydia trachomatis*, *C. psittaci*, *C. pecorum*, and *C. pneumoniae*. *C. trachomatis* includes the organisms causing trachoma, inclusion conjunctivitis, lymphogranuloma venerum (LGV), and, genital tract disease and infantile pneumonitis[1]. The three biovars within this species are trachoma, LGV, and murine, but similar organisms have been isolated from swine and ferrets. *C. psittaci* strains infect many avian species and mammals, causing psittacosis, ornithosis, feline pneumonitis, and abortion in cattle[2]. Incidental infections in humans can produce pneumonia and endocarditis. *C. pecorum* has been recovered from ruminants[3] but there is no evidence that it is a human pathogen.

    C. pneumoniae was first isolated from the conjunctiva of a child in Taiwan in 1965[4], and was subsequently associated with an epidemic of mild pneumonia in northern Finland in 1977 by serological testing[5]. However, the first respiratory isolate was from a university student with pharyngitis (designated AR-39)[6]. Since then *C. pneumoniae* has been demonstrated to be primarily a human respiratory pathogen. Other hosts naturally infected with *C. pneumoniae* or a similar organism include the koala, in which the bacterium also causes respiratory infections[7]. The koala biovars of *C. pneumoniae* has also been identified in horses and lung tissue from a sick, free-ranging giant barred frog (*Mixophyes iteratus*) from Australia[8]. *C. pneumoniae* has a similar structure and growth cycle as with other *Chlamydia* species. *Chlamydiae* have cell walls, replicate by binary fission, and contain DNA, RNA, and ribosomes. Heparan sulfate-like glycosaminoglycan is a cellular receptor for *C. pneumoniae*, responsible for adherence to host cells for infection[9]. However, attachment and entry can be mediated by other as yet unidentified receptors, as a background level of *C. pneumoniae* infection can be found in heparan sulfate deficient cell lines[9]. *C. pneumoniae* has less than 10% DNA relatedness to other species[10], and the infectious particles (elementary bodies [EBs]) are pear-shaped rather than round, as seen in *C. trachomatis*. The small dense EB (diameter, 0.25–0.35 μm) is metabolically inactive, has a rigid cell wall and can survive outside the host cell[11]. *C. pneumoniae* EBs first attach to host cells by the pointed end and then secure other binding sites on the host cell wall protrusions, enter host cells by invaginating the host cell membrane, and form vacuolated endocytic vesicles[12], a process similar to receptor-mediated endocytosis. The EB enters the cell in an endosome, where the entire growth cycle is completed. The Chlamydia prevent phagolysosomal fusion. On entering the cell, EB reorganize to form a reticulate body (diameter, 0.5–1 μm) that is richer in RNA than the EB. The metabolically active reticulate body begins dividing by binary fusion after 8 hr and by 18–24 hr after infection, the reticulate bodies reorganize and condense to from EBs. The EBs are then released to initiate another cycle of infection. For many chlamydial diseases, it has been postulated that persistent infection of human cells is a feature[13,14]. In vitro it has been demonstrated that *C. trachomatis* can persist in cell culture and macrophages as viable, aberrant, low metabolically active but non-replicate forms[13,15] (see Figure 5.1). Chlamydia infection of macrophages can induce T-cell apoptosis, and this could explain how persistently infected macrophages escape T-cell surveillance and why Chlamydia-specific T-cell response is diminished during persistent Chlamydiae infection[16]. Epithelial cells infected with *C. pneumoniae* have also been reported to be resistant to apoptosis[17]. Recently, it has also been shown that *C. pneumoniae* can produce an aberrant persistent form in cell culture; and the development of persistence included production of transcripts for DNA replication-related, but not cell division-related, genes[18]. This study provides important new information regarding gene regulation patterns intrinsic to intracellular chlamydial growth. These results also provide new insight of the molecular basis of persistence of *C. pneumoniae* and requirements for reactivation from persistent to productive growth. In this study, high concentration of interferon gamma (IFN-γ) suppressed genes required for bacterial cell division, allowing persistence, but low dose IFN-γ did not[18]. Evidence for persistent infection in animal models of *C. pneumoniae* infection also exists, with reactivation by cortisone therapy[19,20]. Furthermore, persistent infection in humans after acute respiratory illness has also been reported[21].

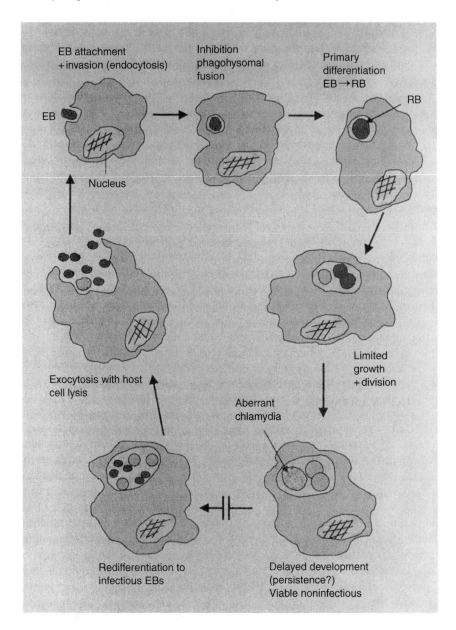

Figure 5.1. The life cycle of *Chlamydia* is shown with the presence of an aberrant, persistent form. Adapted from Beatty et al.[13] with permission of the publishers.

5.2. CHLAMYDIA ANTIGENS

The Chlamydiae possess group (genus-specific), species-specific, and type-specific antigens. It is believed that only a few of the antigens play a role in diagnosis and pathogenesis. The lipopolysaccharide (LPS) is shared by all members of the genus and is the group complement fixation (CF) antigen. It is similar but not as potent as LPS of enteric gram negative bacteria[22]. The major outer membrane protein (MOMP) contains both species- and subspecies-specific antigens[23]. The MOMP is responsible for most of the reactivity seen in the microimmunofluorescence (MIF) test, and can be used for species-specific antibodies. *C. pneumoniae* isolates have 94–100% DNA homology with each other but less than 10% with *C. trachomatis* or *C. psittaci*[10]. All *C. pneumoniae* isolates tested are immunologically similar. Strains (isolates) from different countries and their MOMP are identical[24,25]. Unlike other Chlamydia species, *C. pneumoniae* has only one immunotype or serovar. In *C. trachomatis*, a 60 kDa cysteine-rich structural protein has a high immunogenetic species-specific epitope[26], and a 60 kDa heat-shock protein appears to be important in the immunopathology of human disease[27]. The importance of these proteins in immunity and immunopathology are yet to be demonstrated for *C. pneumoniae* infection.

5.3. EPIDEMIOLOGY OF *CHLAMYDIA PNEUMONIAE* INFECTIONS

C. pneumoniae has a worldwide distribution based on serological studies using the MIF test to detect antibodies to the bacterium[28–36]. Studies of stored sera indicate that *C. pneumoniae* was a cause of acute respiratory infection at least since 1958[33]. *C. pneumoniae* mostly causes endemic respiratory infections but outbreaks of infections have occurred in schools[34], among military recruits[35], in nursing homes[36], and country wide[37]. Infection under 5 years of age is rare but rapidly increases during the school-age and by age 20, approximately 50% of the population is seropositive[38]. The rate of infection continues to increase with age and 75–80% of the elderly have been infected sometime (see Figure 5.2). Reinfection is believed to be common as antibody titers decline with age and high titers in the elderly represent booster effect of antibody response[39].

C. pneumoniae is the third commonest cause of community acquired pneumonia, after *Streptococcus pneumoniae* and *Mycoplasma pneumoniae*, and can also cause bronchitis, sinusitis, and pharyngitis[38]. Since most of the adult population has antibodies to *C. pneumoniae*, it is likely that most

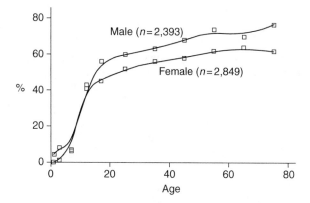

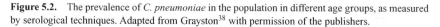

Figure 5.2.   The prevalence of *C. pneumoniae* in the population in different age groups, as measured by serological techniques. Adapted from Grayston[38] with permission of the publishers.

infections are unreorganized and labeled as viral upper respiratory tract infection, or are subclinical to a great extent. The acute respiratory infection with pneumonia is usually mild to moderate in children and healthy young adults with full recovery. However, in the elderly, severe illness with respiratory failure may occur requiring management in the critical care unit, and significant mortality has been reported in the nursing home residents[40,41]. In an outbreak of respiratory infections in three nursing homes in Ontario, Canada, there were 6 deaths among 16 cases of confirmed pneumonia[41]. Also of interest is the association of new onset of asthma, in subjects without previous asthmatic history, with acute *C. pneumoniae* respiratory infection[42,43].

5.4. DIAGNOSIS OF *CHLAMYDIA PNEUMONIAE* INFECTIONS

An acute infection of *C. pneumoniae* can be made by serological assay, culture of the microorganism and by molecular techniques, using polymerase chain reaction (PCR).

5.4.1. Serological Testing

Serological testing, the most widely used method for diagnosis of *C. pneumoniae* infection, has several disadvantages and most often provides a retrospective diagnosis of acute infection and thus not useful for management[44]. A fourfold increase in titer is needed from paired sera to confirm an acute infection, as a single high titer is not reliable. IgM antibodies appear 2–3 weeks after the onset of illness and are generally undetectable after 2–6 months. IgG antibody may not reach high titer until 6–8 weeks after onset of illness; moreover, with reinfection, IgM antibody may not reappear and IgG antibody titer increases within 1–2 weeks[44]. Serological testing is most useful for prevalence of infection in epidemiological studies and in determining the cause of a recent outbreak. However, serology or height of antibody titers has not been shown to predict those subjects with persistent or chronic infection from others with past exposure, and IgA antibodies have not been proven reliable[44].

Currently, the MIF test is the only recommended serological assay and method of choice[44]. It is the only species-specific antibody test available that measures isotype-specific antibody titers to all *Chlamydia* species simultaneously, and its use led to the identification of *C. pneumoniae* as a distinct species of *Chlamydia*[5]. The MIF assay utilizes purified EBs of all three species of *Chlamydia* rather than reticulate bodies that express predominantly genus-specific epitopes. Purified formalinized EBs from *C. pneumoniae*, *C. trachomatis*, and *C. psittaci* are fixed on to glass slides as distinct dots of antigen, and dilutions of sera are placed over the antigen dots and incubated. However, interpretation of the slides is subjective and requires training and experience and is technically difficult. Moreover, the diagnostic criteria and reagents have not been standardized[45]. Recent guidelines for interpretation and quality control has been published[44] and should be adhered to (see Table 5.1). CF, whole-inclusion fluorescence, and enzyme link immunoassay (EIA) are currently not recommended, but have been used in serological studies. The CF test cross reacts with other *Chlamydia* species and other enteric bacteria, and sensitivity for detecting reinfection is low. Whole-inclusion fluorescence tests are not species-specific and have not been widely evaluated. EIA would be an ideal assay because of objective end points and high throughput; however none of the several kits have been approved by the Food and Drug Administration (FDA) of the United States, and large scale studies with comparison with the MIF have not been reported to evaluate and confirm the sensitivity and specificity of the assay[44].

5.4.2. Culture

Culture of *C. pneumoniae* is technically difficult, time consuming and expensive, as it requires cultivation within a eukaryotic host cell; only research

Table 5.1
Recommendations for Use of the Microimmunofluorescence Test

Assay component	Recommendations
Antigen	Renografin-purified elementary bodies resuspended in phosphate-buffered saline that contain 0.02% formalin, combined with 0.5% yolk sac and fixed in acetone
Serum samples	Paired serum samples, obtained 4–8 weeks apart
Testing	Screen at 1:8 or 1:16 and titer at twofold dilutions to end point
	Preabsorb serum samples with anti-IgG before IgM and IgA testing
	Add Evan's blue stain (0.05%) or rhodamine-conjugated bovine albumin stain (at 1/15 volume) as counterstain to fluorescein-conjugated second antibody
Results	Read slides using $\times$ 10 eyepiece and $\times$ 40 plan achromatic objective
Interpretation	Acute infection, IgM of $\geq$1:16 or fourfold increase in IgG
	Possible acute infection, IgG of $\geq$1:512
	Presumed past infection, IgG of $\geq$1:16
Quality assurance	Positive and negative control serum samples in each run
	Check titer of positive control serum sample for reproducibility between runs
	Determine optimal conjugate dilution by titrating with a high-titered serum
	Aliquot undiluted conjugate in small quantities and store at -20 °C until use
	Technician blinded to case/control and acute/convalescent status

Note. Adapted from Dowell et al.[44] with permission of the publishers.

centers and reference centers are capable of culturing the microorganism, and it is not performed by the routine microbiology laboratory. However, culture is the only reliable method of verifying the viability of the organism. Although respiratory secretions and tissues can be used to recover the organisms, the above disadvantages and low sensitivity (when compared to molecular methods) limits its usefulness. Specimens (swabs, secretions, or tissues) should be collected and placed in sucrose-potassium phosphate medium (2SP) and should be processed within 24 hr if held at 4 °C, or -70 °C beyond 24 hr. Processed specimens are centrifuged and inoculated onto human cell lines, Hep-2 or HL cells in multiple-well tissue culture plates or shell vials. The inoculated cells are incubated and are later stained with fluorescent-labeled antibody specific to *Chlamydia* to visualize the bacteria that are growing within the host cells. It has been recommended that respiratory secretions be passaged at least twice before determining results, and tissue

4–6 additional passages be performed to optimize recovery of *C. pneumoniae*[44]. Problems to be aware of are that concentration of cell debris by multiple passage may lead to non-specific staining of the monolayer, sputa frequently inhibits cell growth and may be toxic to the monolayer, and calcified areas of vascular time should be removed before homogenization and suspension in cell culture medium to prevent inhibition of growth. Guidelines for culture of *C. pneumoniae* are summarized in Table 5.2[44].

Table 5.2
Recommendations for Use of Culture for *Chlamydia pneumoniae*

Assay component	Recommendations
Cell type	HEp-2 or HL cells in 6-, 12-, 24-, or 96-well tissue culture plates or shell vials
Media	Eagle's MEM or IMDM supplemented with fetal calf serum (10%), l-glutamine (2 mM), MEM non-essential amino acids, HEPES buffer, gentamicin (10 μg/mL), vancomycin (25 μg/mL), and amphotericin B (2 μg/mL)
Inoculation	Centrifuge the homogenized specimen onto the monolayer at 900–3000 g for 60 min; after centrifugation, replace culture medium with cycloheximide-supplemented medium
Incubation	35 °C with 5% CO_2
Passages	Examine cultures for *C. pneumoniae* on day 3, homogenize duplicate wells, and pass to a fresh cell monolayer twice
Identification of inclusions	Monolayers should be fixed and stained with a genus-specific monoclonal antibody and then with a species-specific monoclonal antibody of confirmation; inclusion-forming units per milliliter should be used for quantifying the number of infectious organisms in the specimen
Quality assurance	Positive controls (cells infected with *C. pneumoniae*) and negative controls (uninfected human cells) should be used in each run
	New lots of swabs, fetal calf serum, and MEM medium should be tested by mock infection and titrated to ensure that they support the growth of *C. pneumoniae*
	Controlling for well-to-well contamination is especially important when using microtiter plates and multiple passages
	Laboratory workers should have sufficient experience and training in interpretation of *C. pneumoniae* microscopic evaluation to differentiate specific staining from the variety of artifacts
	Cell stocks should be routinely tested for *Mycoplasma* contamination by use of a commercially available test or PCR

Note. HEPES, N-2-hydroxyethylpiperazine-N-2-ethane-sulfonic acid; IMDM, Iscove's modified Dulbecco's medium; MEM, minimal essential medium. Adapted from Dowell et al.[44] with permission of the publishers.

5.4.3. Polymerase Chain Reaction

PCR has been used to identify *C. pneumoniae* in clinical respiratory samples[46-48], serum[49], peripheral blood mononuclear cells (PBMC)[50-52], and vascular tissue[53-55]. However, the wide variations in methodology reflect the variations in results from different centers, especially with the detection in vascular tissue and PBMC. The variations in findings may also be due to differences in specimen collection and processing, primer design, nucleic acid extraction, amplification, product detection, or prevention and identification of contamination or false positive and false negative results[44]. There have been at least 18 different PCR assays used in various publications, but none has been commercially standardized or approved by the United States FDA. Moreover, only four widely used protocols have been validated by other laboratories[44]. Furthermore, in a recent multicenter study of DNA extraction methods and PCR assays, for detection of *C. pneumoniae* in endarterectomy specimens wide variations were found among 9 centers employing 16 test methods[56]. There was no consistent pattern of positive results among the various laboratories, and there was no correlation between the detection rates and the sensitivity of the assay used. In order to standardize the PCR methods in different centers, recent recommendations and guidelines for specimen processing, DNA extraction, quality controls for procedures, amplification and interpretation have been published[44]. For acute diagnosis of a respiratory infection, PCR of sputum or bronchial secretion would be the most sensitive and celeritous test that would be most suitable in patient management.

5.4.4. Immunohistochemistry

Besides culture and PCR, *C. pneumoniae* can be detected in tissue specimens by immunohistochemical staining, immunofluorescence, in situ hybridization and electron microscopy. The advantages of these latter techniques include preservation of the tissue morphology and ability to assess the cells involved. Immunohistochemistry (IHC) is the most widely used technique for staining tissues, especially vascular tissues for *C. pneumoniae*. The advantage of this technique is that it has been used by most pathology clinical laboratories for many years to identify various antigen, or specific cell markers in tissue. The major disadvantage is the subjectivity of interpretation and, thus in inexperienced hands can lead to misinterpretation and false positive results. Of major importance in this technique is the utilization of proper negative and positive controls, including isotypic antibodies against

Table 5.3
Recommendations for Standardizing *Chlamydia pneumoniae* Diagnostic Assays

Assay type	Major recommendations
Serological testing	Microimmunofluorescence remains the only currently acceptable approach Acute infection is defined by a fourfold rise in IgG or an IgM titer of ≥16; use of a single elevated IgG titer is discouraged Past exposure is indicated by an IgG titer of ≥16 Neither elevated IgA titers nor any other serologic marker are validated indicators of persisting infection
Culture	Documentation of a positive culture result requires propagation of the isolate or PCR confirmation In the absence of propagation or PCR confirmation, an average of ≥1 inclusion per culture well should be considered a presumptive positive culture The use of serum-free media, multiple centrifugations, or pretreatment of cells is not endorsed
PCR	4 of 18 currently published assays met proposed criteria for optimal validation Each PCR run should include low positive controls (≤1 inclusion-forming units), and water controls every fifth extraction
Immunohistochemistry	Each tissue block should be tested with 2 *Chlamydia* antibodies and 2 control antibodies Each staining run should include 1 positive and 1 negative tissue control, each incubated with the 4 antibodies used on the specimen on interest Intracytoplasmic staining of macrophages, endothelial cells, or smooth-muscle cells in a granular pattern may be considered positive; interpretation of a homogenous staining pattern is controversial

Note. Adapted from Dowell et al.[44] with permission of the publishers.

unrelated rare microorganisms published[44]; see Table 5.3 for a summary of the standardization recommendations of the various diagnostic assays.

5.5. ASSOCIATION OF *C. PNEUMONIAE* INFECTION AND VASCULAR DISEASE

The evidences for association of *C. pneumoniae* infection and cardiovascular disease and stroke include seroepidemiological data, histopathological data, and microbiological evidence. However, the link between infection and a disease process does not prove causality or cause and effect.

5.5.1. Epidemiological Association

Risk factors for a disease entity are often discovered by a hierarchy of studies, with increasing confidence or power in the observations, such as: (1) case reports, (2) case control studies, (3) cross-sectional studies, (4) longitudinal studies, and finally (5) interventional studies. The hypothesis of the infectious etiology of cardiovascular disease, specifically atherosclerotic complications, is not new and was proposed in Europe in the latter part of the 19th century[57]. Saikku et al.[58] in 1988 first reported on the serological association of *C. pneumoniae* infection with coronary heart disease (CHD) and acute myocardial infection in a case control study. Since then numerous seroepidemiological studies have been reported on the association between *C. pneumoniae* infection and cardiovascular disease or stroke. The first major review of this topic by Danesh et al.[59] in 1997, listed 18 epidemiological studies ($\triangle$2 involved cerebrovascular disease, and 3 were prospective), and found an average odds ratio (OR) of 2 to support an association of *C. pneumoniae* infection with CHD and cerebrovascular disease. Problems noted with these studies include different criteria for cases between studies, adjustment for potential confounders to differing degrees and, thus, prone to different biases. Moreover, although most studies used the MIF assay, others used EIA, chlamydial immune complexes (I-C) or antibodies to chlamydial LPS to detect past infection. Furthermore, different end points have been used to determine seropositivity and some noted association with IgG antibodies, and others only with IgM or IgA antibodies or immune complexes (I-C) or antibodies to chlamydial LPS to detect past infection[59].

Since then at least 60 case control or cross-sectional studies on the association of *C. pneumoniae* and vascular diseases and more than 20 prospective or longitudinal studies have been reported. There have been improvements in case definitions and correction for various confounding factors in most of the recent studies, but there are still variability in assays used, end-point definitions of seropositivity and type of antibodies (immunoglobulin) associated with CHD or stroke reported.

Of the 62 retrospective case-control or cross-sectional studies reported up to the spring of 2002, 49 involved cardiovascular disease (CHD)[58,60–103], 10 cerebrovascular disease[104–113], and 2 abdominal aortic aneurysms[114,115] and 1 peripheral vascular disease[116] (see Table 5.4), but only 10 were population-based studies. There were over 18,000 subjects with over 10,000 cases of atherosclerotic vascular diseases. Most of the studies were from Europe and the United States but several studies were from Asia and a few from the Middle East (Israel).

Most studies used serological methods (MIF and EIA) antibodies to *C. pneumoniae*, the majority measured IgG alone or combined with IgA, and

Table 5.4
Retrospective Case Control and Cross-sectional Studies on
Atherosclerotic Vascular Disease and *C. pneumoniae* Infection

---

Cardiovascular disease, N = 49

- Clinical criteria (MI, angina, ECG) = 34 studies
- Angiographic criteria ($\geq 50\%$ stenosis of ≥ 1 coronary artery) = 15 studies
- Cardiac transplant and coronary artery bypass surgery = 1 study
- Population based = 5 studies

Cerebrovascular disease, N = 10

- Clinical criteria (Stroke, TIA) = 3 studies
- Ultrasonic criteria (carotid IMT or $\geq 50\%$ stenosis) = 6 studies
- Population based = 5 studies

Aortic abdominal aneurysms, N = 2

Femoral arteries calcification, N = 1

Summary
No. of vascular studies, *N* = 62
Total no. of cases = 10,539
No. of controls = 9,314

Note. MI, myocardial infarction; ECG, electrocardiogram; TIA, transient ischemic attack; IMT, intima-media thickness.

occasionally IgM. A few studies used immune complex assays[58,60,63], or measured chlamydial-LPS antibodies (genus-specific), or chlamydial heat shock protein-60 (CHSP-60) antibodies[82,100] (see Table 5.5). Seven studies assessed the relationship between *C. pneumoniae* DNA in PBMC and vascular disease[50,51,52,99,103,115,117] and single studies found association with antibodies to specific *C. pneumoniae* antigen by immunoblotting[92] and by cell mediated immune (CMI) response[97]. Overall 38 (63.3%) of the studies using different techniques found a positive association with *C. pneumoniae* infection and atherosclerotic vascular disease.

To date (early 2002) there have been 26 longitudinal, prospective studies on *C. pneumoniae* infection associated with vascular diseases. Twenty-three of these studies assessed mainly cardiovascular endpoints, of which nineteen involved primary events[118–136] and four secondary events[137–140] (subjects with acute myocardial infarction (MI) or unstable angina at entry), see Table 5.6. Only six (26%) of these studies showed an overall positive association with Chlamydia antibodies, two of which involved small high-risk groups: patients with hypertension and additional cardiovascular risk factors[128], or chronic renal failure on dialysis[136]. In addition, another five (21.7%) studies showed correlation with *C. pneumoniae* infection and cardiovascular events in subgroups of patients. For instance, Meittenen et al.[119] found a positive association in East Finland (RR 2.45) but not in West Finland in non-diabetics;

Table 5.5
Assays Used in Retrospective and Cross-sectional Vascular Studies

Serological methods: *specific anti*-C. pneumoniae *antibodies*

1. MIF: 37 studies
   - No. with significant association for any antibody: 26 (70.3%)

2. Enzyme immunoassay (EIA, ELISA) for *C. pneumoniae*: 9 studies
   - 7 used EIA alone (5 positive association)
   - 3 EIA plus MIF (2 correlated positively, 1 both negative)
   - Range of OR 0.8–4.38

3. Indirect immunofluorescent test for *C. pneumoniae*: 4 studies (2 positive association)
   - Range of OR 1.28–3.6

4. Antibodies to specific *C. pneumoniae* antigen by immunoblot: 1 study
   - 98 kDa, OR 2.3
   - 40 kDa, OR 29.4

5. EIA for Chlamydia, LPS antibodies: 4 studies
   - 2 studies sole assay (both no association)
   - 2 plus MIF, all positive association + correlation
   - OR range 0.71–86.1

6. Immune complex with anti-Chlamydial-LPS:
   - 4 studies
   - All 4 studies showed positive association
   - Range of OR 2.0–10.3

7. EIA antibodies to Chlamydia, HSP 60: 2 studies
   - One association, OR 5.4
   - One no association, OR 0.9

C. pneumoniae DNA by PCR in PBMC
   - 7 studies
   - 3 positive association (one in men only OR 3.2)
   - 1 trend OR 2.1 $p = 0.08$
   - OR range 0.9–31.0

Cell-mediated immunity, *LPR to* C. pneumoniae *antigen*
   - One study, strong LPR to EBs in CHD (men)

Total studies: $N = 62$
Association with vascular disease with any test, 40 (64.5%)

Note. LPS, lipopolysaccharide; PBMC, peripheral blood mononuclear cell; HSP, heat shock protein; MIF, microimmunofluorescence; EIA, enzyme immunoassay; LPR, lymphocyte proliferative response.

Glader et al.[135] noted an association with subjects with high Lp(a) (OR 3.8); Strachan et al.[124] found *C. pneumoniae* IgA correlated with fatal CHD (OR 1.68); von Hertzen et al.[121] correlated increased cerebrovascular mortality with high IgG titers >1:512 (hazard ratio 4.93); and Roivainen et al.[134] found anti-*C. pneumoniae* antibodies associated with CHD in those with high C-reactive protein (CRP) (OR 5.4).

Table 5.6

Prospective–Longitudinal Studies on *C. pneumoniae*
Antibodies and Atherosclerotic Vascular Disease

References	Mèthod	Follow-up	Cohort	Results
A. Cardiovascular disease: primary events				
1. Saikku et al. 1992[118]	MIF IgG, A + IC	5 yrs	Case control 103 pairs population based (Helsinki Heart Study)	IgG adj. OR 1.4 (CI 0.5–4.1) IgA OR 2.3 (CI 0.9–6.5) IgA + IC OR 2.6 (CI 1.3–5.2)
2. Meittinen et al. 1996[119]	MIF IgA ≥1:40 IgG ≥1:128	7 yrs	1195 non-diabetic 798 diabetic 202 cases population based	IgG or A, RR 1.8 non-diabetic (CI 0.9–3.73) West Finland NS East Finland, RR 2.45 (CI 1.02–5.90)
3. Ossewaarde et al. 1998[120]	EIA C.pn. IgG + A IC Lps	5 yrs	Case:control 54:108	IgG ≥3200 OR 2.76 (CI 1.3–5.8)
4. von Hertzen et al. 1999[121]	MIF IgG + A	6.5 yrs	67 cases:1196 cohort population >64 yrs	IgG ≥1:32 OR 1.0, IgG ≥1:512 cerebrovascular mortality in men HR 4.93 (CI 1.4–7.3), $p = 0.009$
5. Tavendale et al. 1999[122]	ELISA C.pn. IgG, A + M	3.9 yrs	Case:control 252 pairs	IgG OR 1.45 (NS) IgA OR 1.17 (NS) IgM OR 0.88 (NS)
6. Haider et al. 1999[123]	Unknown	10 yrs	1503 subjects 199 cases population based (Framingham)	IgG >1:128 RR 0.89 (CI 0.66–1.19)
7. Strachan et al. 1999[124]	MIF IgG + A	13 yrs	1733 men 438 cases population based	IgG OR 1.15 (NS) IgA OR 1.14 (NS) but fatal CHD 1.68 (CI 1.15–2.46)
8. Ridker et al. 1999[125]	MIF IgG ≥1:16– 1:256	12 yrs	Case:control 343 pairs (men)	RR 1.1 (CI 0.8–1.5)

Table 5.6

(*continued*)

References	Method	Follow-up	Cohort	Results
9. Ridker et al. 1999[126]	MIF	3 yrs	Case:control 122:244 post-men. women	OR 1.1 (CI 0.7–1.8)
10. Nieto et al. 1999[127]	MIF IgG >1:64	3.3 yrs	Case:control 246:550 population based (ARIC study)	RR 1.2 (NS)— overall RR 3.2 (*p* = 0.02) never smokers
11. Fagerberg et al. 1999[128]	MIF IgG, A + M C.pn. IC	6.5 yrs	Cohort č hypertension + ≥1 risk factor (152 men)	Titer >1:512 RR for CHD events 2.69 *p* = 0.04 Stroke RR 8.58 *p* = 0.04
12. Danesh et al. 2000[129]	Time-resolved fluorimetry	16 yrs	Case:control 496:989 population based	OR 1.22 (CI 0.82–1.82) OR 1.59 (CI 1.17–2.16) before adjusted for childhood social status
13. Wald et al. 2000[130]	Time-resolved fluorimetry C.pn. IgG + A	7 yrs	Case:control 647:1294	IgG OR 1.26 (CI 0.95–1.68) IgA OR 1.09 (CI 0.82–1.43)
14. Siscovick et al. 2000[131]	MIF IgG 1:8 (1024)	5.5 yrs	Case:control 213:405 population ≥65 yrs	IgG ≥1:8 OR 1.1 (NS) ≥1:1024 OR 2.0 (CI 1.1–3.6)
15. Zhu et al. 2001[132]	ELISA C.pn. IgG	3 yrs	Cohort 890 CHD on angio. 167 MI or death	MI-RR 1.47 (CI 0.76–2.8) MI or death RR 1.07 (NS)
16. Rupprecht et al. 2001[133]	Indirect immunofluorescence C.pn. IgG + A	3.1 yrs	Cohort (men) 1010 CHD on angio. MI, death, 78	IgG-RR 0.9 (NS) IgA-RR 0.7 (NS) ≥5 pathogens RR 5.1
17. Roivainen et al. 2000[134]	MIF IgG + A Immune complex (IC)	8.5 yrs	Case:control 241 pairs Helsinki population	anti-C.pn. + low CRP-OR-NS anti-C.pn. + high CRP-OR 5.4 (*p* < 0.05)

Table 5.6

(*continued*)

References	Method	Follow-up	Cohort	Results
18. Glader et al. 2000[135]	MIF + EIA IgG + A C.pn. IC	≃4 yrs	Case:control 78:156 population based	OR −1.0, −1.6 IgG + A (NS) Cp. IC OR 1.4 (C1.8–2–5) Cp. IC + Lp(a) >13 mg OR 3.8 (CI 1.4–10.2)
19. Haubitz & Brunkhorst 2001[136]	MIF IgG ≥1:64 IgA ≥1:80	6 yrs	Cohort of 34 on peritoneal dialysis	IgA-CHD events, OR 7.2, $p < 0.01$ death OR 10.2, $p < 0.005$

Secondary cardiovascular events

20. Gupta et al. 1997[137]	MIF IgG ≥1:64	18 mths	Cohort 213 post. MI	IgG-CHD events OR 4.7 (CI 1.2–15.5) $p = 0.03$
21. Choussat et al. 2000[138]	MIF IgG, A + M	1 yr	Cohort 79 with non-Q wave	IgG ≥1:64 OR 2.3, $p = 0.22$ MI, unstable angina
22. de Maat et al. 2000[139]	EIA C.pn. IgG + A ≥1:3200	18 mths	Cohort 211 unstable angina	IgG OR 0.86–0.9 (NS) IgA OR 1.1–1.49 $p = 0.35$
23. Kähler et al. 2001[140]	EIA IgG + M (anti-LPS)	6 mths	Cohort 1096 unstable angina	IgG OR 0.95 (NS) IgM-NS

B. Cerebrovascular disease studies
Progression of carotid artery disease by ultrasound (IMT and stenosis)

1. Mayr et al. 2000 +Krechl et al. 2001[141,142]	EIA C.pn. IgA >1:16	5 yrs	Cohort 826 (40–79 yrs) Brunek study	Incident atherosclerosis Non-stenotic OR 1.12 $p = 0.02$ Stenotic OR 1.17 $p = 0.03$ New plaque OR 2.0 (CI 1.2–3.0)
2. Sander et al. 2001[143]	MIF C.pn. IgG ≥ 1:64 IgA ≥1:16	3 yrs	Cohort 272 with TIA or 1st stroke	Seropositive 1 MT = 0.12 mm/yr Seronegative 1 MT = 0.07 mm/yr $p < 0.005$

Table 5.6

(*continued*)

References	Method	Follow-up	Cohort	Results
				CHD + CVD events greater in seropositive subjects, anti-C.pn. IgG + CRP < 0.5 mg RR 1.53, $p < 0.05$ anti-C.pn. IgG + CRP > 0.5 mg RR 3.45 (CI, 1.97–9.34) $p < 0.005$
Development of post-angioplasty coronary artery stenosis				
1. Mattila et al. 2001[144]	MIF IgG, A + M EIA for C.pn. IC	6 mths	Cohort 122 post-PTCA	Stenosis or luminal narrowing not related to any antibodies
Progression of abdominal aortic aneurysm				
1. Lindolt et al. 2001[145]	MIF IgG + A	4.1 yrs	Cohort 100 men with AAA	IgG ≥1:128, ≥1 cm expansion/yr OR 12.6 (CI 1.37–293)

Note. CHD, coronary heart disease; C.pn, *C. pneumoniae*; CRP, C-reactive protein; MIF, microimmunofluorescence; EIA, enzyme immunoassay; OR, odd ratio (all adjusted for confounders); RR, relative risk; MI, myocardial infarction; HR, hazard ratio; NS, not significant; IC, immune complex; LPS, lipopolysaccharide; TIA, transient ischemic attack; AAA, abdominal aortic aneurysm; PTCA, percutaneous transluminal coronary angioplasty.

In the two longitudinal studies (one reported twice at different stages) on carotid artery atherosclerosis, using ultrasound to assess progression, there was significant correlation with *C. pneumoniae* infection and increased intima-media thickness (IMT), stenosis, and new plaques compared to seronegative cohorts in both studies[141–143]. In a prospective study on post-coronary angioplasty restenosis there was no correlation with *C. pneumoniae* antibodies[144]. However, in abdominal aortic aneurysm subjects with chlamydial antibodies had greater rate of expansion than those without over an average of 4 years[145]. See Table 5.7 for summary of prospective studies.

Although a recent meta-analysis of *C. pneumoniae* IgG antibody did not find a significant correlation with CHD, there are several criticisms of this study[129]. Since the 15 studies reviewed used several assay methods, with varying cut-off points, this type of analysis may not be valid. Furthermore, this has been confirmed by a recent study by Schumacher et al.[146], who

Table 5.7

Summary of Prospective Studies on *C. pneumoniae* and Vascular Disease

---

Primary cardiovascular events, 19 studies

- Population based 10 (52.6%)
- >3,946 cases and a total of 16,098 subjects
- Mean follow up, 6.8 years
- Overall positive association with *C. pneumoniae* antibodies, 5 studies (26.3%)
- Positive association of subgroups with *C. pneumoniae*, 5 studies (26.3%)

Secondary cardiovascular events, 4 studies

- None population based
- Total cohort, 1,599
- Mean follow up, 13.5 months
- Positive association with *C. pneumoniae*, 1 (25%)

Cerebrovascular disease, progression by ultrasound, 2 studies

- Population based, 1 (50%)
- Total cohort, 1,098
- Mean follow up, 4 years
- Positive association with *C. pneumoniae*, both (100%)

Coronary artery restenosis post-PTCA, 1 study

- 122 subjects
- No association with *C. pneumoniae*

Abdominal aortic aneurysm progression, 1 study

- 100 subjects
- Strongly associated with *C. pneumoniae*

Note. PTCA, percutaneous transluminal coronary angioplasty.

concluded that the choice of serological method had a major impact on evaluating the possible relationship between *C. pneumoniae* and CHD. In addition, in one of the larger prospective study[129], there was a significant correlation with *C. pneumoniae* antibody and CHD after adjustment for standard risk factors and adult socioeconomic status (OR 1.59), but this became insignificant after adjustment for childhood socioeconomic status. Thus, raising the issue of over adjustment[147] as most infectious diseases are greater in lower socioeconomic groups especially in childhood. Making this adjustment, therefore, may mask a real association with infectious diseases.

Comments. In summary, the retrospective and cross-sectional studies strongly support an association with *C. pneumoniae* infection and cardiovascular disease or stroke, but the longitudinal studies are more controversial and overall do not confirm this association. Several reasons may exist for this discrepancy besides inherent biases in retrospective studies and heterogeneity of diagnostic assays and end-points, and this include the lack of any good serological assay to detect persistent or chronic *C. pneumoniae* infections.

If *C. pneumoniae* plays a role in vascular disease, it would probably be in a latent, chronic, persistent state and there is no reliable test to identify this persistent infection. IgA antibodies cannot be used as a measure of chronic infection[44]. It is thus likely that the previous serological studies have a mixture of subjects with past resolved infection and some with chronic, persistent infection producing a gamut of associations. In addition, several studies[148–150] have shown that the present serology or antibody titers do not correlate with the presence or absence of *C. pneumoniae* antigen in atheromatous tissue.

5.5.2. Pathological Evidence of Association

Detection of *C. pneumoniae* in atheromatous plaques, with its absence in normal arteries, is another method of establishing association with atherosclerosis and the disease resulting from subsequent complications. However, this does not prove causality as the organism could be entrapped in the plaques as an "innocent bystander" without causing disease. Over fifty studies have documented the presence of *C. pneumoniae* in vascular tissues by several methods. These include immunocytochemical stain (ICC)[149,151–153], PCR[154–176], combination of the two[54,177–187], rarely immunofluorescence[188,189] alone, or combined with PCR[55,190], or ICC[191] stain, in situ hybridization[192,193], electron microscopy[53,192,194–201] in combination with ICC or PCR, and culture are used much less frequently with other detection methods[184,192,197,202,203]. In general, most of the studies have consistently found evidence of *C. pneumoniae* in atheromatous arteries but not in normal vessels, but at different prevalence rates, see Table 5.8. Only six studies failed to detect, or rarely found *C. pneumoniae* in atheroma, all using PCR techniques[154,157,158,161,174,197]. The negative results in these studies could be due to a combination of factors, including small tissue samples (i.e., atherectomy tissue), tissue inhibitors, calcification, and insensitive techniques. The overall odds ratio for association of *C. pneumoniae* with atherosclerosis, derived from the combined results of the pathological studies is 24.5.

The pathological studies, however, have several limitations. First, tissue PCR results show poor interlaboratory concordance, and only four of the 18 PCR assays used in published reports had been validated by other centers[44]. IHC is prone to interpreter variability and subjectivity, and thus possible false positive results. Second, pathological studies are retrospective or cross-sectional in design (by the nature of the examination) and lack control for confounding risk factors. Most of the pathological studies used controls from normal arteries (usually autopsy specimens) and sometimes from the same subjects as the diseased specimens. By the nature of pathological studies, it is

Table 5.8

Detection of *C. pneumoniae* in Vascular Tissue

Study	Year	Arteries examined	Methods	Proportion positive
1. Shor et al.[194]	1992	Coronary	EM, ICC	5/7
2. Kuo et al.[53]	1993	Coronary	EM, ICC, PCR	20/36
3. Kuo et al.[151]	1993	Aorta	ICC	7/21
4. Weiss et al.[154]	1995	Coronary	PCR	1/36
5. Campbell et al.[195]	1995	Coronary	EM, ICC, PCR	20/38
6. Varghese et al.[177]	1995	Coronary	ICC, PCR	4/40
7. Kuo et al.[178]	1995	Coronary	ICC, PCR	1/22 (ages 15–24)
				7/29 (ages 25–34)
8. Grayston et al.[54]	1995	Carotid	ICC, PCR	37/61
9. Ong et al.[55]	1996	Aorta, iliac	IMF, PCR	19/43
10. Ong et al.[196]	1996	Various	PCR, EM, ICC	36/67
11. Muhlestein et al.[188]	1996	Coronary	IMF	66/90
12. Weiss et al.[197]	1996	Coronary	PCR, EM, culture	1/58
13. Ramirez et al.[192]	1996	Coronary	ICC, PCR, EM, culture, ISH	7/12
14. Blasi et al.[155]	1996	AAA	PCR	26/51
15. Juvonen et al.[198]	1997	AAA	ICC, PCR, EM	12/12
16. Jackson et al.[179]	1997	Coronary, various	ICC, PCR	13/34
17. Gloria-Breceda et al.[189]	1997	Aorta	IMF	2/16
18. Kuo et al.[180]	1997	Femoral, poplital	ICC, PCR	11/23
19. Chiu et al.[149]	1997	Carotid	ICC	54/76
20. Maass et al.[202]	1998	Coronary	PCR, culture	21/70
21. Taylor-Robinson et al.[156]	1998	Aorta, pulmonary	PCR	13/41
22. Shor et al.[199]	1998	Various	ICC, PCR, EM	17/24
23. Paterson et al.[157]	1998	Carotid, coronary	PCR	0/49
24. Daus et al.[158]	1998	Coronary	PCR	0/29
25. Maass et al.[159]	1998	Carotid, coronary	PCR	51/238
26. Davidson et al.[181]	1998	Coronary	ICC, PCR	15/60 raised lesions
				7/60 flat lesions
27. Ouchi et al.[182]	1998	Coronary, iliac	ICC, PCR	25/39
28. Yamashita et al.[152]	1998	Carotid	ICC	11/20
29. Petersen et al.[160]	1998	AAA	PCR	14/40 aneurysm
				2/40 normal aorta
30. Berger et al.[183]	2000	Various, non-coronary	PCR/ICC	33/130
31. Lindholt et al.[161]	1998	AAA	n PCR	0/20
32. Wong et al.[162]	1999	Coronary	PCR	11/33
33. Bauriedel et al.[200]	1999	Coronary	ICC, EM	35/51
34. Esposito et al.[163]	1999	Carotid	PCR, RT-PCR	10/30
35. Blasi et al.[164]	1999	AAA	PCR	17/41
36. Melissano et al.[165]	1999	Carotid	PCR	12/16 untreated
				5/16 treated
37. Wong et al.[166]	1999	Coronary	PCR	26/33 subjects
38. Nadrachal et al.[167]	1999	Carotid, AAA	PCR	8/29 carotid ⎫ 37/60
				3/14 AAA ⎭

Table 5.8

(*continued*)

Study	Year	Arteries examined	Methods	Proportion positive
39. Qavi et al.[168]	2000	Carotid	PCR	7/17
40. Bartels et al.[184]	2000	Coronary, veingraft	PCR/ICC, culture	33/130
41. Mosorin et al.[193]	2000	Carotid	ICC/ISH	11/17
42. Farsak et al.[169]	2000	Various	PCR	12/46
43. Karlsson et al.[203]	2000	AAA	PCR/ICC/culture	20/26
44. Gibbs et al.[170]	2000	Carotid	PCR	25/98
45. Ericson et al.[191]	2000	Coronary	IMF/ICC	36/42 severe ⎫ 37/60 1/18 mild ⎭
46. Ozsan et al.[190]	2000	Coronary	IMF/PCR	11/13
47. Ouchi et al.[185]	2000	Coronary/carotid/ iliac	ICC/PCR	42/67 plaques 2/110 controls
48. Gutierrez et al.[171]	2001	Non-coronary various/aorta	PCR	48/85 samples 44/82 patients
49. Virok et al.[201]	2001	Middle cerebral	N-PCR, EM	5/15
50. La Biche et al.[172]	2001	Carotid	PCR	14/94
51. Vink et al.[186]	2001	Coronary/brachial	PCR, ICC	51/71 CAD ⎫ 59/119 8/48 brachial ⎭
52. Dubrilovic et al.[173]	2001	Carotid	PCR	42/60
53. Ong et al.[174]	2001	Carotid	n PCR	0/40 patients
54. Rassu et al.[187]	2001	Various/aorta	n PCR/ICC	18/18 autopsy subjects 78/90 specimens
55. Radke et al.[175]	2001	Coronary	PCR	17/53
56. Valassina et al.[176]	2001	Carotid	PCR/RT-PCR	13/58
57. Vink et al.[153]	2001	Various	ICC	24/24 autopsy subjects 111/738 arterial segment

not feasible to use healthy vascular tissues from age, sex, and risk factor controls. Moreover, since atherosclerosis is universal among adults and begins in early childhood, it would be difficult to find age-matched controls without atherosclerosis.

Overall *C. pneumoniae* antigen is detected on an average of 40% or more from atheromatous vessels and rarely from normal arteries. However, *C. pneumoniae* DNA has been detected as high as 94.3% in plaques of smokers versus 36% of non-smokers[173]. Jackson et al.[179] have reported on the widespread distribution of *C. pneumoniae* in various tissues from autopsy to test the "innocent bystander" hypothesis, and found *C. pneumoniae* mainly located in vascular tissue and rarely in others. Furthermore, in another study there was an association of *C. pneumoniae* distribution with that of atherosclerosis in the arterial system of individuals at autopsy, and the presence of microorganism correlated with the extent of stenosis of the coronary arteries[153], and *C. pneumoniae* positive coronary lesions more commonly presented with unstable[172] angina. We have also shown that plaques with fresh thrombi are more likely to be *C. pneumoniae* positive than those without thrombi[149], hence suggesting that *C. pneumoniae* may play a role in acute thrombus or ischemic events. However, some studies have not found an association of *C. pneumoniae* presence and the severity of vascular disease (see Table 5.9). Of the studies or

Table 5.9

Correlation of Detection of *C. pneumoniae* and Severity of Disease

Studies	Lesion	Disease	No. positive/No. subjects (%)
1. Kuo et al.[148]	CHD/aorta	Early	16/50 (32)
	Plaques	Advanced	102/184 (55)
			OR 2.64 (95% CI, 1.36–5.12), $p = 0.04$
2. Ong et al.[195]	Various arteries	No to minimal	5/16 (36)
	Infiltrates	Moderate to severe	13/23 (56)
			OR 2.86 (95% CI, 0.74–10.92), NS
3. Chiu et al.[149]	Carotid	No thombus	17/30 (57)
	plaques	Fresh thombus	37/48 (80), $p = 0.04$
4. Bauriedel et al.[200]	Coronary	Stable angina	6/20 (30)
	plaques	Unstable/AMI	26/31 (84), $p = 0.001$
5. Wong et al.[166]	Coronary arteries	Mild (Grade I–III)	27/73 (37)
	Stary grading	Severe (Grade IV–VI)	41/114 (36), NS
6. Ericson et al.[191]	Coronary arteries	Mild	1/18 (6)
	Histological grading	Severe	36/42 (86), $p < 0.01$
7. Gibbs et al.[170]	Carotid atheroma	Emboli	8/26 (26)
	Plaque stability	No emboli	13/44 (30), NS
		Infarction	12/46 (26)
		No infarction	9/24 (37), NS
8. La Biche et al.[172]	Carotid plaques	Asymptomatic	9/57 (16)
	Symptom	Symptomatic	5/37 (14), NS
9. Vink et al.[153]	Various arteries	Cross-sections	C. pn. −mean area of stenosis 13%
	Plaques and stenosis	Area of stenosis	C. pn. +mean area of stenosis 32%, $p < 0.001$

Note. AMI, acute myocardial infarction; NS, not statistically significant; CHD, coronary heart disease.

compilation of studies addressing this issue, five of nine reports showed a significant correlation with severity of vascular lesions (or symptoms) or presence of fresh thrombus with detection of *C. pneumoniae* in tissue.

An important issue is that the wide range of results in detection of *C. pneumoniae* in the vasculature may reflect sampling error, and the absence at one site does not mean that the organism is not present in another atheroma elsewhere in that individual. Two recent studies by Rassu et al.[187] and Vink et al.[153] has addressed this issue. Rassu et al.[187] examined five vascular areas in 18 autopsy subjects, and Vink et al.[153] 33 arterial locations from 24 corpses (738 segments). Both studies found *C. pneumoniae* in all individuals (total 42 subjects)—100% detection rate, but rates of detection in specific arterial locations are similar to previous reports, that is, 33% of coronary arteries, 67% of abdominal aorta but only 2% from cerebral arteries. Moreover, evidence of T-cell immune response in atheromas to *C. pneumoniae* support an active process rather than a passive entrapment. Forty-one percent of established T-cell lines from carotid plaques, and none from control specimens, recognized *C. pneumoniae* as specific T-cell stimulating antigen and CHSP-60 induced specific proliferation in five of seven cases[193]. In addition, when *C. pneumoniae* is present in symptomatic plaques, T-lymphocytes and particularly CD8+ cells are increased, suggesting a specific antigen driven cellular immune response[204].

5.5.3. Culture of *C. pneumoniae* from Plaques

C. pneumoniae is difficult to culture from tissues but a few centers have successfully recovered viable organisms from atheromatous specimens. It is the only microorganism cultured from atheromas, and this establishes the association of viable organisms in plaques and not the mere presence of antigenic particles previously phagocytosed by migrating macrophages. *C. pneumoniae* has been cultured from coronary and carotid arteries, coronary bypass versus grafts, abdominal aortic aneurysms and from a femoral artery noted in seven reports from six different centers, see Table 5.10[184,192,202,203,205–207]. The most successful recovery rates were in 10 of 26 (38%) abdominal aortic aneurysms[203] and in 11 of 70 (16%) atherectomy specimens from coronary arteries and venus bypass grafts[202]. The inability to culture *C. pneumoniae* from vasculature tissues and low recovery rate may be due to small amount of tissue cultured, low concentration of microorganisms, or persistence of the organism in a latent, metabolically inactive and unculturable form. Moreover, optimization of the method may require multiple passage (4–6) before the *Chlamydia* can be isolated. Detection of viable *C. pneumoniae* establishes association with atherosclerosis and suggests a role in pathogenesis, but does

Table 5.10
Studies Reporting Isolation of *C. pneumoniae* from Arteries

Study	Type of artery	Positive culture/total patients, n/n
Ramirez et al.[192]	Coronary	1/10
Jackson et al.[205]	Carotid	1/25
Maass et al.[202]	Coronary + venous grafts	11/70
Bartels et al.[184]	Coronary	7/80
	Venous grafts	5/45
Karlsson et al.[203]	AAA	10/26
Apfalter et al.[206]	Carotid, femoral, AAA	3/38
Walski et al.[207]	coronary	3/3

Note. AAA, abdominal aortic aneurysm.

not prove causality as it is possible that the bacterium can be latently present without inducing disease.

5.6. EVIDENCE OF CAUSALITY

Investigations on evidences to suggest causality or a significant role of *C. pneumoniae* in the pathogenesis of atherosclerosis (and therefore CHD and cerebrovascular disease), include in vitro and in vivo data on biological mechanisms, animal models with induction of atherosclerosis, and human interventional trials.

5.6.1. Biological Mechanisms

There are substantial in vitro data to support biological plausible mechanisms of initiation or acceleration of atherosclerosis by *C. pneumoniae*. *C. pneumoniae* is capable of replicating in human macrophages, endothelial, and smooth-muscle cells derived from human aorta in vitro[208], and can also infect and multiply in lymphocytes[209]. Infection of human endothelial cells can induce proliferation of smooth cells via an endothelial derived soluble factor, and smooth cell proliferation is an integral process in the pathogenesis of atherosclerosis[210]. Endothelial dysfunction and proliferation are early processes in the development of atherosclerosis, and *C. pneumoniae* infected epithelial cells are resistant to apoptosis[211]. Moreover, adhesion of *C. pneumoniae* infected monocytes to endothelium and smooth-muscle cells can allow access to atheromatous lesions. It was recently reported that monocytes infected with viable *C. pneumoniae* adhered preferentially to human coronary artery endothelial and smooth-muscle cells, as compared to uninfected monocytes or monocytes harboring heat inactivated *Chlamydia*[212]. It has also been shown in vitro that *C. pneumoniae* can upregulate RNA expression for genes encoding cytokines (interleukin-1), chemokines (monocyte chemotactic protein 1 and interleukin-8), and cellular growth factors (heparin-binding epidermal-like growth factor, basic fibroblast growth factor and platelet derived growth factor β chain) in human endothelial cells[213]. Production of basic fibroblast growth factor and interleukin-6 by human smooth-muscle cells following infection with *C. pneumoniae* has also been reported[214]. Inflammation is important in the initial phase of atherogenesis, and cytokines are believed to play a key role in the initiation and progression of the inflammation. Acellular components of *C. pneumoniae* are potent stimuli of the pro-inflammatory cytokines production in human blood mononuclear cells[215], and this may play an important role in atherogenesis.

Most importantly, the key elements in the development of atherosclerosis, foam cells and oxidized LDL can be influenced by *C. pneumoniae* in vitro. Kalayoglu and Byrne[216] demonstrated that *C. pneumoniae* induced foam cell formation by human monocyte derived macrophages by causing accumulation of cholesterol esters. The lipid accumulation did not involve scavenger receptors but was blocked by heparin, which blocks binding of LDL to the LDL-receptor, suggesting that the pathogen induced lipid accumulation by dysregulating native LDL uptake or metabolism. Further studies by this group revealed that LPS was the *C. pneumoniae* component responsible for inducing macrophage foam cell formation[217]. In addition, Kalayoglu et al.[218] showed that viable *C. pneumoniae* and chlamydial HSP-60 were able to induce cellular oxidation of LDL—the highly atherogenic form of lipoprotein and the hallmark of atherosclerosis.

Chlamydial HSP-60 also localizes in human atheroma in 47% of endarterectomy specimens and co-localizes with human HSP-60 in plaque macrophages[219]. Chlamydial HSP-60 regulates macrophage tumor necrosis factor-alpha (TNF-α) and matrix metalloproteinase expression, potential mechanisms by which chlamydial infection may promote atherogenesis and precipitate acute ischemic events. Moreover, chlamydial HSP-60 can activate human vascular endothelium, smooth-muscle cells and macrophages[220]. Humoral immune reaction to chlamydial HSP-60 may cross-react with human HSP-60/65 and may play an important role in the process of vascular endothelial injury, a key element in the pathogenesis of atherosclerosis, as antibodies to chlamydial HSP-60 can mediate endothelial cytotoxicity[221]. Other mechanisms by which *C. pneumoniae* may play a role in acute ischemic attacks include induction of the 92 kDa gelatinase by human macrophages, leading to extracellular matrix destruction[222] and, thus, an unstable plaque. Furthermore, *C. pneumoniae* can induce thrombogenicity by upregulation of procoagulant

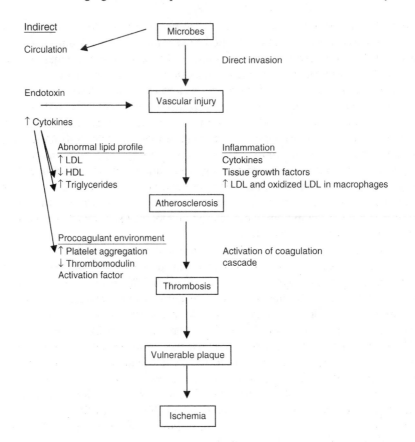

Figure 5.3. A schematic diagram of the potential mechanisms by which an infectious agent (i.e., *C. pneumoniae*) may be involved in atherosclerosis and the vascular complications.

proteins in vitro. Human vascular endothelial cells and smooth-muscle cells infected with *C. pneumoniae* can induce procoagulant protein and proinflammatory cytokine expression such as tissue factor, plasminogen activator inhibitor-1 (PAI-1) and interleukin-6, along with activation of NF-kappa B[223]. The potential mechanisms by which *C. pneumoniae* may play a role in atherogenesis and cardiovascular disease are summarized in Figure 5.3.

5.6.2. Animal Models

The use of animal models in experimentation is crucial to help define causality and possible role of putative factors in the pathogenesis of many diseases. Although results of studies in animals may not be directly applicable to humans, they are often helpful in supporting or refuting cause and effect relationships. The effect of *C. pneumoniae* infection on development of atherosclerosis has been studied mainly in the murine and rabbit models.

Rodents are relatively resistant to development of atherosclerosis and their lipoprotein pattern is different from humans. However, with genetic manipulation gene "knock-out" mice have increased susceptibility to atherosclerosis and they are now commonly used in atherosclerotic research. In initial studies using apolipoprotein (apo) E deficient mice, which spontaneously develop atherosclerosis, *C. pneumoniae* could be recovered from 10–25% of abdominal atherosclerotic aortas within 1–2 weeks after intranasal inoculation, but PCR detected the DNA in 35–100% of aortas up to 8–16 weeks after inoculation[224]. In C57BL/6J mice, which only develop atherosclerosis on an atherogenic diet, *C. pneumoniae* was detected in only 8% of mice 2 weeks after intranasal inoculation[224]. Further studies in apoE deficient mice and LDL-receptor deficient (also prone to atherosclerosis) demonstrated that *C. pneumoniae* infection could enhance and accelerate hypercholesterolemic-induced atherosclerosis[225-227], but did not induce changes by itself in normocholesterolemic mice. In addition, endothelial dysfunction (which is believed to occur in the initial stage of atherosclerosis) can be induced after repeated *C. pneumoniae* infection in apoE-deficient mice[228], and the endothelial nitric oxide pathway is principally involved. *C. pneumoniae* also increased atherosclerotic lesions of wild type mice (C57BL/6J) which were fed a high cholesterol diet by 2.5–3.3-fold after 18–24 weeks, respectively[229]. Furthermore, the enhancing effect of atherosclerosis has been demonstrated only for *C. pneumoniae* and not for *C. trachomatic*[229,230].

On the other hand, two recent studies were unable to demonstrate any increase in atherosclerosis of the aortic root in two strains of apoE-deficient mice after repeated *C. pneumoniae* infection[231], or in a wild type mice (intrinsically resistant to atherosclerosis) fed standard chow[232]. The reasons for the discrepancy in results in the apoE-deficient mice are unclear, but may include different inoculation protocols, different observation periods, failure for infection to take, and less likely different strains of *C. pneumoniae*. Although *C. pneumoniae* has not been shown to produce atherosclerotic changes in wild type mice without hypercholesterolemia, inflammatory changes in the heart and aorta were observed in a small number of chronically infected (C57BL/6J) mice[233].

The rabbit is an established animal model for atherosclerosis, which has been used for almost a century in the study of cholesterol and lipid-rich diet since the landmark studies of Anitschkow in 1913[234]. He demonstrated that cholesterol caused the atherosclerotic changes in the rabbit aortic intima which was very similar to human atherosclerosis. Early changes with fatty streaks and advanced atheromatous plaques were noted, and the amount of cholesterol in the diet was directly proportional to the degree of atherosclerosis. Normally, normocholesterolemic rabbits do not develop changes of atherosclerosis of the aorta spontaneously. We have previously shown that New Zealand White (NZW) rabbits fed standard chow could develop early atherosclerotic-like microscopic lesions (increased foam cells and smooth-muscle cells) in the aorta within 4 weeks of a single nasopharyngeal inoculation with *C. pneumoniae*[235]. Further studies in a larger number of animals with three separate inoculation resulted in more frequent lesion (34%) with more advanced atherosclerotic changes after 12 weeks[236]. Although these de novo lesions were predominantly microscopic in the normocholesterolemic rabbits, some animals demonstrated a few small focal raised visible lesions at the root or arch of the aorta, whereas, sham-infected or *M. pneumoniae* infected rabbits failed to develop any atherosclerotic changes. Histologically the aortic lesions ranged from fatty streaks to fibro-muscular lesions, or calcified fibro-muscular lesions resembling Stary's type I–III and even Grade VII lesions but without luminal narrowing (see Figures 5.4 and 5.5 for normal aorta). The changes in the intima of the aorta closely resembled those produced by a very low cholesterol enriched diet (0.15%), which resulted in serum cholesterol levels (4.1 mmol/L) considered healthy for humans. Finnish investigators have also reported on inflammatory intimal changes of the aorta in NZW rabbits fed standard chow after *C. pneumoniae* infection[237].

C. pneumoniae has also been demonstrated to enhance or accelerate hypercholesterolemic induced atherosclerosis in the rabbit model and these changes were partially reversed by treatment with a new macrolide, azithromycin, when administered early after infection[238]. The exact mechanisms by which *C. pneumoniae* induces de novo changes of atherosclerosis or acceleration in the animal models are not clear. But our ability to detect *C. pneumoniae* by immunostain in the lesions suggest a direct role through stimulation of cytokines and tissue growth factor with increased foam cells and smooth-muscle cells proliferation. However, it is possible that acceleration of hypercholesterolemia-induced atherosclerosis could be by an indirect effect by alteration of the serum lipid profile to a more proatherogenic state. In a recent study performed by our group on NZW rabbit fed a 0.25% cholesterol enriched diet, there was a 57% increase in the area of atherosclerosis of the aorta in *C. pneumoniae* infected rabbits compared to non-infected controls; and these changes were not associated with a significant alteration of the lipid profile except for increased triglyceridemia[239]. However, hypertriglyceridemia in the rabbit model does not enhance atherosclerosis but appears to be protective, as aortic cholesterol is inversely related to plasma

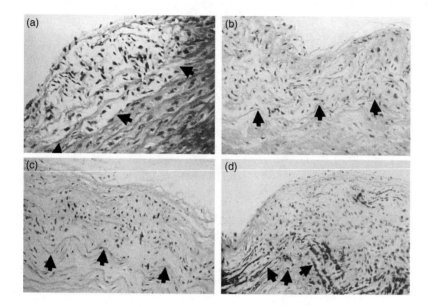

Figure 5.4. The histological changes of atherosclerosis of the aorta are shown in the de novo rabbit model (normocholesterolemic). For comparison to the normal rabbit aorta, see Figure 5.5. *C. pneumoniae*-inoculated rabbit aorta.

(a) Grade I lesion (fatty streak); foamy macrophages (small arrowheads) in the intima. The triangle indicates internal elastic lamina. H&E; original magnification, ×250.

(b) Grade II lesion (advanced fatty streak); mixed foamy macrophages (arrowheads) and spindle smooth-muscle cells. Solid triangles indicate internal elastic lamina. H&E; original magnification, ×250.

(c) Grade III lesion (fibromuscular); smooth-muscle cells in the intima. Arrowheads indicate the internal elastic lamina. H&E; original magnification, ×250.

(d) Grade IV lesion; advanced fibromuscular lesion with smooth-muscle cell proliferation and calcification (indicated by arrowheads). This lesion lacks foam cells, lipid core, and fibrous cap as typical for Stary's Type IV lesion or seen with 0.5% cholesterol. H&E; original magnification, ×250.

Adapted from Fong et al.[236] with permission of the publishers.

triglyceride levels[240]. This study suggests that the acceleration of atherosclerosis seen in rabbits with hypercholesterolemia is probably unrelated to changes in serum lipid profile, but may be more of a direct effect of the inflammatory cytokines in the aorta. However, we cannot exclude functional changes in HDL which could still lead to an indirect effect by decreasing the protective activity of this lipoprotein.

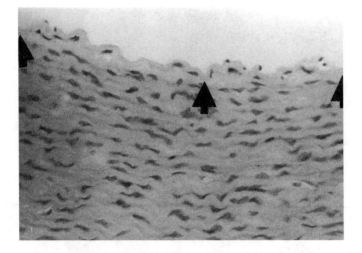

Figure 5.5. The above section of the aorta (magnification ×400) of a normal rabbit, on standard chow, with no changes of atherosclerosis. Arrows indicate the thin layer of the endothelium (intima) which is only one cell larger thick.

5.6.3. Effect of Antimicrobials on Atherosclerosis in Animal Models

Muhlestein et al.[238] first demonstrated that azithromycin 30 mg/kg intra-muscularly daily for 7 days, then twice weekly for 6 weeks largely prevented the enhancing effect of *C. pneumoniae* infection on IMT of the NZW rabbits aorta, fed a 0.25% cholesterol enriched diet. The antibiotic was started imme-diately after the final of a triple inoculation. However, in the apoE-deficient mice, two inoculations of *C. pneumoniae* increased the aortic lesions, but two doses of azithromycin 24 mg/kg by oral suspension administered 2 and 3 weeks after the second inoculation failed to modify the lesions[241].

In the de novo rabbit model without hypercholesterolemia, we demon-strated that early treatment, 5 days after the first of three inoculations, was highly effective but delayed treatment, 2 weeks after the third inoculation, was ineffective in preventing or decreasing early atherosclerotic lesions[242]. Azithromycin 30 mg/kg daily by oral gavage, for 3 days then every 5 days for 4–6 weeks, was used in this experiment to mimic the human dosing in the WIZARD Trial. Further studies with this model using another never macrolide, clarithromycin, with greater in vitro activity but shorter half-life was performed. Acute early treatment with oral clarithromycin 20 mg/kg/day for 8 days starting 5 days after each inoculation was highly effective in mod-ifying development of lesions, but delayed treatment 2 weeks after the third inoculation (6 weeks after initial infection) given daily for 6 weeks was less effective with a trend ($p = 0.07$) to a significant difference compared to the untreated controls[243].

5.6.4. Clinical Trials

Two large retrospective studies on the prophylactic effect of antibiotics in preventing future MI have been published. In a case control study of 3,315 patients with first time acute MI (and free of clinical conditions related to increased risk such as diabetes mellitus, hypertension, etc.), cases were significantly less likely to use tetracycline or quinolone 3 years before compared to 13,139 matched controls[244], indicating a possible protective value of certain prior antibiotics against MI. In another recent study of, 1996 cases with first MI and 4,882 matched controls, there was no difference in the prior use of erythromycin, tetracycline, or doxycycline[245]. This study may not be powered to show a protective effect of antibiotics, owing to the smaller sample size and inclusion of patients with other traditional risk factors for CHD.

A recent large retrospective study on the intake of antichlamydial antibiotics and post-acute myocardial infarction (AMI) prognosis was reported[246]. Three groups of patients were compared: those exposed to (1) antichlamydial antibiotics, (2) sulfa derivative antibiotics, to which *C. pneumoniae* is not sensitive, and (3) neither of the above. Two periods of antibiotic exposure were explored: during 6 months before AMI and during 3 months after AMI. There were 26,195 subjects with AMI in Quebec between 1991 and 1995 that were analyzed in the study. Among individuals treated during 6 months before AMI, the adjusted risk of dying was similar among the three groups. Among patients who were exposed during the three months after AMI and who survived at least 3 months, the one year mortality was similar, 10–11%. However, at 2 years the mortality favored the antichlamydial treated groups (15.9% vs. 23.0% and 20%). In adjusted survival analysis, patients in the sulfa-derivative and nonexposed groups were slightly more likely to die than patients in the antichlamydial group (relative risk 1.38, 95% CI, 1.04–1.82, and 1.29, 93% CI, 1.05–1.59, respectively). Previous preliminary, prospective, randomized small antibiotic trials for secondary prevention of cardiovascular events after AMI suggested a benefit of newer macrolides, azithromycin, and roxithromycin, after AMI or unstable angina in the short term[247,248]. However, the early reduction in secondary events observed at 1 month was lost at 6 months follow up in the larger trail[249]. In another relatively small study of 302 patients with CHD, but no acute syndromes and seropositive for *C. pneumoniae*, no reduction in cardiovascular events at 6 months or 2 years was observed after treatment with azithromycin for

3 months[250,251]. However, there was reduction of a global rank serum score of four inflammatory markers (CRP, IL-1, IL-6, and TNF-α) in the treated group. The size of this study would limit the ability to detect a significant clinical benefit of antibiotics in patients with stable CHD.

In a recent study of 324 patients with AMI or unstable angina, three groups were randomized to receive placebo, or azithromycin with metronidazole and omeprazole, or amoxicillin with metronidazole and omeprazole for 1 week. Both antibiotic regimens reduced secondary cardiac events by 37% compared to placebo after 3 months and a year[252]. This study suggests that bacteria other than *C. pneumoniae*, such as *Helicobacter pylori* or periodontal pathogens may be playing a role in precipitating further cardiac events.

Although there is no good data to suggest that *C. pneumoniae* plays a role in post-percutaneous coronary artery angioplasty (PTCA) stenosis, a recent study has assessed the efficacy of roxithromycin (a new macrolide) in the outcome. In a large (1,010 patients) placebo-controlled study[253] of roxithromycin for 4 weeks after coronary stent placement, no overall effect on restenosis was found after 6 months and a year. In a subgroup of patients with high IgG titers against *C. pneumoniae* ($\geq$1:512), however, there was a significant reduction in restenosis, OR 0.44 (95% CI, 0.19–1.06) $p = 0.038$, and for revascularization 0.332 (95% CI, 0.13–0.81) $p = 0.006$.

It has been postulated that *C. pneumoniae* infection could be involved in the earliest stage of atherogenesis, endothelial dysfunction, which could partly explain our de novo changes in the normocholesterolemic rabbits[236]. As previously mentioned, endothelial dysfunction can be induced in apoE-deficient mice with repeated *C. pneumoniae* infection[228]. Forty male patients with CHD were randomized to received azithromycin or placebo for 5 weeks, and flow-medicated dilatation (FMD) of the brachial artery, E-selectin, von Willebrand factor and CRP levels were measured before and at the end of the treatment period. Azithromycin resulted in significant improvement in FMD (mean change 2.1 + 1.1%, $p < 0.005$), and significant decrease in E-selectin and von Willebrand factor levels[254].

Of interest is a recent pilot study of the use of doxycycline to retard expansion of abdominal aortic aneurysm in a randomized, double-blind study[255]. Thirty-two patients with small aortic abdominal aneurysms (3.0–5.5 cm) were assigned either placebo or doxycycline (150 mg daily) for 3 months and monitored for 18 months with ultrasound. The aneurysm expansion in the treated group was significantly lower than the placebo groups during the 18 month period ($p = 0.01$); and at 6 months the CRP levels were significantly lower than the baseline level in the doxycycline group, $p = 0.01$. This encouraging study needs to be repeated with a much larger sample size and longer follow-up.

Preliminary report of the WIZARD study has just been released at the time of this writing. This is a multicenter, international study of 7,724 patients with previous MI and with *C. pneumoniae* IgG titer of ≥1:16. Patients were randomized to receive either azithromycin 600 mg once daily for 3 days, then once weekly for 3 months or a matching placebo[256]. Unlike previous pilot studies, patients had stable CHD. End-points over the following 2–3 years included recurrent AMI, unstable angina, need for coronary angioplasty or revascularization procedure, stroke, and death. There was no significant reduction in the incidence of secondary cardiovascular events or time to a clinical event. Post hoc analysis revealed a possible early treatment benefit that was not sustained over the observation period[256]. This study result neither confirms nor refutes the hypothesis that *C. pneumoniae* contributes to the incidence of CHD, see discussion in "Future Directions."

5.7. FUTURE DIRECTIONS

It has been argued that further epidemiological studies to assess *C. pneumoniae* infection and atherosclerotic vascular disease are unnecessary, as the association has been established albeit by pathological and microbiological data. Further epidemiological studies cannot establish causality but can only strengthen the association. Certainly, further epidemiological studies using the current serological assays would not be very helpful, and reliable methods that can predict chronic persistent infection or the presence of the bacterium in plaques are needed. Even if further studies confirm that *C. pneumoniae* plays a role in the pathogenesis of atherosclerosis, and therefore CHD and strokes, and find that antimicrobial agents are useful, there would still be a need for a diagnostic test to help select the best candidate for this treatment. It is very unlikely that all patients with CHD or cerebrovascular disease would benefit, and more likely that only a subgroups of patients would need antimicrobial therapy.

Currently there are no established noninvasive techniques to determine the presence of the microorganism in the vasculature. Detection of *C. pneumoniae* in PBMC appears to be a promising technique but lacks standardization and interlaboratory reproducibility. Although, a couple of studies have found the presence of *C. pneumoniae* DNA in PBMC correlated with the presence in atheroma, others have not. Moreover, the number of subjects in these studies is small. Larger studies using a standardized accepted assay are needed to verify the usefulness of this method. Ideally blood should be collected from subjects dying and pathological specimens from multiple arterial sites be examined for *C. pneumoniae* by PCR and IHC. It is possible that in the negative studies the discrepancy in PBMC and atheroma detection is due to sampling error.

Antibody to CHSP-60 may be another useful assay to investigate further. Whereas the standard serological method (MIF or EIA) to *C. pneumoniae* MOMP or LPS does not show any correlation with the presence of the organism in atheroma, anti-CHSP-60 appears to be predictive in a preliminary study. We have recently shown that antibodies to CHSP-60 correlated with the presence of *C. pneumoniae* in carotid endarterectomy specimens in 85 subjects, but the sensitivity of the assay was only 80%[257]. Further large studies from different centers are needed to confirm the usefulness of this assay.

To determine whether or not *C. pneumoniae* plays a role in atherogenesis and cardiovascular disease will require an accumulation of evidence, or "the burden of proof," over time. The animal and in vitro data are very supportive of a causal role but are not sufficiently persuasive, and it is unlikely that Koch's postulate will be fulfilled in such a chronic, largely subclinical disease with so many known risk factors. However, further animal models (other than rodents and rabbits) such as primates, mini-pigs, guinea pigs, etc., need to be investigated. Moreover, enhancement of other risk factors (other than hypercholesterolemia) should be explored in the animal models, that is, hypertension, smoking, diabetes, hyperhomocysteinemia, etc.

Results of large interventional trials on the benefits of antimicrobials on secondary cardiovascular events may or may not establish or disprove causality. The just completed WIZARD study and on going large randomized trials (ACE and MARBLE assessing azithromycin, and PROVE IT study using gatifloxcin) are primarily assessing the precipitating effect of an infectious agent in subjects with known CHD (i.e., the effect on destabilization of a plaque or acute thrombus formation). Negative results from these studies will not disprove a role in initiation and acceleration of atherosclerosis which has been found in animal models. Long-term clinical trials should be planned for younger adults over extended periods of time (10 or more years). However, these studies would be very expensive and difficult to do especially when using clinical end points. More realistically studies could be accomplished using surrogate markers such as progression of abdominal aortic plaques (using magnetic resonance imaging) in apparently healthy middle aged adults. Such an interventional trial would need fewer subjects over a shorter time and would be less expensive.

Another reason that current clinical trials on secondary prevention of cardiovascular events may fail to show an effect include the inability to eradicate *C. pneumoniae* from vascular tissue. There is in vitro data that the persistent state of chlamydia is not very susceptible to antimicrobial agents. It was shown in a continuous cell-culture model of chronic infection that *C. pneumoniae* could not be eliminated by ofloxacin or azithromycin[258]. Despite adequate intra plaque concentration of azithromycin[259] (0.28 µg/ml) and low minimal inhibitory concentration (MIC 0.25–0.125 µg/ml[260]), with high intracellular concentration (at least 200-fold the extracellular level)[261], viable *C. pneumoniae* was recovered from two subjects blood monocytes before and after treatment with azithromycin or rifampin[262]. Also, in patients undergoing experimental treatment with azithromycin for CHD, antibiotics did not inhibit chlamydial growth within monocytes[262]. Furthermore, in experimental mouse pneumonitis with *C. pneumoniae*, there was no difference in eradication rates between controls and azithromycin, but rifampin and azithromycin was significantly more effective[263]. Thus, currently the optimum regimen and duration needed to eliminate chronic *C. pneumoniae* infection from the vasculature is unknown. However, in a small randomized, open study of 32 patients undergoing endartectomy from carotid arteries, 16 subjects received roxithromycin 150 mg twice daily for a man of 26 days, and the other no treatment. In 12 of the 16 non-treated patients, *C. pneumoniae* DNA was detected by PCR but only in 5 of the 16 treated patients, $p = 0.034$[165], thus, suggesting that roxithromycin is effective in reducing the bacterial burden in plaques.

Hence, if *C. pneumoniae* were confirmed to play a major role in atherogenesis, then we should focus on the development of an effective vaccine. Hurdles to overcome, however, include our incomplete understanding of protective immunity in human, and the fact that natural infection with this microorganism does not produce long lasting immunity.

ADDENDUM

Advances in the pathogenesis of chlamydial infection continues in the area of attachment and entry. The dominant process for chlamydial attachment is via heparan sulfate-like compound that serves as a molecular bridge between chlamydial and target cells. The two main candidates for primary chlamydial adhesion are abundant outer membrane proteins present in all chlamydial species: the major outer membrane proteins (MOMP) and 60 kDa cysteine rich protein (OmcB)[264]. The host binding protein for *C. trachomatis* appears to be the mannose receptor, and a recent study also suggests that *C. pneumoniae* can bind to and be internalized by a phosphomannosyl receptor[265]. Recently, an insulin-like growth factor (IGF-2) was shown to enhance infection of endothelial cells by *C. pneumoniae*[266], and the IGF-2 receptor can also bind to mannose 6-phosphate and called the M6P/IGF-2 receptor[265].

It has been previously reported by Reiss et al.[267] that interferon-gamma and immune complexes regulate the expression of an anti-atherogenic cytochrome P450 enzyme, cholesterol-27-hydrolase (C27H). C27H may play a role in the primary defense against the development of atherosclerosis because of its involvement in the reverse transport of cholesterol from the periphery to the liver and its capacity to generate metabolites that inhibit foam cell formation[267,268]. Recently, it was demonstrated that *C. pneumoniae* infection down-regulated the expression of this anti-atherogenic enzyme (C27H) in vitro[269], and thus may play a role in plaque development.

REFERENCES

1. Schacter, J., & Stamm, W. E. (1999) Chlamydia in P. R. Murray, E. J. Baron, M. A. Pfaller, F. C. Tenover, & R. H. Yolken (Eds.) *Manual of clinical microbiology* (7th ed., pp. 795–806) Washington DC: American Society for Microbiology.
2. Storz, J. (1971) *Chlamydia* and *Chlamydia*-induced diseases, Springfield, IL: Charles C. Thomas.
3. Fukushi, H., & Hlrai, K. (1992) Proposal of *Chlamydia pecorum* sp. nov. For *Chlamydia* stains derived from ruminants, *Int. J. Syst. Bacteriol., 42*, 306–308.
4. Kuo, C. C., Chen, H. H., Wang, S. P., & Grayston, J. T. (1986) Identification of a new group of *Chlamydia psittaci* strains called TWAR, *J. Clin. Microbiol., 24*, 1034–1037.
5. Saikku, P., Wang, S. P., Kleemola, M., Brander, E., Rusanen, E., & Grayston, J. T. (1985) An epidemic of mild pneumonia due to an unusual strain of *Chlamydia psittaci, J. Infect. Dis., 151*, 161–168.
6. Grayston, J. T., Kuo, C. C., Wang, S. P., & Altman, J. (1986) A novel *Chlamydia psittaci* strain, TWAR, isolated in acute respiratory tract infections, *N. Engl. J. Med., 315*, 161–168.
7. Jackson, M., White, N., Giffard, P., & Timms, P. (1999) Epizootiology of *Chlamydia* infections in two free-range Koala population, *Vet. Microbiol., 65*, 255–264.
8. Berger, L., Volp, K., Mathews, S., Speare, R., & Timms, P. (1999) *Chlamydia pneumoniae* in a free-ranging giant barred frog (*Mixophyes iteratus*) from Australia, *J. Clin. Microbiol., 37*, 2378–2380.
9. Wuppermann, F. N., Hegemann, J. H., & Jantos, C. A. (2001) Heparan sulphate-like glycosaminoglycan is a cellular receptor for *Chlamydia pneumoniae, J. Infect. Dis., 184*, 181–187.
10. Cox, R. L., Kuo, C. C., Grayston, J. T., & Campbell, L. A. (1988) Deoxyribonucleic acid relatedness of *Chlamydia* sp. strain TWAR to *Chlamydia trachomatis* and *Chlamydia psittaci, Int. J. Syst. Bacteriol., 38*, 265–268.
11. Grayston, J. T., Kuo, C. C., Campbell, L. A., & Wang, S. P. (1989) *Chlamydia pneumoniae* sp. nov. for *Chlamydia* sp. strain TWAR, *Int. Syst. Bacterial., 39*, 88–90.
12. Kuo, C. C., Chi, E. Y., & Grayston, J. T. (1988) Ultrastructural study of entry of *Chlamydia* strain TWAR into Hela cells, *Infect. Immun., 56*, 1668–1672.
13. Beatty, W. L., Morrison, R. P., & Byrne, G. I. (1994) Persistent chlamydia: from cell culture to a paradigm for chlamydial pathogenesis, *Microbiol. Rev., 58*, 686–699.

14. Ward, M. E. (1995) The microbiology and immunopathology of chlamydial infections, *APMIS*, *103*, 769–796.
15. Gerard, H. C., Kohler, L., Branigan, P. J., Zeidler, H., Schumacher, H. R., & Hudson, A. P. (1998) Viability and gene expression in *Chlamydia trachomatis* during persistent infection of cultured human monocytes, *Med. Microbiol. Immunol.*, *187*, 115–120.
16. Jendro, M. C., Deutsch, T., Korber, B., Kohler, L., Kuipers, J. G., Krausse-Opatz, B., Westermann, J., Raum, E., & Zeidler, H. (2000) Infection of human monocyte-derived macrophages with *Chlamydia trachomatis* induces apoptosis of T cells: a potential mechanism for persistent infection, *Infect. Immun.*, *68*, 6704–6711.
17. Rajalingum, K., Al-Younes, H., Muller, A., Meyer, T. F., Sczepek, A. J., & Rudel, T. (2001) Epithelial cells infected with *Chlamydophila pneumoniae* (*Chlamydia pneumoniae*) are resistant to apoptosis, *Infect. Immun.*, *69*, 7880–7888.
18. Byrne, G. I., Ouellette, S. P., Wang, Z., Rao, J. P., Lu, L., Beatty, W. L., & Hudson, A. P. (2001) *Chlamydia pneumoniae* expresses genes required for DNA replication but not cytokinesis during persistent infection of Hep-2 cells, *Infect. Immun.*, *69*, 5423–5429.
19. Laitinen, K., Laurila, A. L., Leinonen, M., & Saikku, P. (1996) Reactivation of *Chlamydia pneumoniae* infection in mice by cortisone treatment, *Infect. Immun.*, *64*, 1488–1490.
20. Malinverni, R., Kuo, C. C., Campbell, L. A., & Grayston, J. T. (1995) Reactivation of *Chlamydia pneumoniae* lung infection in mice by cortisone, *J. Infect. Dis.*, *172*, 593–594.
21. Hammerschlag, M. R., Chirgivin, K., Roblin, P. M., Gelling, M., Dumornay, W., Mandel, L., Smith, P., & Schachter, J. (1992) Persistent infection with *Chlamydia pneumoniae* following acute respiratory illness, *Clin. Infect. Dis.*, *14*, 178–182.
22. Nurminen, M., Leinonen, M., Saikku, P., & Makela, P. H. (1983) The genus-specific antigen of *Chlamydiae* resemblance to the lipopolysaccharide of enteric bacteria, *Science*, *220*, 1279–1281.
23. Caldwell, H. D., & Schachter, J. (1982) Antigenic analysis of the major outer membrane protein of *Chlamydia* spp., *Infect. Immun.*, *35*, 1024–1031.
24. Kaltenboeck, B., Kousoulas, K. G., & Storz, J. (1993) Structures of and allelic diversity and relationships among the major outer membrane protein (OMPA) genes of the four Chlamydial species, *J. Bacteriol.*, *175*, 487–502.
25. Perez Melgosa, M., Kuo, C. C., & Campbell, L. A. (1993) Outer membrane complex proteins of *Chlamydia pneumoniae*, *FEMS Microbiol. Lett.*, *112*, 199–204.
26. Newhall, W. J., Batteiger, B., & Jones, R. B. (1982) Analysis of the human serological response to proteins of *Chlamydia trachomatis*, *Infect. Immun.*, *38*, 1181–1189.
27. Morrison, R. P., Belland, R. J., Lyong, K., & Caldwell, H. D. (1989) Chlamydial disease pathogenesis. The 57-kD chlamydial hypersensitivity antigen is a stress response protein, *J. Exp. Med.*, *170*, 1271–1283.
28. Wang, S. P., & Grayston, J. T. (1986) Microimmunoflorescence serological studies with the TWAR organism, in J. D. Oriel, G. Ridgeway, J. Schacter,

D. Taylor-Robinson, & M. Ward (Eds.) *Chlamydial infections* (pp. 329–332), Cambridge, England: Cambridge University Press.

29. Wang, S. P., & Grayston, J. T. (1990) Population prevalence antibody to *Chlamydia pneumoniae* strain TWAR, in W. R. Bowie, H. D. Caldwell, R. P. Jones, P. A. Mardh, G. L. Ridgeway, J. Shachter, W. E. Stamm, & M. E. Ward (Eds.) *Chlamydial infections* (pp. 402–405), Cambridge, England: Cambridge University Press.

30. Kanamoto, Y., Ouchi, K., Mizui, M., Ushio, M., & Usui, T. (1991) Prevalence of antibody to *Chlamydia pneumoniae* TWAR in Japan, *J. Clin. Microbiol.*, *29*, 816–818.

32. Morton, A., Károlyi, A., & Szalka, A. (1992) Prevalence of *Chlamydia pneumoniae* antibodies in Hungary, *Eur. J. Clin. Microbiol. Infect. Dis.*, *11*, 139–142.

32. Montes, M., Cilia, G., Alcorta, M., & Perez-Trallero, E. (1992) High prevalence of *Chlamydia pneumoniae* infection in children and young adults in Spain, *Pediatr. Infect. Dis. J.*, *11*, 972–973.

33. Karvonen, M., Tuomilethto, J., Naukkarinen, A., & Saikku, P. (1992) The prevalence and regional distribution of antibodies against *Chlamydia psittaci* and *Chlamydia pneumoniae* (strain TWAR) in Finland in 1958, *Int. J. Epidemiol*, *21*, 391–398.

34. Einasson, S., Sigurdsson, H. K., Maynusdottir, S. D., Erlendsdottir, H., Briem, H., & Gudmundsson, S. (1994) Age specific prevalence of antibodies against *Chlamydia pneumoniae* in Iceland, *Scand. J. Infect. Dis.*, *26*, 393–397.

35. Paltiel, O., Kark, J. D., Leinonen, M., & Saikku, P. (1995) High prevalence of antibodies to *Chlamydia pneumoniae*: determinants of IgG and IgA seropositivity among Jerusalem residents, *Epidemiol. Infect.*, *114*, 465–473.

36. Ni, A. P., Lin, G. Y., Yang, L., He, H. Y., Huang, C. W., Liu, Z. J., Wang, R. S., Zhang, J. S., Yu, J. Y., Li, N., Wang, J. B., & Yang, H. Y. (1996) A seroepidemiological study of *Chlamydia pneumoniae, Chlamydia trachomatis*, and *Chlamydia psittaci* in different populations on the mainland of China, *Scand. J. Infect. Dis.*, *28*, 553–557.

37. Grayston, J. T., Mordhorst, C. H., Bruu, A. L., Vene, S., & Wang, S. P. (1989) Countrywide epidemics of *Chlamydia pneumoniae*, strain TWAR, in Scandinavia, 1981–1983, *J. Infect. Dis.*, *159*, 1111–1114.

38. Grayston, J. T. (1992) Infections caused by *Chlamydia pneumoniae* strain TWAR, *Clin. Infect. Dis.*, *15*, 757–763.

39. Patnode, D., Wang, S. P., & Grayston, J. T. (1990) Persistence of *Chlamydia pneumoniae*, strain TWAR microimmunofluorescent antibody, in W. R. Bowie, H. D. Caldwell, R. P. Jones, P. A. Mardh, G. L. Ridgeway, J. Schachter, W. E. Stamm, & M. E. Ward (Eds.) *Chlamydial infections* (pp. 406–409), Cambridge, England: Cambridge University Press.

40. Machi, T., Kazuyama, Y., Kumabashi, I., Matsumoto, Y., & Horita, Y. (1998) Prolonged respiratory failure in *Chlamydia pneumoniae* pneumonia, *Scand. J. Infect. Dis.*, *30*, 620–621.

41. Troy, C. J., Peeling, R. W., Ellis, A. G., Hockin, J. C., Bennett, D. A., Murphy, M. R., & Spika, J. S. (1997) *Chlamydia pneumoniae* as a new source of infectious outbreaks in nursing homes, *JAMA*, *277*, 1214–1218.

42. Hahn, D. L., Dodge, R. W., & Golubjatnikov, R. (1991) Association of *Chlamydia pneumoniae* (strain TWAR) infection with wheezing, asthmatic bronchitis, and adult onset asthma, *JAMA, 266*, 225–230.

43. Emre, U., Roblin, P. M., Gelling, M., Dumornay, W., Rao, M., Hammerschlag, M. R., & Schachter, J. (1994) The association of *Chlamydia pneumoniae* infection and reactive airway disease in children, *Arch. Pediatr. Adolesc. Med., 148*, 727–732.

44. Dowell, S. F., Peeling, R. W., Boman J., Carlone, G. M., Fields, B. S., Guaner, J., Hammerschlag, M. R., Jackson, L. A., Kuo, C. C., Maas, M., Messmer, T. O., Talkington, D. F., Tondella, M. L., Zaki, S. R., & the *C. pneumoniae* workshop participants (2001) Standardizing *Chlamydia pneumoniae* assays: recommendations from the Centers for Disease Control and Prevention (USA) and the Laboratory Centre for Disease Control (Canada), *Clin. Infect. Dis., 33*, 492–502.

45. Peeling, R. W., Wang, S. P., Grayston, J. T., Blasi, F., Boman, J., Clad, A., Freidank, H., Gaydos, C. A., Gnarpe, J., Hagiwara, T., Jones, R. B., Orfila, J., Persson, K., Poukkainen, M., Saikku, P., & Schachter, J. (2000) *Chlamydia pneumoniae* serology: interlaboratory variation in microimmunoflorescence assay results, *J. Infect. Dis., 181*(Suppl. 3), S426–S429.

46. Tong, C., & Sillis, M. (1993) Detection of *Chlamydia pneumoniae* and *Chlamydia psittaci* in sputum samples by PCR, *J. Clin. Pathol., 46*, 313–317.

47. Bowman, J., Allard, A., Persson, K., Lundborg, M., Juts, P., & Waddell, G. (1997) Rapid diagnosis of respiratory *Chlamydia pneumoniae* infection by nested touch down polymerase chain reaction compared with culture and antigen detection by EIA, *J. Infect. Dis., 175*, 1523–1526.

48. Gaydos, C. A., Roblin, P. M., Hammeschlag, M. R., Hyman, C. L., Eiden, J. J., Schacter, J., & Quinn, T. L. (1994) Diagnostic utility of PCR, enzyme immunoassay, culture and serology for detection of *Chlamydia pneumoniae* in symptomatic and asymptomatic patients, *J. Clin. Microbiol., 32*, 903–905.

49. Naidu, B. R., Ngeow, Y. F., Kannan, P., Jeyamalar, R., Khir, A., Khoo, K. L., & Pang, T. (1997) Evidence of *Chlamydia pneumoniae* infection obtained by the polymerase chain reaction (PCR) in patients with acute myocardial infection and coronary heart disease, *J. Infect., 35*, 199–200.

50. Bowman, J., Södenberg, S., Forsberg, J., Birgander, L. S., Allard, A., Persson, K., Jidell, E., Kumlin, U., Juto, P., Waldenström, A., & Wadell, G. (1998) High prevalence of *Chlamydia pneumoniae* DNA in peripheral blood mononuclear cells in patients with cardiovascular disease and in middle-aged blood donors, *J. Infect. Dis., 178*, 247–277.

51. Wong, Y. K., Dawkins, K. D., & Ward, M. E. (1999) Circulating *Chlamydia pneumoniae* DNA as a predictor of coronary artery disease, *J. Am. Coll. Cardiol., 34*, 1440–1443.

52. Kaul, R., Uphoff, J., Wiederman, J., Yadlapalli, S., & Wenman, W. M. (2000) Detection of *Chlamydia pneumoniae* DNA and CD3+ lymphocytes from healthy blood donors and patients with coronary artery disease, *Circulation, 102*, 2341–2346.

53. Kuo, C. C., Shor, A., Campbell, L. A., Fukushi, H., Panton, D. L., & Grayston, J. T. (1993) Demonstration of *Chlamydia pneumoniae* in atherosclerotic lesions of coronary arteries, *J. Infect. Dis, 167*, 841–849.

54. Grayston, J. T., Kuo, C. C., Coulson, A. S., Campbell, L. A., Lawrence, R. D., Lee, M. J., Strandness, E. D., & Wang, S. P. (1995) *Chlamydia pneumoniae* (TWAR) in atherosclerosis of the carotid artery, *Circulation, 92*, 3397–3400.

55. Ong, G., Thomas, B. J., Mansfield, A. O., Davidson, B. R., & Taylor-Robinson, D. (1996) Detection and widespread distribution of *Chlamydia pneumoniae* in the vascular system and possible implications, *J. Clin. Pathol., 49*, 102–106.

56. Apfalter, P., Blasi, F., Boman, J., Gaydos, C. A., Kundi, M., Maass, M., Makristathis, A., Meijer, A., Nadrchal, R., Persson, K., Rotter, M. L., Tong, C. Y., Stanek, G., & Hirschl, A. M. (2001) Multicenter comparison trial of DNA extraction methods and PCR assays for detection of *Chlamydia pneumoniae* in endarterectomy specimens, *J. Clin. Microbiol., 39*, 519–524.

57. Neito, F. J. (1998) Infection and atherosclerosis: new clues from an old hypothesis, *Am. J. Epidemiol., 148*, 937–947.

58. Saikku, P., Leinonen, M., Maitlla, K., Ekman, M. R., Neiminen, M. S., Makela, P. H., Huttunen, J. K., & Valtonen, V. (1988) Serological evidence of an association of a novel *Chlamydia* TWAR, with chronic coronary heart disease and acute myocardial infarction, *Lancet, 2*, 983–986.

59. Danesh, J., Collins, R., & Peto, R. (1997) Chronic infection and coronary heart disease: is there a link? *Lancet, 350*, 430–436.

60. Leinonen, M., Linnamaki, E., Matilla, K., Nieminen, M. S., Valtonen, V., Leirsalo-Repo, M., & Saikku, P. (1990) Circulating immune complexes containing Chlamydial lipopolysaccharide in acute myocardial infarction, *Microb. Pathog., 9*, 67–73.

61. Thom, D. H., Wang, S. P., Grayston, J. T., Siscovick, D. S., Stewart, D. K., Kronmal, R. A., & Weiss, N. S. (1991) *Chlamydia pneumoniae* strain TWAR antibody and angiographically demonstrated coronary artery disease, *Arterioscl. Thromb., 11*, 547–551.

62. Thom, D. H., Grayston, J. T., Siscovik, D. S., Wang, S. P., Weiss, N. S., & Daling, J. R. (1992) Association of prior infection with *Chlamydia pneumoniae* and angiographically demonstrated coronary artery disease, *JAMA, 268*, 68–72.

63. Linnamaki, E., Leinonen, M., Matilla, K., Nieminen, M. S., Valtonen, V., & Saikku, P. (1993) *Chlamydia pneumoniae* specific circulating immune complexes in patients with chronic coronary heart disease, *Circulation, 87*, 1130–1134.

64. Dahlen, G. H., Boman, J., Birgander, L. S., & Lindblom, B. (1995) Lp (a) lipoprotien, IgG, IgA, and IgM antibodies to *Chlamydia pneumoniae* and ItLA class II genotype in early coronary artery disease, *Atherosclerosis, 114*, 165–174.

65. Mendall, M. A., Carrington, D., Strachan, D., Patel, P., Molineaux, N., Levi, J., Toosey, T., Camm, A. J., & Northfield T. C. (1995) *Chlamydia pneumoniae*: risk factors for seropositivity and association with coronary heart disease, *J. Infect., 30*, 121–128.

66. Patel, P., Mendall, M. A., Carrington, D., Strachan, D. P., Leutham, E., Molineaux, N., Levy, J., Blakeston, C., Seymour, C. A., & Camm, A. J. (1995) Association of *Helicobacter pylori* and *Chlamydia pneumoniae* infections with coronary heart disease and cardiovascular risk factors, *BMJ, 311*, 711–714 [Erratum] 1995, *311*, 985.

67. Thomas, G. N., Scheel, D., Koehler, A. P., Bassett, D. C., & Cheng, A. F. (1997) Respiratory chlamydial infections in a Hong Kong teaching hospital and associations with coronary heart disease, *Scand. J. Infect. Dis. Suppl., 104*, 30–33.

68. Blasi, F., Cosentini, R., Raccanelli, R., Massori, F. M., Arosio, C., Tarsia, P., & Allegra, L. (1997) A possible association of *Chlamydia pneumoniae* infection and acute myocardial infarction in patients younger than 65 years of age, *Chest, 112*, 309–312.

69. Kark, J. D., Leinonen, M., Paltiel, O., & Saikku, P. (1997) *Chlamydia pneumoniae* and acute myocardial infarction in Jerusalem, *Int. J. Epidemiol., 26*, 730–738.

70. Mazzoli, S., Tofani, N., Fantini, A., Senplici, F., Bandini, F., Salvi, A., & Vergassola, R. (1998) *Chlamydia pneumoniae* antibody response in patients with acute myocardial infarction and their follow up, *Am. Heart J., 135*, 15–20.

71. Anderson, J. L., Carlquist, J. F., Muhlestein, J. B., Horne, B. D., & Elmer, S. P. (1998) Evaluation of C-reactive protein, an inflammatory marker, and infectious serology as risk factors for coronary artery disease and myocardial infarction, *J. Am. Coll. Cardiol., 32*, 35–41.

72. Gabriel, A. S., Gnarpe, H., Gnarpe, J., Hallander, H., Nyquist, O., & Martinsson, A. (1998) The prevalence of chronic *Chlamydia pneumoniae* infection as detected by polymerase chain reaction in pharyngeal samples from patients with ischaemic heart disease, *Eur. Heart J., 19*, 1321–1327.

73. Miyashita, N., Toyota, E., Sawayama, T., Matsumoto, A., Mikami, Y., Kawai, N., Takada, K., Niki, Y., & Matsushima, T. (1998) Association of chronic infection of *Chlamydia pneumoniae* and coronary heart disease in the Japanese, *Inter. Med., 37*, 913–916.

74. Altman, R., Rouvier, J., Scazziota, A., Absi, R. S., & Gonzalez, C. (1999) Lack of association between prior infection with *Chlamydia pneumoniae* and acute or chronic coronary artery disease, *Clin. Cardiol., 22*, 85–90.

75. Danesh, J., Wong, Y., Ward, M., & Muir, J. (1999) Chronic infection with *Helicobacter pylori, Chlamydia pneumoniae*, or cytomegalovirus: population based study of coronary heart disease, *Heart, 81*, 245–247.

76. Sessa, R., Di Pietro, M., Santino, I., del Piano, M., Varveri, A., Dagianti, A., & Penc, M. (1999) *Chlamydia pneumoniae* infection and atherosclerotic coronary disease, *Am. Heart J., 137*, 1116–1119.

77. Cellesi, C., Sansoni, A., Casini, S., Migliorini, L., Zacchini, F., Gasparini, R., Montomoli, E., Bonacci, A., & Bravi, A. (1999) *Chlamydia pneumoniae* antibodies and angiographically demonstrated coronary artery disease in a sample population from Italy, *Atherosclerosis, 145*, 81–85.

78. Leowattana, W., Mahanonda, N., Bhuripumyo, K., Leelarasamee, A., Pokum, S., & Suwimol, B. (1999) The prevalence of *Chlamydia pneumoniae* antibodies in Thai patients with coronary artery disease, *J. Med. Assoc. Thai., 82*, 792–797.

79. Nobel, M., De Torrente, A., Peter, O., & Genne, D. (1999) No serological evidence of association between *Chlamydia pneumoniae* infection and acute coronary heart disease, *Scand. J. Infect. Dis., 31*, 261–264.

80. Kaykov, E., Abbou, B., Friedstrom, S., Hermoni, D., & Roguin, N. (1999) *Chlamydia pneumoniae* in ischaemic heart disease, *Israel Med. Assoc. J.*, *1*, 225–227.

81. Hoffmeister, A., Rothenbacher, D., Wanner, P., Bode, G., Persson, K., Brenner, H., Hombach, V., & Koenig, W. (2000) Seropositivity to chlamydial lipopolysaccharide and *Chlamydia pneumoniae*, systemic inflammation and stable coronary artery disease: negative results of a case-control study, *J. Am. Coll. Cardiol.*, *35*, 112–118.

82. Jantos, C. A., Knombach, C., Wuppermann, F. N., Gardemann, A., Bepler, S., Asslan, H., Hegemann, J. H., & Haberbosch, W. (2000) Antibody response to the 60-kDa heat-shock protein of *Chlamydia pneumoniae* in patients with coronary artery disease, *J. Infect. Dis.*, *181*, 1700–1705.

83. Song, Y. G., Kwon, H. M., Kim, J. M., Hong, B. K., Kim, D. S., Huh, A. J., Chang, K. H., Kim, H. Y., Kang, T. S., Lee, B. K., Choi, D. H., Jang, Y. S., & Kim, H. S. (2000) Serologic and histopathologic study of *Chlamydia pneumoniae* infection in atherosclerosis: a possible pathogenetic mechanism of atherosclerosis induced by *Chlamydia pneumoniae*, *Yonsei Med. J.*, *41*, 319–327.

84. Zhu, J., Quyyumi, A. A., Norman, J. E., Csako, G., Waclawiw, M. A., Shearer, G. M., & Epstein, S. E. (2000) Effects of total pathogen burden on coronary artery disease risk and C-reactive protein levels, *Am. J. Cardiol.*, *85*, 140–146.

85. Di Tano, G., Picerno, I., Calisto, M. L., Delia, S. A., Lagana, P., & Spataro, P. (2000) *Chlamydia pneumoniae* and *Helicobacter pylori* infections in acute myocardial infarction, *Italian Heart J.*, *1*(Suppl. 12), 1576–1581.

86. Kosaka, C., Hora, K., Komiyama, Y., & Takahashi, H. (2000) Possible role of chronic infection with *Chlamydia pneumoniae* in Japanese patients with acute myocardial infarction, *Jpn. Circ. J.*, *64*, 819–824.

87. Romeo, F., Martuscelli, E., Chiireolo, G., Cerabino, L. M., Ericson, K., Saldeen, T. G., & Mehta, J. L. (2000) Seropositivity against *Chlamydia pneumoniae* in patients with coronary atherosclerosis, *Clin. Cardiol.*, *23*, 327–330.

88. Kaftan, A. H., & Kaftan, O. (2000) Coronary heart disease and infection with *Chlamydia pneumoniae*, *Jpn. Heart J.*, *41*, 165–172.

89. Ashkenazi, H., Rudensky, B., Paz, E., Raveh, D., Balkin, J. A., Tzivoni, D., & Yinnon, A. M. (2001) Incidence of immunoglobulin G antibodies to *Chlamydia pneumoniae* in acute myocardial infarction patients, *Israel Med. Assoc. J.*, *3*, 818–821.

90. Stollberger, C., Molzer, G., Finsterer, J. (2001) Seroprevalence of antibodies to microorganisms known to cause arterial and myocardial damage in patients with or without coronary stenosis, *Clin. Diag. Lab. Immunol.*, *8*, 997–1002.

91. Tsai, C. T., Kao, J. H., Hsu, K. L., Chiang, F. T., Tseng, C. D., Liau, C. S., Tseng, Y. Z., & Hwang, J. J. (2001) Relation of *Chlamydia pneumoniae* infection in Taiwan to angiographically demonstrated coronary artery disease and to the presence of acute myocardial infarction or unstable angina pectoris, *Am. J. Cardiol.*, *88*, 960–963.

92. Maass, M., & Gieffers, J. (1997) Cardiovascular risk from prior *Chlamydia pneumoniae* infection can be related to certain antigens recognized in the immunoblot profile, *J. Infect.*, *35*, 171–176.

93. Mendis, S., Arseculeratne, Y. M., Withana, N., & Samitha, S. (2001) *Chlamydia pneumoniae* infection and its association with coronary heart diseases and cardiovascular risk factors in a sample South Asian population, *Int. J. Cardiol.*, *79*, 191–196.

94. Momiyama, Y., Hirano, R., Taniguchi, H., Nakamura, H., & Ohsuzn, F. (2001) Effects of interleukin-1 gene polymorphism on the development of coronary artery disease associated with *Chlamydia pneumoniae* infection, *J. Am. Coll. Cardiol.*, *38*, 712–717.

95. Chandra, H. R., Choudhary, N., O'Neill, C., Boura, J., Timmis, G. C., & O'Neill, W. W. (2001) *Chlamydia pneumoniae* exposure and inflammatory markers in acute coronary syndrome, *Am. J. Cardiol.*, *88*, 214–218.

96. Shimada, K., Daida, H., Mokuno, H., Watanabe, Y. Sawano, M., Iwama, Y., Seki, E., Kurata, T., Sato, H., Ohashi, S., Susuki, H., Miyauchi, K., Takaya, J., Sakurai, H., & Yamaguchin, H. (2001) Association of seropositivity for antibody to *Chlamydia*-specific lipopolysaccharide and coronary artery disease in Japanese men, *Jpn. Circ. J.*, *65*, 182–187.

97. Halme, S., Syrjala, H., Bloigu, A., Saikku, P., Leinonen, M., Airaksinen, J., & Surcel, H. M. Lymphocyte responses to *Chlamydia* antigens in patients with coronary heart disease, *Eur. Heart J.*, *18*, 1095–1101.

98. Fang, J. C., Kinlay, S., Kundsin, R., & Ganz, P. (1998) *Chlamydia pneumoniae* is frequent but not associated with coronary arteriosclerosis in cardiac transplant recipients, *Am. J. Cardiol.*, *82*, 1479–1483.

99. al-Amro, A. A., al-Jafari, A. A., al-Fagih, M. R., Tajeldin, M., & Qavi, H. B. (2001) Frequency of occurrence of cytomegalovirus and *Chlamydia pneumoniae* in lymphocytes of atherosclerotic patients, *Central Eur. J. Public Health*, *9*, 106–108.

100. Burian, K., Kis, Z., Virok, D., Endresz, V., Prohaszka, Z., Duba, J., Berencsi, K., Boda, K., Horvath, L., Romics, C., Fust, G., & Gonczol, E. (2001) Independent and joint effects of antibodies to human heat-shock protein 60 and *Chlamydia pneumoniae* infection in the development of coronary atherosclerosis, *Circulation*, *103*, 1503–1508.

101. Gattone, M., Iacoviello, L., Colombo, M., Castelnuovo, A. D., Soffiantino, F., Gramoni, A., Piuo, D., Benedetta, M., & Giannuzzi, P. (2001) *Chlamydia pneumoniae* and cytomegalovirus seropositivity inflammatory markers, and the risk of myocardial infarction at a young age, *Am. Heart J.*, *142*, 633–640.

102. Pieniazek, P., Karczewska, E., Stepien, E., Tracz, W., & Konturek, S. J. (2001) Incidence of *Chlamydia pneumoniae* infection in patients with coronary artery disease subjected to angioplasty or bypass surgery, *Med. Sci. Monitor*, *7*, 995–1001.

103. Smeija, M., Chong, S., Natarajam, M., Petrich, A., Rainen, L., & Mahony, J. B. (2001) Circulating nucleic acids of *Chlamydia pneumoniae* and cytomegalovirus in patients undergoing coronary angiography, *J. Clin. Microbiol.*, *39*, 596–600.

104. Melnick, S. L., Shahar, E., Folsom, A. R., Grayston, J. T., Sorlie, P. D., Wang, S. P., & Szklo, M. (1993) Past infection by *Chlamydia pneumoniae* strain TWAR and asymptomatic carotid atherosclerosis. Atherosclerosis risk in communities (ARIC) study investigators, *Am. J. Med.*, *95*, 499–504.

105. Wimmer, M. L., Sandmann-Strupp, R., Saikku, P., & Haberl, R. L. (1996) Association of chlamydial infection with cerebrovascular disease, *Stroke, 27,* 2207–2210.

106. Lindberg, G., Rastam, L., Lundblad, A., Sorlie, P. D., & Folsom, A. R. (1997) The association between serum sialic acid and asymptomatic carotid atherosclerosis is not related to antibodies to herpes type viruses or *Chlamydia pneumoniae.* The atherosclerosis risk in communities (ARIC) study investigators, *Int. J. Epidemiol., 26,* 1386–1391.

107. Elkind, M. S., Lin, I. F., Grayston, J. T., & Sacco, R. L. (2000) *Chlamydia pneumoniae* and the risk of first ischaemic stroke: the northern Manhattan stroke study, *Stroke, 31,* 1521–1525.

108. Heuschmann, P. U., Neureiter, D., Guesslein, M., Craiovan, B., Maass, M., Faller, G., Beck, G., Neundoefer, B., & Kolominsky-Rabas, P. L. (2001) Association between infection with *Helicobacter pylori* and *Chlamydia pneumoniae* and risk of ischaemic stroke subtypes: results from a population based case control study, *Stroke, 32,* 2253–2258.

109. Linares-Palomino, J., Gutierrez, J., Lopez-Espada, C., Ros, E., Moreno, J., Perez, T., Rodriquez, M., & Maroto, M. C. (2001) *Chlamydia pneumoniae* and cerebrovascular disease, *Revita de neurologia, 32,* 201–206.

110. Coles, K. A., Plant, A. J., Riley, T. V., Smith, D. W., McQuillan, B. M., & Thompson, P. L. (1999) Lack of association between seropositivity to *Chlamydia pneumoniae* and carotid atherosclerosis, *Am. J. Cardiol., 84,* 825–828.

111. Markus, H. S., Sitzer, M., Carrington, D., Mendall, M. A., & Steinmetz, H. (1999) *Chlamydia pneumoniae* infection and early asymptomatic carotid atherosclerosis, *Circulation, 100,* 832–837.

112. Espinola-Klein, C., Rupprecht, H. J., Blankenberg, S., Bickel, C., Kopp, H., Rippen, G., Hafner, G., Pfeifer, U., & Meyer, J. (2000) Are morphological or functional changes in the carotid artery wall associated with *Chlamydia pneumoniae, Helicobacter pylori,* cytomegalovirus, or herpes simplex virus infection? *Stroke, 31,* 2127–2133.

113. Cook, P. J., Honeybourne, D., Lip, G. Y., Beevers, D. G., Wise, R., & Davies, P. (1998) *Chlamydia pneumoniae* antibody titers are significantly associated with acute stroke and transient cerebral ischaemic: the West Birmingham stroke project, *Stroke, 29,* 404–410.

114. Blanchard, J. F., Armerian, H. K., Peeling, R., Friesen, P. P., Shen, C., & Brunham, R. C. (2000) The relation between *Chlamydia pneumoniae* infection and abdominal aortic aneurysm: case-control study, *Clin. Infect. Dis., 30,* 946–947.

115. Maratha, B., den Heijer, M., Wullink, M., van der Zee, A., Bergmans, A., Verbakel, H., Kerver, M., Graafsma, S., Kranendonk, S., & Peeters, M. (2001) Detection of *Chlamydia pneumoniae* DNA in buffy-coat samples of patients with abdominal aortic aneurysm, *Eur. J. Clin. Microbiol. Infect. Dis., 20,* 111–116.

116. Lehto, S., Niskanen, L., Suhonen, M., Ronnemaa, T., Saikku, P., & Laakso, M. (2002) Association between *Chlamydia pneumoniae* antibodies and intimal

calcification in femoral arteries of nondiabetic patients, *Arch. Intern. Med.*, *162*, 594–599.

117. Sessa, R., Di Pietro, M., Schiavoni, G., Santini, I., Cipriani, P., Romano, S., Penco, M., & del Piano, M. (2001) Prevalence of *Chlamydia pneumoniae* in peripheral blood mononuclear cells in Italian patients with acute ischaemic heart disease, *Atherosclerosis*, *159*, 521–525.

118. Saikku, P., Leinonen, M., Tenkanen, L., Linnanmaki, E., Ekman, M. R., Manninen, V., Mänttäri, M., Trick, M. H., & Huttunen, J. K. (1992) Chronic *Chlamydia pneumoniae* infection as a risk factor for coronary heart disease in Helsinki Heart study, *Ann. Intern. Med.*, *116*, 273–278.

119. Meittinen, H., Lehto, S., Saikku, P., Haffner, S. M., Ronnemaa, T., Pyorala, K., & Laakso, M. (1996) Association of *Chlamydia pneumoniae* and acute coronary heart disease events in non-insulin dependent diabetic and non-diabetic subjects in Finland, *Eur. Heart J.*, *17*, 682–688.

120. Ossewaarde, J. M., Feskens, E. J., De Vries, A., Vallinga, C. E., & Kromhout, D. (1998) *Chlamydia pneumoniae* is a risk factor for coronary heart disease in symptom-free elderly men, but *Helicobacter pylori* and cytomegalovirus was not, *Epidemiol. Infect.*, *120*, 93–99.

121. von Hertzen, L., Isoaho, R., Kivalä, S. L., & Saikku, P. (1999) Relation of Finnish study finds significant association between raised IgG, but not IgA, titers and mortality, *BMJ*, *319*, 1575–1577.

122. Tavendale, R., Parratt, D., A'Brook, R., & Tunstall-Pedoe, H. (1999) Antibodies to *Chlamydia pneumoniae* do not predict subsequent coronary heart disease in the Scottish Heart Health and MONICA studies, *Eur. Heart J.*, *20*(Abstract Suppl.), 425.

123. Haider, A. W., Wilson, P. W. F., Larson, M. G., Sutherland, P., Evans, J. C., O'Donnell, C. J., Wolf, P. A., Michelson, E. L., Levy, D., Astra, P., Wayne, P. A., & Framingham Heart Study (1999) *Chlamydia*; *H. pylori*, and cytomegalovirus seropositivity and risk of cardiovascular disease: the Framingham heart study, *J. Am. Coll. Cardiol.*, *33(Suppl. A), 314A [Abstract 892–6]*.

124. Strachan, D. P., Corrington, D., Mendall, M. A., Ballam, L., Morris, J., Butlard, B. K., Sweetnan, P. M., & Elwood, P. C. (1999) Relation of *Chlamydia pneumoniae* serology to mortality and incidence of ischaemic heart disease over 13 years in the Caerphilly prospective heart disease study, *BMJ*, *318*, 1035–1039.

125. Ridker, P. M., Kundsin, R. B., Stampfer, M. J., Poulin, S., & Hennekens, C. H. (1999a) Prospective study of *C. pneumoniae* IgG seropositivity and risks of future myocardial infarction, *Circulation*, *99*, 1161–1164.

126. Ridker, P. M., Hennekens, C. H., Buring, J. E., Kundsin, R., & Shih, J. (1999b) Baseline IgG antibody titers to *Chlamydia pneumoniae, Helicobacter pylori*, herpes simplex virus, and cytomegalovirus and the risk for cardiovascular disease in women, *Ann. Intern. Med.*, *131*, 573–577.

127. Neito, F. J., Folsom, A. R., Sorlie, P. D., Grayston, J. T., Wang, S. P., & Chambless, L. E. (1999) *Chlamydia pneumoniae* infection and incident coronary heart disease: the atherosclerotic risk in communities study, *Am. J. Epidemiol.*, *150*, 149–156.

128. Fagerberg, B., Gnarpe, J., Gnarpe, H., Agewall, S., & Wikstrand, J. (1999) *Chlamydia pneumoniae* but not cytomegalovirus antibodies are associated with future risk of stroke and cardiovascular disease: a prospective study in middle-aged to elderly men with treated hypertension, *Stroke, 30*, 299–305.

129. Danesh, J., Whincup, P., Walker, M., Lennon, L., Thompson, A., Appleby, P., Wong, Y., Bernardes-Silva, M., & Ward, M. (2000) *Chlamydia pneumoniae* IgG titers and coronary heart disease: prospective study and meta-analysis, *BMJ, 321*, 208–213.

130. Wald, N. J., Law, M. R., Morris, J. K., Zhou, X., Wong, Y., & Ward, M. E. (2000) *Chlamydia pneumoniae* infection and morality from ischemic heart disease: large prospective study, *BMJ, 321*, 204–207.

131. Siscovick, D., Schwartz, S. M., Corey, L., Grayston, T., Ashley, R., Wang, S. P., Pasty, B. M., Tracy, R. P., Kuller, L. H., & Kronmal, R. A. (2000) *Chlamydia pneumoniae*, herpes simplex virus Type I, and cytomegalovirus and incident myocardial infarction and coronary heart disease death in older adults, *Circulation, 102*, 2335–2340.

132. Zhu, J., Nieto, F. J., Horne, B. D., Anderson, J. L., Muhlestein, J. B., & Epstein, S. E. (2001) Prospective study of pathogen burden and risk of myocardial infarction or death, *Circulation, 103*, 45–51.

133. Rupprecht, H. J., Blankenberg, S., Bickel, C., Rippin, G., Hafner, G., Prellwitz, W., Schulumberger, W., & Meyer, J., for the Athero-gene Investigators (2001) Impact of viral and bacterial infectious burden on long-time prognosis in patients with coronary artery disease, *Circulation, 104*, 25–31.

134. Roivainen, M., Viik-Kajander, M., Palosuo, T., Toivanen, P., Leinonen, M., Saikku, P., Tenkanen, L., Manninen, V., Hovi, T., & Mantari, M. (2001) Infections, inflammations, and the risk of coronary heart disease, *Circulation, 101*, 252–257.

135. Glader, C. A., Boman, J., Saikku, P., Stenlund, H., Weinehall, L., Hallmanns, G., & Dahken, G. H. (2000) The proatherogenic properties of lipoprotein (a) may be enhanced through the formation of circulating immune complexes containing *Chlamydia pneumoniae*-specific IgG antibodies, *Eur. Heart J., 21*, 639–646.

136. Haubitz, M., & Brunkhorst, R. (2001) C-reactive protein and chronic *Chlamydia pneumoniae* infection—long-term predictors for cardiovascular disease and survival in patients on peritoneal dialysis, *Nephrol. Dial. Transplant., 16*, 809–815.

137. Gupta, S., Leatham, E. W., Corrington, D., Mendall, M. A., Kaski, J. C., & Camm, A. J. (1997) Elevated *Chlamydia pneumoniae* antibodies, cardiovascular events, and azithromycin in mate survivors of myocardial infarction, *Circulation, 96*, 404–407.

138. Choussat, R., Montalescot, G., Collet, J. P., Jardel, C., Ankri, A., Fillet, A. M., Thomas, D., Raymond, J., Bastard, J. P., Drobinski, G., Orfila, J., Agut, H., & Thomas, D. (2000) Effect of prior expense to *Chlamydia pneumoniae, Helicobacter pylori*, or cytomegalovirus on the degree of inflammation and one-year prognosis of patients with unstable, angina pectoris or non-Q wave acute myocardial infarction, *Am. J. Cardiol., 86*, 379–384.

139. de Maat, M. P. M., Ossewaarde, J. M., Verheggen, P. W. H. M., Kluft, C., Cats, V. M., & Haverkate, F. (2000) Antibodies to *Chlamydia pneumoniae* and

clinical course in patients with unstable angina pectoris, *Atherosclerosis, 153*, 499–504.

140. Kähler, J., Gerth, S., Schäfer, P., Boersma, E., Koster, R., Terres, W., Simons, M. L., Berger, J., Mienertz, T., & Hamm, C. W. (2001) Antibodies to chlamydial lipopolysaccharides in unstable angina pectoris, *Am. J. Cardiol., 87*, 1150–1153.

141. Mayr, M., Kiechl, S., Willeit, J., Wick, G., & Xu, Q. (2000) Infections, immunity and atherosclerosis: associations of antibodies to *Chlamydia pneumoniae, Helicobacter pylori*, and cytomegalovirus with immune reactions to heat-shock protein 60 and carotid or femeral atherosclerosis, *Circulation, 102*, 833–839.

142. Kiechl, S., Egger, G., Mayr, M., Wiedermann, C. J., Bonora, E., Oberhollenzer, F., Muggeo, M., Xu, Q., Wick, G., Poewe, W., & Willeit, J. (2001) Chronic infections and the risk of carotid atherosclerosis: prospective results from a large population study, *Circulation, 103*, 1064–1070.

143. Sander, D., Winbeck, K., Klingelhofer, J., Etgen, T., & Conrad B. (2001) Enhanced progression of early carotid atherosclerosis is related to *Chlamydia pneumoniae* (Taiwan acute respiratory) seropositivity, *Circulation, 103*, 1390–1395.

144. Mattila, K. J., Juvonen, J. T., Kotamäki, M. T., & Saikku, P. A. (2001) *Chlamydia pneumoniae* and luminal narrowing after coronary angioplasty, *J. Intern. Med., 250*, 67–71.

145. Lindholt, J. S., Ashton, H. A., & Scott, A. P. (2001) Indications of infection with *Chlamydia pneumoniae* are associated with expansion of abdominal aortic aneurysm, *J. Vasc. Surg., 34*, 212–215.

146. Schumacher, A., Lerkerof, A. B., Seljeflot, I., Sommervoll, L., Holme, I., Otterstad, J. E., & Arresen, H. (2001) *Chlamydia pneumoniae* serology: importance of methodology in patients with coronary heart disease and healthy individuals, *J. Clin. Microbiol., 39*, 1859–1864.

147. West, R. (2000) Commentary: adjustment for potential confounders may have been taken too far, *BMJ, 321*, 213.

148. Kuo, C. C., & Campbell, L .A. (2000) Detection of *Chlamydia pneumoniae* in arterial tissues. *J. Infect. Dis., 181*(Suppl. 3), S432–S436.

149. Chiu, B., Viira, E., Tucker, W., & Fong, I. W. (1997) *Chlamydia pneumoniae*, cytomegalovirus and herpes simplex virus in atherosclerosis of the carotid artery, *Circulation, 96*, 2144–2148.

150. Maass, M., Gieffers, J., Krause, E., Engel, P. M., Bartels, C., & Solback, W. (1998) Poor correlation between microimmunofluorescence serology and polymerase chain reaction for detection of vascular *Chlamydia pneumoniae* infection in coronary artery disease patients, *Med. Microbiol. Immunol., 187*, 103–106.

151. Kuo, C. C., Gown, A. M., Benditt, E. P., & Grayston, J. T. (1993) Detection of *Chlamydia pneumoniae* in aortic lesions of atherosclerosis by immunocytochemical stain, *Arterioscler. Thromb., 13*, 1501–1504.

152. Yamashita, K., Ouchi, K., Shiirai, M., Gondo, T., Nakazawa, T., & Ito, H. (1998) Distribution of *Chlamydia pneumoniae* infection in the atherosclerotic carotid artery, *Stroke, 29*, 773–778.

153. Vink, A., Poppen, M., Schoneveld, A. H., Roholl, P. J. M., de Kleijn, D. V. P., Borst, C., & Pasterkamp, G. (2001) Distribution of *Chlamydia pneumoniae* in

the human arterial system and its relation to the local amount of atherosclerosis within the individual. *Circulation, 103*, 1613–1617.

154. Weiss, S. M., Roblin, P. M., & Gaydos, G. A. (1994) Failure to detect *Chlamydia pneumoniae* (Cp.) in coronary atheromas of patients undergoing atherectomy, in: J. Orfila, G. I. Byrne, & M. A. Chernesky (Eds.) *Chlamydia infections* (pp. 220–223), Bologna, Italy: Societa Editrice Esculapio.

155. Blasi, F., Denti, F., Erba, M., Cosentini, R., Raccanelli, R., Rinaldi, A., Fagetti, L., Esposito, G., Ruberti, U., & Alegra, L. (1996) Detection of *Chlamydia pneumoniae* but not *Helicobacter pylori* in atherosclerotic plaques of aortic aneurysms, *J. Clin. Microbiol., 34*, 2766–2769.

156. Taylor-Robinson, D., Ong, G., Thomas, B. J., Rose, M. L., & Yacoub, M. Y. (1998) Detection of *Chlamydia pneumoniae* in vascular tissues from heart transplant donors aged four months to sixty years, *Lancet, 351*, 1255.

157. Paterson, D. L., Hall, J., Rasmussen, S. J., & Timms, P. (1998) Failure to detect *Chlamydia pneumoniae* in atherosclerotic plaques of Australian patients, *Pathology, 51*, 812–817.

158. Daus, H., Ozbek, C., Saage, D., Scheller, B., Schieffer, H., Pfreundschuh, M., & Gause, A. (1998) Lack of evidence for a pathogenic role of *Chlamydia pneumoniae* and cytomegalovirus infection in coronary atheroma formation, *Cardiology, 90*, 83–88.

159. Maass, M., Bartels, C., Kruger, S., Krause, E., Engel, P. M., & Dalhoff, K. (1998) Endovascular presence of *Chlamydia pneumoniae* DNA is a generalized phenomenon in atherosclerotic vascular tissue, *Atherosclerosis, 140*(Suppl. 1): S25–30.

160. Petersen, E., Boman, J., Persson, K., Arnerlov, C., Wadell, G., Juto, P., Eriksson, A., Dahlen, G., & Angquist, K. A. (1998) *Chlamydia pneumoniae* in human abdominal aortic aneurysms, *Eur. J. Vasc. Endovasc. Surg., 15*, 138–142.

161. Lindholt, J. S., Ostergard, L., Henneberg, E. W., Fasting, H., & Anderson, P. (1998) Failure to demonstrate *Chlamydia pneumoniae* in symptomatic abdominal aortic aneurysm by a nested polymerase chain reaction (PCR), *Eur. J. Vasc. Endovasc. Surg., 15*, 161–164.

162. Wong, Y., Thomas, M., Tsang, V., Gallagher, P. J., & Ward, M. E. (1999) The prevalence of *Chlamydia pneumoniae* in atherosclerotic and nonatherosclerotic blood vessels of patients attending for redo and first time coronary artery bypass graft surgery, *J. Am. Coll. Cardiol., 33*, 152–156.

163. Esposito, G., Blasi, F., & Allegra, L. (1999) Demonstration of viable *Chlamydia pneumoniae* in atherosclerotic plaques of carotid arteries by reverse transcriptase polymerase chain reaction, *Ann. Vasc. Surg., 13*, 421–425.

164. Blasi, F., Boman, J., Esposito, G., Malissano, G., Chelsea, R., Consentini, R., Tarsia, P., Tshomba, Y., Betti, M., Alessi, M., Morelli, W., & Allegra, L. (1999) *Chlamydia pneumoniae* DNA detection in peripheral blood mononuclear cells is predictive of vascular infection, *J. Infect. Dis., 180*, 2074–2076.

165. Melissano, G., Blasi, F., Esposito, G., Tarsia, P., Dordoni, L., Arosio, C., Tshomba, Y., Fagetti, L., Allegra, L., & Chelsea, R. (1999) *Chlamydia pneumoniae* eradication from carotid plaques. Results of an open, randomized treatment study, *Eur. J. Vasc. Endovasc. Surg., 18*, 355–359.

166. Wong, T. M., Thomas, D., Ajaz, M., Tsang, V., Gallagher, P. J., & Ward, M. E. (1999) Relation between direct detection of *Chlamydia pneumoniae* DNA in human coronary arteries at post mortem examination and histological severity (Stary grading) of associated atherosclerotic plaque, *Circulation*, *99*, 2733–2736.

167. Nadrachal, R., Makristathis, A., Apfalter, P., Rotter, M., Trubel, W., Huk, I., Polterauer, P., & Hirschl, A. M. (1999) Detection of *Chlamydia pneumoniae* in atheromatous tissues by polymerase chain reaction, *Wiener Klinische Wochenschrift*, *111*, 153–156.

168. Qavi, H. B., Melnick, J. L., Adam, E., & Debakey, M. E. (2000) Frequency of coexistence of cytomegalovirus and *Chlamydia pneumoniae* in atherosclerotic plaques, *Central Eur. J. Public Health*, *8*, 71–73.

169. Farsak, B., Yildirir, A., Akyon, Y., Pinar, A., Oc, M., Boke, E., Kes, S., & Tokgozoglu, L. (2000) Detection of *Chlamydia pneumoniae* and *Helicobacter pylori* DNA in human atherosclerotic plaques by PCR, *J. Clin. Microbiol.*, *38*, 4408–4411.

170. Gibbs, R. G., Sian, M., Mitchell, A. W., Greenhalgh, R. M., Davies, A. H., & Corey, N. (2000) *Chlamydia pneumoniae* does not influence atherosclerotic plaque behavior in patients with established carotid artery stenosis, *Stroke*, *31*, 2930–2935.

171. Gutierrez, J., Linares-Palomino, J., Lopez-Espada, C., Rodriguez, M., Ros, E., Piedrola, G., & Maroto, M. C. (2001) *Chlamydia pneumoniae* DNA in the arterial wall of patients with peripheral vascular disease, *Infection*, *29*, 196–200.

172. La Biche, R., Koziol, D., Quinn, T. C., Gaydos, C., Azhar, S., Ketron, G., Sood, S., & DeGraba, T. J. (2001) Presence of *Chlamydia pneumoniae* in human symptomatic and asymptomatic carotid atherosclerotic plaque, *Stroke*, *32*, 855–860.

173. Dobrilovic, N., Vadlamani, L., Meyer, M., & Wright, C. B. (2001) *Chlamydia pneumoniae* in atherosclerotic carotid artery plaques: high prevalence among heavy smokers, *Am. Surgeon*, *67*, 589–593.

174. Ong, G. M., Coyle, P. V., Barros D'Sa, A. A., McCluggage, W. G., Duprex, W. P., O'Neill, H. J., Wyatt, D. E., Bamford, K. B., O'Loughlin, B., & McCaughey, C. (2001) Non-detection of Chlamydia species in carotid atheroma using generic primers by nested PCR in a population with a high prevalence of *Chlamydia pneumoniae* antibody, *BMC Infect. Dis.*, *1*, 12 (http://www.biomed-central.com/1471-2334/1/12).

175. Radke, P. W., Merkelbach-Bruse, S., Messner, B. J., vomDahl, J., Dorge, H., Naami, A., Vogel, G., Handt, S., & Hanrath, P. (2001) Infectious agents in coronary lesions obtained by endatherectomy: pattern of distribution, co-infection, and clinical findings, *Coronary Art. Dis.*, *12*, 1–6.

176. Valassina, M., Migliorini, L., Sansoni, A., Sani, A., Sani, G., Corsaro, D., Cusi, M. G., Valensin, P. E., & Cellesi, C. (2001) Search for *Chlamydia pneumoniae* genes and their expression in atherosclerotic plaques of carotid arteries, *J. Med. Microbiol.*, *50*, 228–232.

177. Varghese, P. J., Gaydos, C. A., Arumugham, S. B., Pham, D. G., Quinn, T. C., & Tuazon, C. U. (1995) Demonstration of *Chlamydia pneumoniae* in coronary atheroma specimens from young patients with normal cholesterol from southern part of India, *Clin. Infect. Dis.*, *21*, 728 [Abstract 53].

178. Kuo, C. C., Grayston, J. T., Campbell, L. A., Goo, Y. A., Wissler, R. W., & Benditt, E. P. (1995) *Chlamydia pneumoniae* (TWAR) in coronary arteries of young adults (15–34 years old), 1995, *Proc. Natl. Acad. Sci. USA, 92,* 6911–6914.

179. Jackson, L. A., Campbell, L. A., Schmidt, R. A., Kuo, C. C., Cappuccio, A. L., Lee, M. J., & Grayston, J. T. (1997) Specificity of detection of *Chlamydia pneumoniae* in cardiovascular atheroma: evaluation of the innocent bystander hypothesis, *Am. J. Pathol., 150,* 1785–1790.

180. Kuo, C. C., Coulson, A. S., Campbell, L. A., Cappuccio, A. L., Lawrence, R. D., Wang, S. P., & Grayston, J. T. (1997) Detection of *Chlamydia pneumoniae* in atherosclerotic plaques in the walls of arteries of lower extremities from patients undergoing bypass operation for arterial obstruction, *J. Vasc. Surg., 26,* 29–31.

181. Davidson, M., Kuo, C. C., Middaugh, J. P., Campbell, L. A., Wang, S. P., Newman, W. P., Finley, J. C., & Grayston, J. T. (1998) Confirmed previous infection with *Chlamydia pneumoniae* (TWAR) and its presence in early coronary atherosclerosis, *Circulation, 98,* 628–633.

182. Ouchi, K., Fujii, B., Kanamoto, Y., Karita, M., Shirai, M., & Nakazawa, T. (1998) *Chlamydia pneumoniae* in coronary and iliac arteries of Japanese patients with atherosclerotic cardiovascular diseases, *J. Med. Microbiol., 47,* 907–913.

183. Berger, M., Schroder, B., Daeschlein, G., Schneider, W., Busjahn, A., Buchwalow, I., Luft, F. C., & Haller, H. (2000): *Chlamydia pneumoniae* DNA in non-coronary atherosclerotic plaques and circulating monocytes, *J. Lab. Clin. Med., 136,* 194–200.

184. Bartels, C., Maass, M., Bein, G., Brill, N., Bechtel, M., Leyh, R., & Sievers, H. H. (2000) Association of serology with the endovascular presence of *Chlamydia pneumoniae* and cytomegalovirus in coronary artery and vein graft disease, *Circulation, 101,* 137–141.

185. Ouchi, K., Fugii, B., Kudo, S., Shirai, M., Yamashita, K., Gondo, T., Ishihara, T., Ito, H., & Nakazawa, T. (2000) *Chlamydia pneumoniae* in atherosclerotic and nonatherosclerotic tissue, *J. Infect. Dis., 181*(Suppl. 3), 5441–5443.

186. Vink, A., Posterkamp, G., Poppen, M., Schoneveld, A. H., de Kleijn, P. V., Roholl, P. J. M., Fontijn, J., Plomp, S., & Borst, C. (2001) The adventitia of atherosclerotic coronary arteries frequently contains *Chlamydia pneumoniae*, *Atherosclerosis, 157,* 117–112.

187. Rassu, M., Cazzavillan, S., Scagnelli, M., Peron, A., Bevilacqua, P. A., Facco, M., Bertoloni, G., Lauro, F. M., Zambello, R., & Bonoldi, E. (2001) Demonstration of *Chlamydia pneumoniae* in atherosclerotic arteries from various vascular regions, *Atherosclerosis, 158,* 73–79.

188. Muhlestein, J. B., Hammond, E. H., Carlquist, J. F., Radicke, E., Tompson, M. J., Karagonnis, L. A., Woods, M. L., & Anderson, J. L. (1996) Increased incidence of *Chlamydia* species within the coronary arteries of patients with symptomatic atherosclerosis versus other forms of cardiovascular disease, *J. Am. Coll. Cardiol., 27,* 1555–1561.

189. Gloria-Breceda, F., Meaney-Mediolea, E., Valero-Elizondo, G., & Vela-huerta, A. (1997) The relationship between *Chlamydia pneumoniae* and atherosclerotic lesions of the aorta, *Arch. Inst. Cardiol. Mex., 67,* 17–23.

190. Ozsan, M., Gungor, C., Kahraman, M., Ozkul, A., Cinel, L., Tezcaner, T., Yorgancioglu, C., & Suzer, K. (2000) Chlamydia and atherosclerotic coronary arterial disease in Turkey, *Acta Cardiol., 55*, 295–300.

191. Ericson, K., Saldeen, T. G., Linquist, O., Pahlson, G., & Mehta, J. L. (2000) Relationships of *Chlamydia pneumoniae* infection to severity of human coronary atherosclerosis, *Circulation, 101*, 2568–2571.

192. Ramirez, J. A., *Chlamydia pneumoniae*/Atherosclerosis Study Group (1996) Isolation of *Chlamydia pneumoniae* from the coronary artery of a patient with coronary atherosclerosis, *Ann. Intern. Med., 125*, 979–982.

193. Mosorin, M., Surcel, H. M., Laurila, A., Lehtinen, M., Kattunen, R., Juvonen, J., Paavonen, J., Morrison, R. P., Saikku, P., & Juvonen, T. (2000) Detection of *Chlamydia pneumoniae*-reactive T lymphocytes in human atherosclerotic plaques of carotid artery, *Arterioscler. Thromb. Vasc. Biol., 20*, 1061–1067.

194. Shor, A., Kuo, C. C., & Patton, D. L. (1992) Detection of *Chlamydia pneumoniae* in coronary arterial fatty streaks and atheromatous plaques, *S. Afr. Med. J., 82*, 158–161.

195. Campbell, L. A., O'Brien, E. R., Cappuccio, A. L., Kuo, C. C., Wang, S. P., Stewart, D., Patton, D. L., Cummings, P. K., & Grayston, J. T. (1995) Detection of *Chlamydia pneumoniae* TWAR in human coronary atherectomy tissues, *J. Infect. Dis., 172*, 585–588.

196. Ong, G., Thomas, B., Mansfield, A. O., Davidson, B. R., & Taylor-Robinson, D. (1996) *Chlamydia pneumoniae* in vascular tissue, in A. Stary (Ed.), *Proceedings of the Third Meeting of the European Society for Chlamydia Research* (p. 222) Vienna.

197. Weiss, S. M., Roblin, P. M., Gaydos, C. A., Cummings, P., Patton, D. L., Schulhoff, N., Shani, J., Frankel, R., & Penney, K. (1996) Failure to detect. *Chlamydia pneumoniae* in coronary atheromas of patients undergoing atherectomy, *J. Infect. Dis., 173*, 957–962.

198. Juvonen, J., Juvonen, T., Laurila, A., ala Karppa, H., Lounatmaa, K., Surcel, H. M., Leinonen, M., Kairaluoma, P. I., & Saikku, R. (1997) Demonstration of *Chlamydia pneumoniae* in the walls of the abdominal aortic aneurysms, *J. Vasc. Surg., 25*, 499–505.

199. Shor, A., Phillips, J. I., Ong, G., Thomas, B. J., & Taylor-Robinson, D. (1998) *Chlamydia pneumoniae* in atheroma: consideration of criteria for causality, *J. Clin. Pathol., 51*, 812–817.

200. Bauriedel, G., Welsch, U., Likungu, J. A., Welz, A., & Luderitz, B. (1999) *Chlamydia pneumoniae* in coronary plaques: increased detection with acute coronary syndrome, *Dtsch. Med. Wochenschr., 124*, 375–380.

201. Virok, D., Kis, Z., Karai, L., Intzedy, L., Burian, K., Szabo, A., Ivanyi, B., & Gonczol, E. (2001) *Chlamydia pneumoniae* in atherosclerotic middle cerebral artery, *Stroke, 32*, 1973–1978.

202. Maass, M., Bartels, C., Engel, P. M., Mamat, U., & Sievers, H. H. (1998) Endovascular presence of viable *Chlamydia pneumoniae* is a common phenomenon in coronary artery disease, *J. Am. Coll. Cardiol., 31*, 827–832.

203. Karlsson, L., Gnarpe, J., Naas, J., Olsson, G., Lindholm, J., Steen, B., & Gnarpe, H. (2000) Detection of viable *Chlamydia pneumoniae* in abdominal aortic aneurysms, *Eur. J. Vasc. Endovasc. Surg., 19*, 630–635.

204. Nadareishvilli, Z. G., Koziol, D. E., Szekely, B., Ruetzler, B. A., La Biche, R., McCarron, R., & DeGraba, T. J. (2001) Increased CD8 + T cells associated with *Chlamydia pneumoniae* in symptomatic carotid plaque, *Stroke, 32*, 1966–1972.
205. Jackson, L. A., Campbell, L. A., Kuo, C. C., Rodriques, D. L., Lee, A., & Grayston, J. T. (1997) Isolation of *Chlamydia pneumoniae* from carotid endarterectomy specimens, *J. Infect. Dis., 176*, 292–295.
206. Apfalter, P., Loidl, M., Nadrchal, R., Makristathis, A., Rotter, M., Bergmann, M., Polterauer, P., & Hirschl, A. M. (2000) Isolation and continuous growth of *Chlamydia pneumoniae* from atherectomy specimens, *Eur. J. Clin. Microbiol. Infect. Dis., 19*, 305–308.
207. Walski, M., Podsiadly, E., Walczak, E., Celary-Walska, R., Dabrowski, M., Tylewska-Wierzbanowska, S., Ruzytlo, W., Witkowski, A., & Slysz, A. (1999) The presence of *Chlamydia pneumoniae* in atherosclerotic plaques—a report of three cases of ischaemic heart disease, *Pol. J. Pathol., 50*, 93–97.
208. Gaydos, C. A., Summergill, J. T., Sahney, N. N., Ramirez, J. A., & Quinn, T. C. (1996) Replication of *Chlamydia pneumoniae* in vitro in human macrophages, endothelial and aortic artery smooth muscle cells, *Infect. Immun., 64*, 1614–1620.
209. Haranaga, S., Yamaguchi, H., Friedman, H., Izumi, S. T., & Yamamoto, Y. (2001) *Chlamydia pneumoniae* infects and multiplies in lymphocytes in vitro, *Infect. Immun., 69*, 7753–7759.
210. Coombes, B. K., & Mahony, J. B. (1999) *Chlamydia pneumoniae* infection of human endothelial cells induces proliferation of smooth muscle cells via an endothelial cell derived soluble factor(s), *Infect. Immun., 67*, 2909–2915.
211. Rajalingan, K., Al-Younes, H., Muller, A., Meyer, T. F., Szczepek, A. J., & Rudel, T. (2001) Epithelial cells infected with *Chlamydophila pneumoniae* (*Chlamydia pneumoniae*) are resistant to apoptosis, *Infect. Immun., 69*, 7880–7888.
212. Kaul, R., & Wenman, W. M. (2001) *Chlamydia pneumoniae* facilitates monocyte adhesion to endothelial and smooth muscle cells, *Microb. Pathol., 30*, 149–155.
213. Coombes, B. K., & Mahony, B. (2001) c DNA array analysis of altered gene expression in human endothelial cells in response to *Chlamydia pneumoniae* infection, *Infect. Immun., 69*, 1420–1427.
214. Rodel, J., Woytas, M., Groh, A., Schmidt, K. H., Hartmann, M., Lehmann, M., & Straube, E. (2000) Production of basic fibroblast growth factor and interleukin 6 by human smooth muscle cells following infection with *Chlamydia pneumoniae*, *Infect. Immun., 68*, 3635–3644.
215. Netea, M. G., Selzman, C. H., Kullberg, B. J., Galama, J. M., Weinberg, A., Stalenhoef, A. F., Van der Meer, J. W., & Dinarello, C. A. (2000) Acellular components of *Chlamydia pneumoniae* stimulate cytokine production in human blood mononuclear cells, *Eur. J. Immunol., 30*, 541–549.
216. Kalayoglu, M. V., & Byrne, G. I. (1998) Induction of macrophages foam cell formation by *Chlamydia pneumoniae*, *J. Infect. Dis., 177*, 725–729.
217. Kalayoglyu, M. V., & Byrne, G. I. (1998) A *Chlamydia pneumoniae* component that induces macrophage foam cell formation is chlamydial lipopolysaccharide, *Infect. Immun., 66*, 5067–5072.

218. Kalayoglu, M. V., Hoerneman, B., LaVerda, D., Morrison, S. G., Morrison, R. P., & Byrne, G. I. (1999) Cellular oxidation of low density lipoprotein by *Chlamydia pneumoniae, J. Infect. Dis., 180,* 780–790.

219. Kol, A., Sukhova, G. K., Lichtman, A. H., & Libby (1998) Chlamydial heat shock protein-60 localizes in human atheroma and regulates macrophage tumor necrosis factor alpha and matrix metalloproteinase expression, *Circulation, 98,* 300–307.

220. Kol, A., Boucier, T., Lichtman, A. H., & Libby, P. (1999) Chlamydial and human heat shock protein-60's activate human vascular endothelial smooth muscle cells and macrophages, *J. Clin. Invest., 103,* 571–577.

221. Mayr, M., Metzler, B., Kiechl, S., Willeit, J., Schett, G., Xu, Q., & Wick, G. (1999) Endothelial cytotoxicity mediated by serum antibodies to heart shock proteins of *Escherichia coli* and *Chlamydia pneumoniae*: immune reactions to heart shock proteins as a possible link between infection and atherosclerosis, *Circulation, 99,* 1560–1566.

222. Vehmaan Kreula, P., Puolakkainen, M., Sarvas, M., Welgus, H. G., & Kovanen, P. T. (2001) *Chlamydia pneumoniae* proteins induces secretion of the 92-kDa gelatinase by human monocyte-derived macrophages, *Arterioscler. Thromb. Vasc. Biol., 21,* E1–8.

223. Dechend, R., Maas, M., Gieffers, J., Dietz, R., Scheridereit, C., Leutz, A., & Gulba, D. C. (1999) *Chlamydia pneumoniae* infection of vascular smooth muscle and endothelial cells activates NF-kappa B and induces tissue factor and PAI-1 expression: a potential link to accelerated atherosclerosis, *Circulation, 100,* 1369–1373.

224. Moazed, T. C., Kuo, C. C., Grayston, J. T., & Campbell, L. A. (1997) Murine models of *Chlamydia pneumoniae* infection and atherosclerosis, *J. Infect. Dis., 175,* 833–890.

225. Moazed, T. C., Campbell, L. A., Rosenfield, M. E., Grayston, J. T., & Kuo, C. C. (1999) *Chlamydia pneumoniae* infection accelerates the progression of atherosclerosis in apolipoprotein E-deficient mice, *J. Infect. Dis., 180,* 238–241.

226. Burnett, M. S., Gaydos, C. A., Madico, G. E., Gilad, S. M., Palgen, B., Quinn, T. C., & Epstein, E. (2001) Atherosclerosis in APOE knockout mice infected with multiple pathogens, *J. Infect. Dis., 183,* 226–231.

227. Hu, H., Pierce, G. N., & Zhang, G. (1999) Atherogenic effect of *Chlamydia* are dependent or serum cholesterol and specific to *Chlamydia pneumoniae, J. Clin. Invest., 103,* 747–753.

228. Liuba, P., Karnani, P., Pesonen, E., Paakkari, I., Forslid, A., Johansson, L., Persson, K., Wadstrom, T., & Laurini, R. (2000) Endothelial dysfunction after repeated *Chlamydia pneumoniae* infection in apolipoprotein E- knockout mice, *Circulation, 102,* 1039–1044.

229. Blessing, E., Campbell, L. A., Rosenfeld, M. E., Chough, N., & Kuo, C. C. (2001) *Chlamydia pneumoniae* infection accelerates hyperlipidemia induced atherosclerotic lesion development in C57 BL/6J mice, *Atherosclerosis, 158,* 13–17.

230. Blessing, E., Nagano, S., Campbell, L. A., Rosenfield, M. E., & Kuo, C. C. (2000) Effect of *Chlamydia trachomatis* infection on atherosclerosis in apolipoprotein E-deficient mice, *Infect. Immun., 68,* 7195–7197.

231. Aalto-Setälä, K., Laitinen, K., Erkkilä, L., Leinonen, M., Jauhiainen, M., Ehnholm, C., Tamminen, M., Poulakkainen, M., Perntilä, I., & Saikku, P. (2001) *Chlamydia pneumoniae* does not increase atherosclerosis in the aortic root of apolipoprotein E-deficient mice, *Arterioscler. Thromb. Vasc. Biol., 21*, 578–584.
232. Caligiuir, G., Rottenberg, M., Nicoletti, A., Wigzell, H., & Hansson, G. K. (2001) *Chlamydia pneumoniae* infection does not induce or modify atherosclerosis in mice, *Circulation, 103*, 2834–2838.
233. Blessing, E., Lin, T. M., Campbell, L. A., Rosenfeld, M. E., Lloyd, D., Kuo, C. C. (2000) *Chlamydia pneumoniae* induces inflammatory changes in the heart and aorta of normocholesterolenic C57Bl/6J mice, *Infect. Immun., 68*, 4765–4768.
234. Finging, G., & Hanke, H. (1997) Nikolai, Nikolajewitsch Anitschkow (1885–1964) established the cholesterol fed rabbit as a model for atherosclerosis research, *Atherosclerosis, 135*, 1–7.
235. Fong, I. W., Chiu, B., Viira, E., Fong, M. W., Jang, D., & Mahony, J. B. (1997) Rabbit model for *Chlamydia pneumoniae* infection, *J. Clin. Microbiol., 35*, 48–52.
236. Fong, I. W., Chiu, B., Viira, E., Jang, D., & Mahony, J. B. (1999) De novo induction of atherosclerosis by *Chlamydia pneumoniae* in a rabbit model, *Infect. Immun., 7*, 6048–6055.
237. Lautinen, K., Laurila, A., Pyhala, L., Leinonen, M., & Saikku, P. (1997) *Chlamydia pneumoniae* infection induces inflammatory changes in the aortas of the rabbits, *Infect. Immun., 65*, 4832–4835.
238. Muhlestein, J. B., Anderson, J. L., Hammond, E. H., Zhao, L., Trehan, S., Schwobe, E. P., & Carlquist, J. F. (1998) Infection with *Chlamydia pneumoniae* accelerates the development of atherosclerosis and treatment with azithromycin prevents it in a rabbit model, *Circulation, 97*, 633–636.
239. Fong, I. W., Chiu, B., Mahony, J. B., Jang, D., Coombes, B., Dunn, P., Caterini, J., & Murdin, A. (2002) *C. pneumoniae* enhancing effect on atherosclerosis and relationships with lipid profile and fibrinogen in a rabbit model, *Tenth International Symposium on Human Chlamydia Infections*, Antalya, Turkey.
240. Van Heek, M., & Zilversmit, D. B., (1988) Evidence for an inverse relation between plasma triglyceride and aortic cholesterol in the coconut oil/cholesterol-fed rabbit, *Atherosclerosis, 71*, 185–192.
241. Rothstein, N. M., Quinn, T. C., Madico, G., Gaydos, C. A., & Lowerstein, C. J. (2001) Effect of azithromycin on murine arteriosclerosis exacerbated by *Chlamydia pneumoniae, J. Infect. Dis., 183*, 232–238.
242. Fong, I. W., Chiu, B., Viira, E., Jang, D., Fong, M. W., Peeling, R., & Mahony, J. B. (1999) Can an antibiotic (macrolide) prevent *Chlamydia pneumoniae*-induced atherosclerosis in a rabbit model? *Clin. Diag. Lab. Immun., 6*, 891–894.
243. Fong, I. W., Chui, B., Viira, E., Jang, D., & Mahony, J. B. (2002) The influence of clarithromycin on early atherosclerotic lesions after *Chlamydia pneumoniae* infection in a rabbit model, *Antimicrob. Agents Chemother., 46*, 2321–2326.
244. Meier, C. R., Derby, L. E., Jick, S. S., Vasilakis, C., & Jick, H. (1999) Antibiotics and risk of subsequent first time acute myocardial infarction, *JAMA, 287*, 427–431.

245. Jackson, L. A., Smith, N. L., Heckbert, S. R., Grayston, J. T., Siscovick, D. S., & Psatty, M. B. (1999) Lack of association between first myocardial infarction and past use of erythromycin, tetracycline or doxycycline, *Emerging Infect. Dis.*, 5, 281–284.

246. Pilote, L., Green, L., Joseph, L., Richard, H., & Eisenberg, M. J. (2002) Antibiotics against *Chlamydia pneumoniae* and prognosis after acute myocardial infarction, *Am. Heart J.*, 143, 294–300.

247. Gupta, S., Leatham, E. W., Carrington, D., Mendall, M. A., Kaski, J. C., & Camm, A. J. (1997) Elevated *Chlamydia pneumoniae* antibodies, cardiovascular events and azithromycin, in male survivors of acute myocardial infarction, *Circulation*, 96, 404–407.

248. Gurfinkel, E., Bozovich, G., Doroca, A., Beck, E., & Mautner, B., for the Roxis Study Group (1997) Randomized trail of roxithromycin in non-Q wave coronary syndromes: Roxis pilot study, *Lancet*, 350, 404–407.

249. Gurfinkel, E., Bozovich, G., Beck, E., Testa, E., Livellara, B., & Mautner, B. (1999) Treatment with the antibiotic roxithromycin in patients with acute non-Q wave coronary syndrome. Final report of the Roxis study, *Eur. Heart J.*, 20, 121–127.

250. Anderson, J. L., Muhlestein, J. B., Carlquist, J., Allen, A., Trehan, S., Nielson, C., Hall, S., Brady, J., Egger, M., Horne, B., & Lim, T. (1999) Randomized secondary prevention trial of azithromycin in patients with coronary artery disease and serological evidence for *Chlamydia pneumoniae* infection: the azithromycin in coronary artery disease elimination of myocardial infarction with *Chlamydia* academic study, *Circulation*, 99, 1538–1539.

251. Muhlestein, J. B., Anderson, J. L., Carlquist, J. F., Salunkhe, K., Horne, B. D., Pearson, R. R., Burch, T. J., Allen, A., Trehan, S., & Nielson, C. (2000) Randomized secondary prevention trial of azithromycin in patients with coronary artery disease: primary clinical results of the academic study, *Circulation*, 102, 1755–1760.

252. Stone, A. F. M., Mendall, M. A., Kaski, J., Edger, T. M., Gupta, S., Polonieiki, J., Camm, A. J., & Northfield, T. C. (2001) The South Thames trial of antibiotics in myocardial infarction and unstable angina (Stamina Trial), *Eur. Heart J.*, 22(Abstract Suppl.), 643.

253. Neumann, F. J., Kastrati, A., Mitehke, T., Pogalsa-Murray, G., Mehilli, J., Valina, C., Jogethaei, N., de Costa, C. P., Wagner, H., & Schomig, A. (2001) Treatment of *Chlamydia pneumoniae* infection with roxithromycin and effect on neointima proliferation after coronary stent placement (ISAR-3): a randomized, double-blind, placebo-controlled trail, *Lancet*, 357, 2085–2089.

254. Parchure, N., Zouridakis, E. G., & Kaski, J. C. (2002) Effect of azithromycin treatment on endothelial function in patients with coronary artery disease and evidence of *Chlamydia pneumoniae* infection, *Circulation*, 105, 1298–1303.

255. Mosorin, M., Juvonen, J., Biancari, F., Surcel, H. M., Leinonen, M., Saikku, P., & Juvonen, T. (2001) Use of doxcycline to decrease the growth rate of abdominal aortic aneurysms: a randomized double-blind placebo-controlled pilot study, *J. Vasc. Surg.*, 34, 757–758.

256. Dunne, M., O'Connor, C., Pfeiffer, M., Muhlstein, B., Gupta, S., & Yao, L., for the WIZARD Investigators (2002) Weekly intervention with azithromax for

atherosclerosis and its related disorders (The WIZARD Study), *Am. Coll. Cardiol. Conf. Atlanta*, Georgia, March 18, Session 405, Late Breaking Clinical Trails 1.

257. Fong, I. W., Chiu, B., Viira, E., Tucker, W., & Peeling, R. (2002) Correlation of chlamydial heat shock protein-60 (CHS P-60) and presence of *C. pneumoniae* antigen in carotid plaques, *J. Infect. Dis.* (in press).

258. Kutlin, A., Roblin, P. M., & Hammerschlag, M. R. (1999) In vitro activities of azithromycin and ofloxacin against *Chlamydia pneumoniae* in a continuous-infection model, *Antimicrob. Agents Chemother.*, *43*, 2268–2272.

259. Schneider, C. A., Diedrichs, H., Riedel, K. D., Zimmermann, T., & Hopp, H. W. (2000) In vivo uptake of azithromycin in human coronary plaques, *Am. J. Cardiol.*, *86*, 789–791.

260. Hammerschlag, M. R., Qumei, K. K., & Roblin, P. M. (1992) In vitro activities of azithromycin, clarithromycin, L-ofloxacin and other antibiotics against *Chlamydia pneumoniae*, *Antimicrob. Agents Chemother.*, *36*, 1572–1574.

261. Rukita, R. M. (1998) Intracellular activity, potential clinical uses of antibiotics, *ASM News*, *64*, 570–575.

262. Gieffers, J., Fullgraf, H., Jahn, J., Klinger, M., Dalhoff, K., & Katus, H. A. (2001) *Chlamydia pneumoniae* infection in circulating human monocytes is refractory to antibiotic treatment, *Circulation*, *103*, 351–356.

263. Wolf, K., & Malinverni, R. (1999) Effect of azithromycin plus rifampin versus that of azithromycin alone on eradication of *Chlamydia pneumoniae* from lung tissue in experimental pneumonitis, *Antimicrob. Agents Chemother.*, *43*, 1491–1493.

264. Rockey, D. P. (2002) Chlamydial interactions with host cells: recent progress and remaining issues, in J. Schachter, G. Christiansen, I. N. Clarke, M. Hammerschlag, B. Kaltenboeck, C. C. Kuo, R. G. Rank, P. Saikku, W. E. Stamm, R. S. Stephens, J. T. Summersgill, P. Timms, & P. B. Wyrick (Eds.) *Chlamydial infections* (pp. 35–44), Proceedings of the Tenth International Symposium on Human Chlamydial Interactions, Antalya, Turkey, Grafmat Basim ve Reklam Sanayi Tic. Ltd. Sti, Istanbul.

265. Puolakkainen, M., Kuo, C. C., & Campbell, L. A. (2002) Mannose 6-phosphate inhibits growth of *Chlamydia pneumoniae* in human arterial endothelial cells, in J. M. Schachter, G. Christiansen, I. N. Clarke, M. Hammerschlag, B. Kaltenboeck, C. C. Kuo, R. G. Rank, P. Saikku, W. E. Stamm, R. S. Stephens, J. T. Summersgill, P. Timms, & P. B. Wyrick, (Eds.) *Chlamydial infections* (pp. 53–56), Proceedings of the Tenth International Symposium on Human Chlamydial Infections, Antalya, Turkey, Grafmat Basin ve Reklam Sanayi Tic. Ltd. Sti, Istanbul.

266. Lin, T. M., Campbell, L. A., Rosenfeld, M. E., & Kuo, C. C. (2001) Human monocyte-derived insulin-like growth factor-2 enhances the infection of human arterial endothelial cells by *Chlamydia pneumoniae*, *J. Infect. Dis.*, *183*, 1368–1372.

267. Reiss, A. B., Awadallah, N. W., Malhotra, S., Montesinos, M. C., Chan, E. S., Javitt, N. B., & Cronstein, B. N. (2001) Immune complexes and the IFN-gamma

decrease cholesterol 27-hydroxylase in human arterial endothelium and macrophages, *J. Lipid Res.*, *42*, 1913–1922.

268. Reiss, A. B., Awadallah, N. W., Roblin, P. M., Chan, E. S., Montesinos, M. C., Khoa, N. D., Crostein, B. N., & Hammerschlag, M. R. (2001) Immune modulation of cholesterol homeostasis, *Recent Res. Devel. Protein Eng.*, *1*, 23–28.

269. Hammerschlag, M. R., Roblin, P. M., Reiss, A. B., Awadallah, N. W., Kutlin, A., Chan, E. S. L., & Cronstein, B. N. (2002) Chlamydia decreases expression of anti-atherogenic enzyme, cholesterol 27-hydrolase, in vitro, in J. Schachter, G. Christiansen, I. N. Clarke, M. R. Hammerschlag, B. Kaltenboeck, C. C. Kuo, R. G. Rank, G. L. Ridgway, P. Saikku, W. E. Stamm, R. S. Stephens, J. T. Summersgill, P. Timms, & P. B. Wyrick (Eds.) *Chlamydial infections* (pp. 85–88), Proceedings of the Tenth International Symposium on Human Chlamydial Infections, Antalya, Turkey, Gramat Basim ve Reklam Sanayi Tic. Ltd. Sti, Istanbul.

6

Periodontal Disease and the Cardiovascular System

6.1. INTRODUCTION

For years dental clinicians have noticed that there are certain characteristics that are common in patients with periodontal disease and cardiovascular disease. Both these conditions are more likely to occur in older persons, males, of lower educational status, with fewer financial resources, who smoke, have stress, and are socially isolated. The classical risk factors for cardiovascular disease—hypertension, diabetes, hypercholesterolemia and cigarette smoking can only account for about one half to two thirds of all cases. In the past decade, there have been several reports linking periodontitis with coronary heart disease (CHD) and stroke. The current data and state of our understanding of this new paradigm will be reviewed in this chapter.

6.2. PERIODONTAL DISEASE

Periodontal disease refers to a diverse group of diseases that affect the periodontium. The periodontium is the supporting structure of the tooth and includes the cementum, the periodontal membrane, the bones of the jaw, and the gingivae (gums). The gingivae is the tissue covered by mucous membrane that surrounds the necks of teeth and covers the jaw. Disease is initiated by the formation of subgingival plaque, the plaque that forms at the dentogingival margin and extends down into the gingival tissue. Recent evidence shows that

179

Porphyromonas (formerly bacteroides) *gingivalis* is the main species in this plaque and is responsible for the tissue breakdown through the production of several proteases. The result is an initial inflammatory reaction known as periodontitis, which is caused by the host's immune response to both the plaque, bacteria, and the tissue destruction. This leads to swelling of the tissue and the formation of periodontal pockets. Bacteria colonize these pockets and cause more inflammation, which leads to periodontal abscess, bone destruction or periodontosis, inflammation of the gingivae or gingivitis, and general tissue necrosis. If the condition is not treated, the tooth may fall out of its socket. Periodontitis in moderate to severe form affects roughly 15% of the North American population over the age of 18, and similar or higher prevalence is seen in most countries[1]. The prevalence among middle age and older adults may be as high as 30–40%, and periodontal disease is the most frequent cause of loss of dentition in adults and the process usually begins in early adulthood.

6.2.1. Microbial Etiology

Periodontal diseases are infections in nature. Over 300 species and serotypes of bacteria can be found in the oral cavity, and a dozen or more species have been implicated to one extent or another in the causation of periodontitis in humans[2]. However, experts have recently concluded that three species, all of which are gram-negative anaerobes or facultative, account for most cases of periodontitis. These include *P. gingivalis, Bacteroides forysthus*, and *Actinobacillus actinomycetemcomitans*, the latter found mostly in cases of juvenile periodontitis[3]. Spirochaetes may also play a significant role[4].

After cleaning the teeth becomes coated with a glycoprotein from saliva to form a pellicle. Adhesions from gram-positive bacteria bind to pellicle to mediate colonization and growth of supragingival plaque. Gram-negative bacteria colonize and bind to the gram-positive bacteria by specific receptors. Subsequently, if left unchecked, tightly adherent microbial plaques become visible at the gingival margin of the tooth surface, and an acute inflammation or gingivitis develops.

In susceptible individuals, plaques bacteria extend into the gingival sulcus and form subgingival plaques which are tightly adherent to the tooth surface. These plaques have all the characteristics of biofilms[5], which are matrix-enclosed bacterial populations adherent to each other and to the surfaces or intersurfaces[6]. The biofilm concept is important in understanding the pathobiology of periodontitis and its relation to systemic disease. Subgingival plaques are extraordinarily persistent and difficult to eliminate as with biofilms in general. Gingival fluid, which contains complement, antibodies, and other substances in blood for controlling and preventing infection, flows through the periodontal pocket, continuously bathing the biofilm. The subgingival biofilms constitute an enormous and continuing bacterial load. A pocket will contain over 10^7–10^8 bacteria per milliliter, with the three major gram-negative pathogens shedding vesicles rich in lipopolysaccharide (LPS) in continuous contact with periodontal tissue and the circulation.

There is evidence that viable gram-negative bacteria, LPS, and other soluble bacterial components have easy access to the connective tissues and enter the circulation frequently. About 55% of subjects with severe periodontitis have positive blood cultures after chewing[7], and tooth brushing, flossing, and procedures such as scaling result in bacteremia and humoral immune responses[8–10]. *P. gingivalis* can block the initial steps in local inflammatory response, by blocking induction of E-selectin by other gram-negative bacteria in the subgingival biofilm, that normally limit and control microbial overgrowth of itself and other bacteria in the periodontal pockets[11].

6.2.2. Pathobiology of Periodontal Disease

Major advances have been made recently in the understanding of the pathogenesis and the natural history of periodontitis. A new paradigm for the pathobiology of periodontitis is illustrated in Figure 6.1, and recently

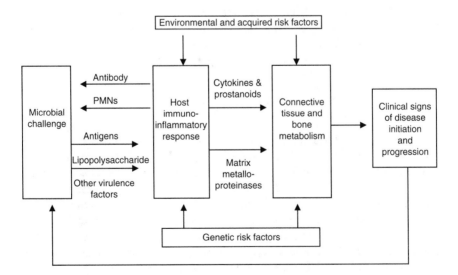

Figure 6.1. A schematic diagram of the pathogenesis of periodontitis is shown. Adapted from Page[13] with permission of the publishers.

reviewed by Page[12,13]. Bacteria are essential, but insufficient to cause disease; a susceptible host and host factors are necessary and determinative. Periodontitis is a complex of related diseases that differs in etiology, disease progression, natural history, and response to therapy, but with a common pathway for tissue destruction[14,15].

The basic pathologic mechanism is the same that leads to connective tissue and bony destruction, as well as ultra structural changes, healing, and regeneration. The proinflammatory cytokines tumor necrosis factor alpha (TNF-α), interleukin-1β (IL-1β), interferon gamma (IFN-γ) induce and enhance production of prostaglandin E_2 (PGE$_2$) and matrix metalloproteinases (MMP), and these molecules mediate destruction of the extracellular matrix of the gingiva and periodontal ligament and resorption of alveolae[13].

Proinflammatory cytokines and prostaglandins accumulate and reach high concentrations in periodontitis affected tissues and may serve as a reservoir for these mediators which can enter the circulation and induce or perpetuate systemic effects. IL-1β can influence coagulation and thrombosis and retard fibrinolysis[16]. IL-1, TNF-α, and thromboxane can cause platelet aggregation and adhesion, and may play a role in foam cell formation and cholesterol deposition.

The pathobiology of periodontal disease is influenced by disease modifiers or risk factors—genetic, environmental or acquired which may differ with the stages or form of disease[17]. The modifying factors may affect the age of disease onset, pattern of observed bone and tissue destruction, rates of disease progression, severity and frequency of recurrences, and even response to therapy. These modifying factors, include hereditary factors, stress, tobacco smoking, diet, and diabetes mellitus. However, periodontitis itself may influence the course of diabetes mellitus and worsen the disease[17].

6.2.3. Risk Factors for Periodontal Disease

Although bacteria are essential for the causation of periodontitis, other factors may be equally as important. Genetic factors may be very important both in early onset juvenile periodontitis and adult onset disease. Twin studies of adult periodontitis have shown greater susceptibility for periodontitis among monozygotic compared to dizygotic twins. It is estimated that 50% of the enhanced risk for severe periodontitis can be accounted for by genetic or hereditary predisposition alone[18]. In families with early onset periodontitis and in some with adult onset disease specific gene loci are linked to enhanced susceptibility for periodontitis[19], and the linkage with juvenile periodontitis has been demonstrated on a major autosomal gene locus[20].

Studies of families with juvenile onset periodontitis have linked disease susceptibility to a region on chromosome 6 on the immune response genes[21]. The major antibody produced in response to periodontitis is IgG_2[22] which is genetically determined. Other genetic predisposition to periodontitis include polymorphism for IL-1 gene family[23], trisomy 21 and traits that lead to abnormalities of neutrophil function or number[19].

Other risk factors for periodontitis include advancing age, male gender, tobacco smoking, systemic disease such as diabetes mellitus, drugs and disease that impair host defense, poor oral hygiene, and lack of dental care (the latter two conditions being more common in lower socioeconomic groups and minorities). Recent studies suggest that tobacco smoking is equally or more important as a disease determinant than the bacteria alone[24], and stress also has been documented to be a significant risk factor[25].

6.3. PERIODONTAL DISEASE AND CARDIOVASCULAR DISEASE AND ATHEROSCLEROSIS

During the past decade several reports have suggested a relationship between chronic oral infection (i.e., periodontitis) or tooth loss with cardiovascular disease, but others have not. Most of the data available is from epidemiological studies on association of periodontitis and CHD or cerebrovascular disease, but there are a few studies on the pathological association and biological plausible mechanisms.

6.3.1. Epidemiological Evidence

Since Matilla et al.[26] first reported on the association of total dental index and acute myocardial infarction in a case control study in 1989, there has been considerable interest in this area. The dental index, used in all of Matilla's reports, is the sum of carious lesions, probing depth measures (pockets), and the presence or absence of periodontitis. These index scores showed that patients had worse dental health than controls. Logistic regression analysis indicated that the poor dental health and CHD was independent of age, total cholesterol, high-density lipoprotein (HDL), triglycerides, C peptide, hypertension, diabetes, and smoking[26]. Subsequently there have been a total of 12 retrospective case control[27–33] or cross-sectional studies[34–37] reported (see Table 6.1). As noted, some of these studies used a composite of caries, periodontal disease, oral tooth loss; others tooth loss or edentulous state

Table 6.1
Retrospective Studies of Periodontitis and Atherosclerotic Vascular Disease

Study	Cases	Measure of periodontitis	Vascular end point	Result	Comments
Mattila et al. 1989[26]	100 cases 102 controls	Clinical and radiological	Acute MI	OR 1.3 ($p = 0.004$)	Assessed dental health in cases and controls
Syrjanen et al. 1989[27]	40 cases (CVA) 40 controls <50 yrs	Clinical and radiological	Acute ischemic stroke	OR 12.8 ($p \leq 0.02$)	Assessed severe dental infections in CVA cases and controls
Mattila et al. 1993[28]	100	Radiological	Coronary artery stenosis	OR 1.4 ($p = 0.003$)	Assessed severity of dental infections and coronary atherosclerosis by angiogram
Paunio et al. 1993[35]	1384 cohort male (45–64 yrs)	Number of missing teeth	Nonfatal CHD	RR 2.3 ($p = 0.04$)	Correlate missing teeth with CHD in cohort
Grau et al. 1997[29]	166 cases (CVA) 166 controls	Clinical and radiological	Cerebrovascular ischemia (nonfatal)	RR = 2.6 (95% CI, 1.18–5.7)	Determined total dental index in cases and controls
Ziegler et al. 1998[30]	66 CVA cases 60 controls	Clinical and radiological	Acute cerebral ischemia/stroke	RR = 2.4 (95% CI, 1.09–5.1)	No association in young, assessed total dental index in cases and controls
Loesche et al. 1998[31]	320 males ≥ 60 yrs	Clinical indices (1–14 versus 0 teeth)	History of CHD	RR = 2.64 (93% CI, 1.26–5.56)	Compared CHD in dentate subjects (no. of teeth), and edentulous subjects

Study	Sample	Measure	Outcome	Result	Comments
Loesche et al. 1998[32]	401 cohort males >60 yrs	Clinical indices, plaque index >1	Cerebrovascular ischemia	OR 2.28 $p = 0.032$ (higher plaque index in subjects)	Dentate subjects with 15–28 teeth, compared oral hygiene and plaque index
Arbes et al. 1999[36]	5564 cohort	% periodontal attachment loss	Self-reported history of heart attack	OR = 3.8 (95% CI, 1.5–9.7) for >67% loss	Incremental increase of greater loss
Emingil et al. 2000[33]	60 AMI 60 CCHD	Clinical exam	Acute MI	Logistic regression analysis $p < 0.05$	Compared periodontal disease in AMI patients and those with stable CCHD
Takata et al. 2001[37]	697 cohort >80 yrs	Number of teeth	ECG: ST, T- or Q-wave abnormalities	RR 0.402 (95% CI, 0.228–0.706) $p \leq 0.005$ <19 vs. >20 teeth	Compared ECG abnormalities with number of teeth
Mattila et al. 2000[34]	85 CHD 53 controls	Clinical exam (dental index)	CHD	OR 1.0 (NS) (clinical and radiology sum score)	Compared dental pathology in older subjects with CHD and controls
Beck et al. 2001[38]	6017 cohort	% periodontal attachment loss	Carotid intima-media thickness ≥1 mm	OR = 1.31 (95% CI, 1.03–1.66)	Periodontal disease correlated with atherosclerosis of carotid artery by ultrasound

Note. CI, confidence interval; ECG, electrocardiogram; MI, myocardial infarction; AMI, acute myocardial infarction; CHD, coronary heart disease; CCHD, chronic coronary heart disease; CVA, cerebrovascular accidents (stroke); Exam, examination.

alone, or periodontal disease alone with different criteria. The large majority of these retrospective studies showed an association with poor dental health and CHD or cerebrovascular disease. Also, in a large cohort periodontal disease was associated with increased carotid artery intima-media thickness (IMT)[38].

Limitations of these studies included biases from the retrospective nature of the investigations; it is possible that the associations in the previous studies merely reflect the fact that people who are more health conscious are at lower risk of CHD and have better dental health[39]. Loss of dentition may be related to a number of factors besides periodontal disease or caries, such as financial status or dental insurance. Some of the studies failed to adequately adjust for other confounders such as physical activity, diet, smoking and the amount, and socioeconomic status. In cross-sectional studies, part of the reported associations may be attributed to confounding factors[39].

Large prospective or longitudinal studies should give a clearer picture of the relationship between chronic periodontitis and atherosclerotic vascular disease and the complications. There have been 11 prospective cohort studies on periodontitis and CHD or cerebrovascular disease (stroke) link[40-50], and one on the association with peripheral vascular disease (PVD)[51], see Table 6.2. The associated increased risk of atherosclerotic vascular disease with periodontitis or oral health vary substantially from one study to the next (Table 6.2). Of the 11 studies on CHD or stroke, the increased maximal risk reported was 170%[44] and the lowest risk a 3% decrease[50]. Four of those studies showed a small increase in risk (25–70%), three others a moderated increased risk (111–170%) and four no increased risk. One study on PVD[51] detected an increased risk of 127% associated with alveolar bone loss. Of note all four of the negative studies adjusted for smoking dose and two for health awareness, whereas only three of the eight studies with increased risk adjusted for smoking dose and none for health awareness. Since there were significant differences in methods of measurement of periodontal disease or oral health and design of the studies, including population at risk, a meta-analysis of these studies would not be valid or reliable.

There are two other prospective studies not included in Table 6.2, which addressed special issues in specific groups of subjects. Hujoel et al.[52], as part of the National Health and Nutrition Examination Survey (NHANES-1)[46], examined prospectively a cohort of 4,027 people over 17 years to compare the rates of CHD events in edentulous subjects (cured of any periodontal disease) with those with periodontitis. After adjustment for confounders there was no significant difference in CHD events, indicating that elimination of chronic dental infection may not reduce cardiovascular risk. In the other study two groups of diabetics, with and without severe periodontal disease (39 case–control pairs) were followed for 6 years[53]. Significantly higher prevalence of vascular complications such as myocardial infarction, angina, stroke, and intermittent claudication were found in the case group.

Table 6.2

Prospective, Longitudinal Studies of Periodontitis and Atherosclerotic Vascular Disease

Study	Cohort/cases	Methods	End point	Control for		% Risk change (95% CI)	Size of risk of increase
				Smoking dose	Health awareness		
1. DeStefano et al. 1993[40]	9,760/556 25–74 yrs	Clinical exams, 14 yrs follow up	CHD mortality	No	No	+25% (6–48%) Men < 50 yrs +71%	Small Small-moderate
2. Mattila et al. 1995[41]	214/52 all CHD, <65 yrs	Clinical exams and radiology, 7 yr follow up	Fatal and nonfatal fatal CHD events	No No	No No	+21% (8–36%)	Small
3. Beck et al. 1996[42]	1,147 men/207 CHD 40 strokes	Clinical exam and radiology, 18 yr follow up	CHD, stroke mortality	No	No	+50% (4–114%)	Small
4. Joshipura et al. 1996[43]	44,119 men/757	Self-reported dental disease and tooth loss, 6 yrs follow up	CHD	Yes	Yes	+4% (−14–25%)	No assoc.
5. Genco et al. 1997[44]	1,372/68 Native Indians <60 yrs	Bone loss (radiology), 10 yr follow up	CHD	No	No	+168% (30–45%)	Moderate
6. Morrison et al. 1999[45]	11,251/466 34–84 yrs	Clinical exam, 21 yr follow up	CHD, stroke mortality	Yes	No	+37% (−20–135%)	Small
7. Hujoel et al. 2000[46]	8,032/1,265 25–74 yrs	Clinical exam, (periodontal index), 21 yrs follow up	CHD	Yes	No	+14% (−4–36%)	Small ns

Table 6.2
(*continued*)

Study	Cohort/cases	Methods	End point	Control for		% Risk change (95% CI)	Size of risk of increase
				Smoking dose	Health awareness		
8. Wu et al. 2000[47]	9,962/803 24–74 yrs	Clinical exam, 18 yr follow up	Stroke TIA/mortality	No	No	All stroke +66% (15–139%) non-hem stroke- +111% (30–242%)	Small–moderate
9. Howell et al. 2001[48]	22,037/797 male physicians	Self-reported periodontal disease, 12.3 yr follow up	CHD/strokes CVS mortality	Yes	Yes	+1% (−14–15%)	No assoc.
10. Jansson et al. 2001[49]	1,393/162 18–66 yrs	Clinical exam and radiology (Russel's index), 26 yrs follow up	Fatal CHD	Yes	No	+170% $p = 0.04$ <45 yrs	Moderate
11. Hujoel et al. 2002[50]	653/352 prior CHD	17 yrs follow up	CHD sec. events	Yes	No	−+3% (−28–31%)	No assoc.
12. Mendez et al. 1998[51]	1,110/80 21–80 yrs males	Radiology alveolar bone loss, 25 yrs follow up	Peripheral vasc. dis. (PVD)	Yes	No	+127% (32–290%)	Moderate

6.3.2. Pathological Evidence

A few studies have reported on the presence of oral bacteria in atheromatous plaque by immunostain or by polymerase chain reaction (PCR). Using a polyclonal antibody for immunostain at least two bacteria, *P. gingivalis* (42%) and *Streptococcus sanguis* (12%) were identified in the periphery of plaques by immunostain[54]. However, further studies using specific monoclonal antibodies would need to verify these results.

Investigations from the University of Buffalo had identified multiple oral bacteria from carotid endarterectomy specimens using PCR for 16S ribosomal RNA of oral pathogens, 44% of 50 atheromas were positive for at least one periodontal pathogen—*B. forysthus* was detected in 30%, *P. gingivalis* in 26%, *A. actinomycetemcomitans* in 18%, and *Prevotella intermedia* in 14%[55]. The same group also reported on finding one or more periodontal organisms from 39% of 96 carotid atheromas from a German population, using the same technique[56]. These findings have to be considered unproven until several studies from other centers have confirmed these results. As noted by Shor[57] "it seems improbable that pathologists examining these lesions (atheromas) could overlook such large organisms," especially with electron microscopic examinations.

6.4. BIOLOGICAL MECHANISMS

The biological basis for link between periodontal disease and atherosclerosis, CHD and stroke is illustrated in Figure 6.2, as proposed by Beck et al.[42] Cells of the monocytic lineage and the proinflammatory cytokines play a critical role in initiating and propagating both atheroma formation and periodontal disease. In their model, certain individuals with hyper-responsive monocytes (producing 3–10-fold greater amounts of mediators such as TNF-α, IL-1β, and prostaglandin E_2 (PGE_2) in response to LPS challenge than normal individuals) are at risk for early onset or refractory periodontitis, atherosclerosis, CHD, and insulin dependent diabetes mellitus[43,58–60].

LPS is released as extracellular blebs from microorganisms within periodontal pockets and may enter the circulation bound to LPS binding protein (LBP). When LPS is bound to LBP it is then able to bind to CD14 receptors, either soluble or on endothelium or on monocytes or macrophages, resulting in cellular activation. Cellular activation can produce upregulation of adhesion molecules and cytokine and chemokine release. These effects may result in subintimal leukocyte infiltration and proliferation of smooth-muscle cells in the blood vessel—initiating or enhancing atherosclerosis. Fibrinogen and white blood cell increases noted in periodontitis patients may be a secondary

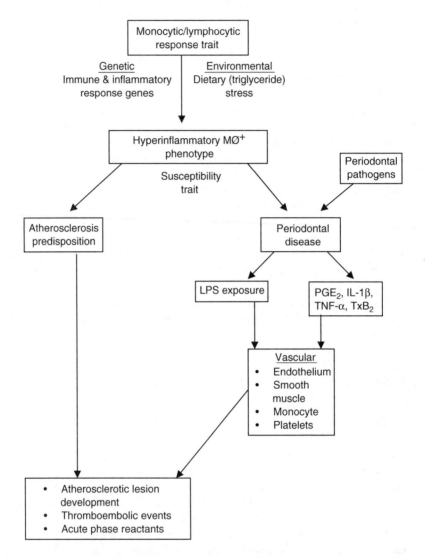

Figure 6.2. A biological basis for the link between periodontitis and atherosclerosis is illustrated as proposed by Beck et al.[42], adapted with the permission of the publishers.

effect of the proinflammatory cytokine activation or a constitutive feature of those at risk of both cardiovascular disease and periodontitis[61]. Soluble CD14 (SCD14) which mediates the response to LPS in cells lacking membrane-bound CD14 is increased in the sera of patients with periodontitis, probably due to chronic exposure to LPS[62].

It has been shown that cell-free pool of CD14 mediates activation of nuclear transcription factor NF-kB by LPS in human endothelial cells[63]. NF-kB controls the expression of many genes linked to atherogenesis including those involved in inflammation. It has been proposed the NF-kB is a key step that links the inflammatory state that accompanies periodontitis and atherogenesis[64]. The chronic and intense inflammatory response accompanying periodontal disease produces an excess of circulating mediators of inflammation that initiate or exacerbate the inflammatory components of atherosclerosis.

C-reactive protein (CRP), an acute response protein, is a well-established marker of inflammation and predictor of current and future cardiovascular events[65,66]. The blood levels may increase by 500-fold or more in response to severe infection or inflammation, and this is a host response to microbial invasion. CRP has anti-infective properties by binding to phosphocholine on microbe surfaces and marking them for killing by complement and phagocytes. It has been postulated that CRP may play a role in atherogenesis as this protein binds lipids of damaged cell membrane and fixes complement—thus, inducing a proinflammatory response. Hence CRP may enhance uptake of cholesterol by macrophages to help form fatty streaks. CRP may also play a role in precipitating acute ischemic attacks by stimulating tissue factor from monocytes to produce a procoagulant environment. There is evidence that CRP elevation occurs in periodontitis patients and the height of the increase is related to the severity of the disease[67,68]. Furthermore, specific treatment for periodontitis can reduce CRP concentration[69]. In an analysis of 10,000 participants of the Third National Health and Nutrition Survey, CRP and fibrinogen showed significant relation with poor periodontal status, but there was no significant association with total cholesterol or HDL cholesterol[70].

Thrombogenesis is intimately related to atherogenesis, and hypercoagulable or prothrombotic environment can precipitate or predispose to acute ischemic events. Infections can lead to a procoagulant state by several mechanisms, including increasing serum fibrinogen, platelet aggregation, and activation of blood coagulation factors. *P. gingivalis* and *Streptococcus sanguis* have been shown to induce platelet aggregation in vitro[71,72]. Adherence of the bacteria to platelet may be facilitated by *P. gingivalis* fimbriae and outer membrane vesicles possess potent platelet aggregating—inducing activity[72]. Furthermore, proteinases (gingipain—Rs) from *P. gingivalis* can cause activation of the blood coagulation factor X[73]. A potential mechanism by which periodontitis could play a role in atherogenesis is by direct invasion of the subintima of the arterial wall, leading to an inflammatory response, by periodontal pathogens. Oral bacteria frequently enter the blood circulation after chewing, brushing, or flossing the teeth especially in the presence of gingivitis and periodontitis. It has been shown that periodontal pathogens, especially *P. gingivalis*, are capable of invading bovine and human endothelial cells[74] and more specifically human coronary artery endothelial and smooth-muscle cells[75]. *A. actinomycetemcomitans*, another periodontal pathogen, has also been shown to be capable of invading human vascular endothelial cells via the receptor for platelet-activating factor[76]. *P. gingivalis* may survive intracellularly by evading the endocytic pathway to lysosomes and instead traffics to the autophagosome[77]. In addition *P. gingivalis* fimbrillin-specific peptides, LPS, or heat killed whole organisms can stimulate modest IL-8 and monocyte chemotactic protein-1(MCP-1) in human endothelial cells[78]. However, coculture with live *P. gingivalis* abolished the IL-8 and MCP-1 response, indicating that the organism can temporally modulate chemokine response in endothelial cells.

P. gingivalis and several other oral bacteria were recently shown to induce foam cell formation (a key characteristic of early lesions in atherogenesis) in the murine macrophage line[79]. This property appears to be mediated by LPS fraction of the cell, and it was demonstrated that *P. gingivalis* could degrade fibrous caps of atheromas from autopsy samples. Moreover, *P. gingivalis* could strongly induce MMD activity, implicated in plaque rupture, and enhance MCP-1 and NADH oxidose expression from endothelial cells[79].

6.4.1. Animal Models

Animal models are critical in the investigation of disease pathogenesis and establishing cause and effect relationships. There are only a few studies on periodontitis and animal models, and even less on the relationship with cardiovascular disease. *S. sanguis*, a supragingival plaque organism can increase platelet aggregation by expressing platelet aggregating associated protein (PAAP)[71,80] and may increase the risk of acute thrombosis. In a rabbit model, infusion of PAAP-positive *S. sanguis* resulted in acute electrocardio-graphic changes indicative of ischemia that are not seen with the PAAP-negative strain[80]. However, this model is substantially different from natural periodontal disease and explores the relationship with an acute bacteremic load and acute thrombosis.

The systemic effects of periodontitis in a non-human primate model has also been studied[81]. Ligature-induced periodontitis in *Macaca fascicularis* was produced over a four-month period, clinical measures of gingivitis and periodontitis were evaluated, and the serum levels of lipids, lipoprotein, endo-toxin, and acute phase reactants were measured. Increased levels above base-line were noted during the periodontitis stage for endotoxin ($p < 0.008$), fibrinogen (10-fold), and IL-8 and equivocal for CRP, but in the gingivitis stage, only IL-8 increased and CRP decreased. In 13 monkeys fed a normal chow diet, there was a trend toward increased total and LDL-cholesterol,

HDL-cholesterol showed little change but the apoA 1 levels were slightly decreased during both gingivitis and periodontitis stages[81]. ApoA-1 is an important component of the anti-atherogenic characteristics of HDL and is inversely related to CHD. Thus, in the animal model, periodontitis is capable of inducing mild changes of dyslipoproteinemia.

P. gingivalis repeated systemic inoculation, once a week for 24 weeks, have recently been reported to accelerate progression of atherosclerosis in a heterozygous apolipoprotein (apo)-E deficient murine model[82]. At 24 weeks after inoculation, proximal aorta lesion size quantified by histomorphometry was nine fold greater in regular chow fed mice inoculated with *P. gingivalis* than in non-inoculated mice ($p < 0.001$), and was two fold greater in the infected versus noninfected high fat diet fed mice ($p < 0.001$). *P. gingivalis* DNA was also found in the aortas and hearts 24 weeks after inoculation.

In a pilot study using five pigs (genetically predisposed to atherosclerosis) there was a trend to increased lesion area of the aorta and coronary artery compared to a control noninfected pig after initial immunization with heat killed *P. gingivalis*, followed by systemic inoculation of live organisms three times a week for 5 months[83]. Further experiments with a larger number of animals are needed to confirm these preliminary findings and demonstrate statistical significance.

The findings of these animal models are interesting and certainly suggest that periodontal pathogens, particularly *P. gingivalis*, are capable of accelerating atherosclerosis in animal models prone to the disease. However, the data would be more convincing if the same could be shown in animals using a periodontitis model to mimic human disease.

6.4.2. Clinical Trails

There are no reports of randomized interventional trial in patients with periodontitis to assess subsequent development of cardiovascular events. However, there is a preliminary report on short-term interventional study to detect changes in rheological risk factors for atherosclerotic disease following periodontal therapy[84]. Forty patients with periodontitis were recruited and of the thirty three subjects completing periodontal therapy, there were significant rises in clotting factors VII and VIII after treatment ($p < 0.05$), and a trend for Factor IX ($p = 0.06$). There was also a decrease in enzyme activity of platelet activating factor-acetylhydrolase (PAF-AH) after treatment, $p < 0.001$[84]. This preliminary analysis suggests that within 6–8 weeks of periodontal therapy there is a reduction in systemic PAF-AH activity and a perturbation of clotting factors VII, VIII, and IX. Another study looked at the effect of full mouth tooth extraction (the final cure for advanced periodontitis) on hemostatic risk factors before and after the procedure in 25 patients[85]. There was a 25% reduction in plasminogen activator inhibitor (PAI-1), $p = 0.009$, and a trend to reduced tissue plasminogen activator antigen (ePA), $p = 0.08$, and fibrinogen level, $p = 0.07$[85]. However, there was no change in CRP level. Thus, dental extraction (a cure for severe periodontitis) could modify systemic, thrombotic risk, a potential mechanism by which periodontal disease might be causally linked to cardiovascular disease. In another small pilot study, periodontal therapy/oral hygiene instructions, scaling and root planning reduced fibrinogen level by 15.3% and leukocytes by 6.4% 1–2 months after treatment in 20 patients[86]. Elevated fibrinogen and leukocytes are predictors of present and future cardiovascular disease.

6.5. FUTURE DIRECTIONS

Although the results of prospective studies on gingivitis and periodontal disease relationships with cardiovascular disease and stroke have been conflicting, large interventional trials are warranted. The data on biological mechanisms and the early animal models are sufficiently convincing to sanction the next major step in the investigation of this link. Randomized, longitudinal trials over several years need to be accomplished with standardized methods of examination, diagnosis, and treatment intermittently, in well-balanced groups of subjects. Adjustment for various confounding factors will need to be considered such as diet, physical activity, social economic status, smoking dose, comorbid illness such as diabetes, hypertension, etc.

Currently, a relatively large interventional trail is about to start but mainly powered to assess surrogate cardiovascular markers such as CRP, fibrinogen, cytokines, and adhesion molecules in subjects with periodontitis randomized to receive standard care versus intensive management (personal communication with Robert Genco).

Expansion of animal model data is also necessary to help elucidate any cause and effect relationship between oral health and atherosclerosis. These investigations should include usage of other models such as rabbits, guinea pigs, mini-pigs and more nonhuman primate animals if possible. Application of the periodontitis model for acceleration or initiation of atherosclerosis would also be necessary, rather than just systemic inoculation of periodontal pathogens.

In conclusion there is suggestive data that periodontitis and possibly gingivitis could play a role in the pathogenesis of atherosclerosis and the complicating diseases (myocardial infarction and stroke), but much more data are needed and the "jury is still undecided."

REFERENCES

1. Brown, L. J., & Löe, H. (1993) Prevalence, extent, severity and progression of periodontal disease, *Periodontol. 2000*, *2*, 57–71.
2. Haffajee, A. D., & Socransky, S. S. (1994) Microbial etiologic agents of destructive periodontal disease, *Periodontol. 2000*, *5*, 78–111.
3. Consensus report on periodontal disease, 1996, Pathogenesis and microbial factors, *Ann. Serotypes*, *1*, 926–932.
4. Socransky, S. S., Haffajee, A. D., Cugiri, M. A., Smith, C., & Kent, R. L. (1997) Microbial complexes in subgingival plaque, *J. Dent. Res.*, *76*(Special issue), *51* [Abstract 302].
5. Darveau, R. P., Tanner, A., & Page, R. C. (1997) The microbial challenge in periodontitis, *Periodontol. 2000*, *14*, 12–32.
6. Costerston, J. W., Lewandowski, Z., DeBeer, D., Caldwell, D., Korber, D., & James, G. (1994) Biofilms, the customized microniche, *J. Bacteriol.*, *176*, 2137–2142.
7. Murray, M., & Moonsrick, F. (1941) Incidence of bacteremia in patients with dental plaque, *J. Lab. Clin. Med.*, *26*, 801–802.
8. Sconyers, J. R., Crawford, J. J., & Moriarty, J. D. (1973) Relationships of bacteremia to tooth brushing in patients with periodontitis, *J. Am. Dent. Assoc.*, *87*, 616–622.
9. Carroll, G. C., & Sebor, R. J. (1980) Flossing and its relationships to transient bacteremia, *J. Periodontol.*, *51*, 691–692.
10. Chen, H. A., Johnson, B. D., Sims, T. J., Darveau, R. P., Moncla, B. J., Whitney, C. W., Engel, D., & Page, R. C. (1991) Humoral immune responses to *Porphyromonas gingivalis* before and following therapy in rapidly progressive periodontitis patients, *J. Periodontol.*, *62*, 781–791.
11. Reife, R. A., Shapiro, R. A., Bamber, B. A., Berry, K. K., Mick, G. E., & Darveau, R. P. (1995) *Porphyromonas gingivalis* lipopolysaccharide is poorly recognized by molecular components of innate host defense in a mouse model of early inflammation, *Infect. Immun.*, *63*, 4686–4694.
12. Page, R. C., & Kornmann, K. S. (1997) Pathogenesis of periodontitis. An introduction, *Periodontol. 2000*, *14*, 216–246.
13. Page, R. C. (1998) The pathobiology of periodontal diseases may affect systemic diseases: Inversion of a paradigm, *Ann. Periodontol.*, *3*, 108–120.
14. Page, R. C., Offenbacher, S., Schroeder, H. E., Seymour, G. J., & Kornman, R. S. (1997) Advances in the pathogenesis of periodontitis. Summary of developments, clinical implications and future directions, *Periodontol. 2000*, *14*, 216–248.
15. Page, R. C., & Schroeder, H. E. (Eds.) (1982) *Periodontitis in man and other animals*, Basel, Switzerland: S. Karger Publishers.
16. Clinton, S. K., Fleet, J. C., Loppnow, H., Salomon, R. N., Clark, B. D., Cannon, J. G., Shaw, A. R., Dinarello, C. A., & Libby, P. (1991) Interleukin 1 gene expression in rabbit vascular tissue in vivo, *Am. J. Pathol.*, *138*, 1005–1014.
17. Page, R. C., & Beck, J. D. (1997) Risk assessment for periodontal diseases, *Int. Dent. J.*, *47*, 61–67.

18. Michalowicz, B. S., Aeppli, D., Virag, J. G., Klump, D. G., Hinrichs, J. E., Segal, N. L., Bouchard, T. J. Jr., & Pihlstrom, B. L. (1991) Periodontal findings in adult twins, *J. Periodontol.*, *62*, 293–299.
19. Hart, T., & Kornman, K. S. (1997) Genetic factors in the pathogenesis of periodontitis, *Periodontol. 2000*, *14*, 202–215.
20. Marazita, M. L., Burmeister, J. A., Gimsolley, J. C., Koertge, T. E., Lake, K., & Schenkein, H. A. (1994) Evidence for autosomal dominant inheritance and race-specific heterogeneity in early-onset periodontitis, *J. Periodontol*, *65*, 623–630.
21. Wang, S., Sun, C., Gillanders, E., Wang, Y. F., Duffy, B., Bock,C., Freas-Lutz, D., Zhang, Y. J., Lopez, N., Schenkein, H., & Diehl, S. (1996) Genome scan for susceptibility loci to the complex disorder early onset periodontitis, *Am. J. Hum. Genet.*, *59*, 1386.
22. Whitney, C., Ant, J., Monela, B., Johnson, B., Page, R. C., & Engel, D. (1992) Serum immunoglobulin G-antibody to *Porphyromonas gingivalis* in rapidly progressive periodontitis, titer, avidity and subclass distribution, *Infect. Immun.*, *609*, 2194–2200.
23. Kornman, K. S., Crane, A., Wang, H. Y., di Giovine, F. S., Newman, M. G., Pirk, F. W., Wilson, T. G. Jr., Higginbottom, F. L., & Duff, G. W. (1997) The interleukin-1 genotype as a severity in adult periodontal disease, *J. Clin. Periodontol.*, *24*, 72–77.
24. Grossi, S. A., Zambon, J. J., Ho, A. W., Koch, G., Dunford, R. G., Machtei, E. E., Nordeyd, O. M., & Genco, R. J. (1994) Assessment of risk for periodontal disease. I. Risk indicators for attachment loss, *J. Periodontol.*, *65*, 260–267.
25. Genco, R. J., Ho, A. W., Kopman, J., Grossi, S. G., Dunford, R. G., & Tedesco, L. A. (1998) Models to evaluate the role of stress in periodontal disease, *Ann. Periodontol.*, *3*, 288–302.
26. Mattila, K. J., Nieminen, M. S., Valtonen, V. V., Rasi, V. P., Kesaniemi, Y. A., Syrjala, S. L., Jungell, P. S., Isoluoma, M., Hietaniemi, K., & Jokinen, M. (1989) Association between dental health and acute myocardial infarction, *BMJ*, *298*, 779–781.
27. Syrjanen, J., Peltola, J., Valtonen, V., Iivanainen, M., Kaste, M., & Huttunen, J. K. (1989) Dental infections in association with cerebral infarction in young and middle-aged men, *J. Intern. Med.*, *225*, 179–184.
28. Mattila, K. J., Valle, M. S., Nieminen, M. S., Valtonen, V. V., & Hietaniemi, K. L. (1993) Dental infections and coronary atherosclerosis, *Atherosclerosis*, *103*, 205–211.
29. Grau, A. J., Buggle, F., Ziegler, C., Schwartz, W., Meuser, J., Tasman, A. J., Buhler, A., Benesch, C., Becher, H., & Hacke, W. (1997) Association between acute cerebrovascular ischemia and chronic and recurrent infection, *Stroke*, *28*, 1724–1729.
30. Ziegler, C. M., Schwartz, W., Grau, A., Buggle, F., Hassfeld, S., & Muehling, J. (1998) Odontogener Fokus als Ursache Zerebraler Ischaemien, *Mund Kiefer Gesichts Chir*, *2*, 316–319.
31. Loesche, W. J., Schork, A., Terpenning, M. S., Chen, Y. M., Dominguez, B. L., & Grossman, N. (1998a) Assessing the relationships between dental infections and coronary heart disease in elderly US veterans, *JADA*, *129*, 301–311.

32. Loesche, W. J., Schork, A., Terpenning, M. S., Chen, Y. M., Kerr, C., & Dominguez, B. L. (1998b) The relationship between dental disease and cerebral vascular accidents, *Ann. Periodontol., 3,* 161–174.

33. Emingil, G., Buduneli, E., Aliyev, A., Akilli, A., & Atilla, G. (2000) Association between periodontal disease and acute myocardial infarction, *J. Periodontol., 71,* 1882–1886.

34. Mattila, K. J., Asikainen, S., Wolf, J., Jousimies-Somer, H., Valtonen, V., & Nieminen, M. (2000) Age, dental infections, and coronary heart disease, *J. Dent. Res., 79,* 756–760.

35. Paunio, K., Impivaara, O., Tiekso, J., & Maki, J. (1993) Missing teeth and ischaemic heart disease in men aged 45–64 years, *Eur. Heart J., 14*(Suppl K), 54–56.

36. Arbes, S. J. Jr., Slade, G. D., & Beck, J. D. (1999) Association between extent of periodontal disease and attachment loss and self-reported history of heart attack: an analysis of NHANES III data, *J. Dent. Res., 78,* 1777–1782.

37. Takata, Y., Ansai, T., Matsumura, K., Awano, S., Hamasaki, T., Sonoki, K., Kusaba, A., Akifusa, S., & Takehara, T. (2001) Relationship between tooth loss and electrocardiographic abnormalities in octogenarians, *J. Dent. Res., 80,* 1648–1652.

38. Beck, J. D., Elter, J. R., Heiss, G., Couper, D., Mauriello, S. M., & Offenbacher, S. (2001) Relationship of periodontal disease to carotid artery intima-media wall thickness: the atherosclerotic risk in communities (ARIC) study, *Arterioscler. Thromb. Vasc. Biol., 21,* 1816–1822.

39. Joshipura, K. J., Douglass, C. W., & Willett, W. C. (1998) Possible explanations for the tooth loss and cardiovascular disease relationship, *Ann. Periodontol., 3,* 175–183.

40. DeStefano, F., Anda, R. F., Kahn, H. S., Williamson, D. F., & Russell, C. M. (1993) Dental disease and risk of coronary heart disease and mortality, *BMJ, 306,* 688–691.

41. Mattila, K. J., Valtonen, V. V., Neiminen, M., & Huttunen, J. K. (1995) Dental infection and the risk of new coronary events: prospective study of patients with documented coronary artery disease, *Clin. Infect. Dis., 20,* 588–592.

42. Beck, J., Garcia, R., Heiss, G., Vokonas, P. S., & Offenbacher, S. (1996) Periodontal disease and cardiovascular disease, *J. Periodontol., 67*(Suppl 10), 1123–1137.

43. Joshipura, K. J., Rimm, E. B., Douglass, C. W., Trichopoulas, D., Ascherio, A., & Willett, W. C. (1996) Poor oral health and coronary heart disease, *J. Dent. Res., 75,* 1631–1636.

44. Genco, R., Chadda, S., Grossi, S., Dunford, R., Taylor, G., & Knowler, W. (1997) Periodontal disease is a predictor of cardiovascular disease in a Native North American population, *J. Dent. Res., 76* [Abstract 3158] (special issue), 408.

45. Morrison, H. I., Ellison, L. F., & Taylor, G. W. (1999) Periodontal disease and risk of fatal coronary heart and cerebrovascular disease, *J. Cardiovasc. Risk, 6,* 7–11.

46. Hujoel, P. P., Drangsholt, M., Spiekerman, C., & De Rouen, T. A. (2000) Periodontal disease and coronary heart disease risk, *JAMA, 284,* 1406–1410.

47. Wu, T., Trevisan, M., Genco, R. J., Dorn, J. P., Falkner, K. L., & Sempos, C. T. (2000) Periodontal disease and risk of cerebrovascular disease: the first National health and nutritional examination survey and its follow up study, *Arch. Intern. Med.*, *160*, 2749–2755.

48. Howell, T. H., Ridker, P. M., Ajani, U. A., Hennekens, C. H., & Christen, W. G. (2001) Periodontal disease and risk of subsequent cardiovascular disease in US male physicians, *J. Am. Coll. Cardiol.*, *37*, 445–450.

49. Jansson, L., Lavstedt, S., Frithiof, L., & Theobald, H. (2001) Relationship between oral health and mortality in cardiovascular diseases, *J. Clin. Periodontol.*, *28*, 762–768.

50. Hujoel, P. P., Drangsholt, M., Spiekerman, C., & De Rouen, T. A. (2002) Pre-exiting cardiovascular disease and oral periodontitis: a follow-up study, *J. Dent. Res.*, *81*, 186–191.

51. Mendez, M. V., Scott, T., LaMorte, W., Vokonas, P., Menzoian, J. O., & Garcia, R. (1998) An association between periodontal disease and peripheral vascular disease, *Am. J. Surg.*, *176*, 153–157.

52. Hujoel, P. P., Drangsholt, M., Spiekerman, C., & DeRouen, T. A. (2001) Examining the link between coronary heart disease and the elimination of chronic dental infections, *JADA*, *132*, 883–889.

53. Thorstensson, H., Kuylenstierna, J., & Hugoson, A. (1996) Medical status and complications in relation to periodontal disease experience in insulin-dependent diabetics, *J. Clin. Periodontol.*, *23*, 194–202.

54. Chiu, B. (1999) Multiple infections in carotid atherosclerotic plaques, *Am. Heart J.*, *138*, S534–S536.

55. Haraszthy, V. I., Zambon, J. J., Trevisan, M., Zeid, M., & Genco, R. J. (2000) Identification of periodontal pathogens in atheromatous plaques, *J. Periodontol.*, *71*, 1554–1560.

56. Haraszthy, V. I., Jordan, S. F., Zambon, J. J., Zafiropoulos, G. G., Mastragelopulos, N., & Genco, R. J. (2001) Periodontal pathogens in atheromas from a German population, *Ann. Periodontal.*, *6*, 64 [Abstract].

57. Shor, A. (2001) A pathologist's view of organisms and human atherosclerosis, *J. Infect. Dis.*, *183*, 1428–1429.

58. Shapira, L., Soskolne, W. A., Sela, M. N., Offenbacher, S., & Barak, V. (1994) The secretion of PGE_2 and IL-1β, IL-6 and TNFα by monocytes from early onset periodontitis patients, *J. Periodontol.*, *65*, 139–146.

59. Offenbacher, S., Heasman, P. A., & Collins, J. G. (1993) Modulation of most PGE_2 secretion as a determinant of periodontal disease expression, *J. Periodontol.*, *64*, 432–444.

60. Yalda, B., Collins, J. B., Arnold, R. R., & Offenbacher, S. (1994) Monocytic and crevicular fluid PGE_2 and IL-1β in diabetic patients, *J. Dent. Res.*, *73* (special issue), 394 [Abstract 2337].

61. Kweider, M., Lowe, G. D. O., Murray, G. D., Kinane, D. F., & McGowan, D. A. (1993) Dental disease, fibrinogen and white cell count: links with myocardial infarction? *Scot. Med. J.*, *38*, 73–74.

62. Hayashi, J., Masaka, T., & Ishikawa, I. (1999) Increased levels of soluble CD14 in sera of periodontitis patients, *Infect. Immun.*, *67*, 417–420.

63. Read, M. A., Cordle, S. R., Veach, R. A., Carlisle, C. D., & Hawiger, J. (1993) Cell-free pool of CD14 mediates activation of transcription factor NF-kβ by lipopolysaccharide in human endothelial cells, *Proc. Natl. Acad. Sci. USA, 90*, 9887–9891.

64. Nicols, T. C., Fischer, T. H., Deliargyris, E. N., & Baldwin, A. S., Jr. (2001) Role of nuclear factor kappa B (NF-kB) in inflammation, periodontitis, and atherogenesis, *Ann. Periodontol., 6*, 20–29.

65. Danesh, J., Collins, R., Appleby, P., & Peto. R. (1998) Fibrinogen, C-reactive protein, albumin or white blood cell count: meta-analyses of prospective studies of coronary heart disease, *JAMA, 279*, 1477–1482.

66. Ridker, P. M., Hennekens, C. H., Buring, J. E., & Rifai, N. (2000) C-reactive protein and other markers of inflammation in the prediction of cardiovascular disease in women, *N. Engl. J. Med., 342*, 836–843.

67. Noack, B., Genco, R. J., Trevisan, M., Grossi, S., Zamban, J. J., & De Nardin, E. (2001) Periodontal infections contribute to elevated systemic C-reactive protein level, *J. Periodontol., 72*, 1221–1227.

68. Slade, G. D., Offenbacher, S., Beck, J. D., Heiss, G., & Pankow, J. S. (2000) Acute-phase inflammatory response to periodontal disease in the US population, *J. Dent. Res., 79*, 49–57.

69. Ebersole, J. L., Machen, R. L., Steffen, M. L., & Willmann, D. E. (1997) Systemic acute phase reactants, C-reactive protein and haptoglobin, in adult periodontitis, *Clin. Exp. Immunol., 107*, 347–352.

70. Wu, T., Trevisan, M., Genco, R. J., Falkner, K. L., Dorn, J. P., & Sempos, C. T. (2000) Examination of the relation between periodontal health status and cardiovascular risk factors; serum total and high density lipoprotein cholesterol, C-reactive protein, and plasma fibrinogen, *Am. J. Epidemiol., 151*, 273–282.

71. Erikson, P. R., & Herzberg, M. C. (1987) A collagen-like immunodeterminant on the surface of *Streptococcus sanguis* induces platelet aggregation, *J. Immunol., 138*, 3360–3366.

72. Sharma, A., Novak, E. K., Sojar, H. T., Swank, R. T., Kuramitsu, H. K., & Genco, R. J. (2000) *Porphyromonas gingivalis* platelet aggregation activity: outer membrane vesicles are potent activators of murine platelets, *Oral Microbiol. Immunol., 15*, 393–396.

73. Imamura, T., Potempa, J., Tanase, S., & Travis, J. (1997) Activation of blood coagulation factor X by arginine-specific cysteine proteinases (gingipain-RS) from *Porphyromonas gingivalis*, *J. Biol. Chem., 272*, 16062–16067.

74. Deshpande, R. G., Khan, M. B., & Genco, C. A. (1998) Invasion of aortic and heart endothelial cells by *Porphyromonas gingivalis*, *Infect. Immun., 66*, 5337–5343.

75. Dorn, B. R., Dunn, W. A. Jr., & Progulske-Fox, A. (1999) Invasion of human coronary artery cells by periodontal pathogens, *Infect. Immun., 67*, 5792–5798.

76. Schienkein, H. A., Barbour, S. E., Berry, C. R., Kipps, B., & Tew, J. G. (2000) Invasion of human vascular endothelial cells by *Actinobacillus actinomycetemcomitans* via the receptor for platelet-activating factor, *Infect. Immun., 68*, 5416–5419.

77. Dorn, B. R., Dunn, W. A., & Progulske-Fox, A. (2001) *Porphyromonas gingivalis* traffics to autophagosomes in human coronary artery endothelial cells, *Infect. Immun.*, *69*, 5698–5708.
78. Nassar, H., Chou, H. H., Khlgatian, M., Gibson, F. C. 3rd, Van Dyke, T. E., & Genco, C. A. (2002) Role for fimbriae and lysine-specific cysteine proteinase gingipain K in expression of interleukin-8 and monocyte chemoattractant protein in *Porphyromonas gingivalis* infected endothelial cells, *Infect. Immun.*, *70*, 268–270.
79. Kuramitsu, H. K., Qi, M., Kang, I. C., & Chen, W. (2001) Role for periodontal bacteria in cardiovascular disease, *Ann. Periodontol.*, *6*, 41–47.
80. Herzberg, M. C., & Meyer, M. W. (1998) Dental plaque, platelets and cardiovascular disease, *Ann. Periodontol.*, *3*, 151–160.
81. Ebersole, J. L., Cappelli, D., Mott, G., Kesavalu, L., Holt, S. C., & Stinger, R. E. (1999) Systemic manifestations of periodontitis in the non-human primate, *J. Periodontal. Res.*, *34*, 358–362.
82. Li, L., Messas, E., Batista, E. L., Jr., Levine, R. A., & Amar, S. (2002) *Porphyromonas gingivalis* infection accelerates the progression of atherosclerosis in a heterozygous apolipoprotein E-deficient murine model, *Circulation*, *105*, 861–867.
83. Brodala, B., Madianos, P. N., Geva, S., Offenbacher, S., Beck, J. D., Fischer, T., Smith, S., Bellinger, D. A., & Nichols, T. C. (2001) Recurrent *Porphyromonas gingivalis* bacteremia induces atherosclerosis in susceptible pigs, *Ann. Periodontol.*, *6*, 63 [Abstract].
84. Marshall, G. J., Kinane, D. F., Lowe, G. D. O., Lösche, W., Rumley, A., & Apatzidou, D. (2001) Changes in rheological cardiovascular risk factors after periodontal therapy, *Ann. Periodontol.*, *6*, 59 [Abstract].
85. Taylor, B., Tofler, G., Philcox, S., Carey, H., Champion, H., Elliot, M., Kull, A., Morel-Kopp, M. C., & Schenck, K. (2001) Full-mouth tooth extraction lowers hemostatic risk: periodontal cardiovascular study (PERICAR), *Ann. Periodontol.*, *6*, 61 [Abstract].
86. Hermans, M., Daelemans, P., El Mahi, T., Le Roux, B., & Sauvêtre, E. (2001) Reduction of the plasma fibrinogen level and the white blood cell count after initial periodontal therapy, *Ann. Periodontol.*, *6*, 63 [Abstract].

7

Cytomegalovirus and Herpes Simplex Virus in Cardiovascular Disease

7.1. INTRODUCTION

Interest in the herpes group of viruses as causally associated with atherosclerosis and cardiovascular disease was evident from the 1970s. Subsequently, interest waned over the years, but has been renewed in the past decade with rising interest of infectious agents and cardiovascular disease relationship that has been widely publicized.

7.2. MICROBIOLOGY

7.2.1. Cytomegalovirus

Human cytomegalovirus (HCMV) is a β herpes virus and the largest virus to infect human beings. Its genome encodes 230 proteins many of which play a significant role in downregulation of the immune system[1]. The CMV genome is a linear double-stranded DNA molecule of 230 million Da that has been completely sequenced[2]. Like all human herpes viruses, it encodes DNA polymerase gene and genes needed for its own DNA replication. The viral DNA polymerase is a target for antiviral drugs and the current therapies inhibit this enzyme as the final target[3]. The CMV genome also encodes a protein phosphotransferase enzyme, whose role in DNA replication is not well understood[3]. CMV is able to evade immune control by production of several proteins that downregulate the host immune system. One of the most important CMV proteins prevents HLA-1 molecule from reaching the cell surface and thus, impairs recognition and destruction of the virus by CD8 lymphocytes[4], there by avoiding immune destruction of the virus and allowing a persistent latent infection. The double-stranded DNA is wrapped in a nucleoprotein core, surrounded by matrix proteins, the pp65 antigen of CMV, which is important for diagnosis of CMV and can be detected in cells by immunofluorescence, immunoperoxidase, and other antigen detection methods[5].

The specific cellular protein receptor for CMV entry has not been identified but virus infects and enters the cell by endocytosis. The CMV genome is uncoated within the cell and the DNA core is transported to the nucleus, where replication occurs following synthesis of DNA polymerase. A large eosinophilic nuclear inclusion appears (representing aggregates of replicating CMV nucleoprotein cores), which is valuable in establishing the diagnosis of CMV infection in patients[6].

CMV, like other herpes viruses, can remain latent in the cells after infection and persistence of the genome and antigen can be detected in many tissues (including vascular tissue) and circulating leukocytes[7]. The mechanisms controlling latency are unknown but the ability to evade immune destruction by downregulating cell surface markers such as HLA-1, may contribute to the capacity of the virus to remain undetected[4].

The replication of the virus is relatively slow and newly made infectious particles are first detected in 48–72 hr after infection. The maturation of viral particles appear to be inefficient, hence the yield of infectious virus in tissue cultures is low and as many as 10^6 particles are needed to initiate infection of tissue culture. Virus has been isolated and propagated only in human fibroblasts, and cultivated epithelial cells are not infected in vitro, despite prominent involvement in disease. Although initially labeled as salivary gland virus, cytomegalovirus can affect many organs such as the brain, heart, eye, kidneys, liver, lungs, adrenal, and tissues such as lymph nodes, vasculature, the gut, endothelial, and epithelial tissue. Although many species of animals are infected with their specific cytomegaloviruses (e.g., murine cytomegalovirus), no laboratory animal has proved susceptible to infection with HCMV.

The laboratory diagnosis of CMV infection can be made by culturing the virus from body fluids, urine, or tissues; by direct detection of antigen (matrix protein pp65) in neutrophils (using a monoclonal antibody) which has been useful in immunosuppressed hosts[8]; or by detection of intranuclear inclusion in tissues or DNA by PCR[9] in body fluids or tissues. Acute and convalescent sera with a fourfold rise in titer, or elevated IgM antibody can be used to diagnose acute infection in normal hosts.

7.2.2. Herpes Simplex Virus

Herpes simplex virus (HSV), also a member of the herpes viruses family is also a DNA virus that replicates in the cell nucleus, and like other members of the family has special affinity for cells of ectodermal origin and tends to produce latent infections, a characteristic that would be suitable in atherogenesis. The morphology of all herpes viruses is similar. They consist of a DNA-containing core approximately 760 Å in diameter, an icosahedral capsid 950–1050 Å in diameter, a surrounding granular zone, an encompassing envelope possessing periodic short projections. The envelope appears to contain both host cell and viral components. The envelope is important for adsorption to susceptible host cells and HS virions are agglutinated by antibodies to uninfected cells. Several receptors for viral attachment have been identified, including heparan sulfate and members of the tumor necrosis factor (TNF) family of proteins[10,11].

Although HSV is cytopathic to cells that harbor the full replication cycle, infection of some neuronal cells does not result in cell death. Instead the viral genomes are maintained by the cell in a repressed latent state. Latency is associated with transcription of a limited number of virus encoded proteins[12]. With reactivation of the virus there is release of the virus from the neuron and subsequent entry into epithelial cells with resulting viral replication[13]. The molecular mechanisms of latency of HSV are not well understood.

Two immunological variants, types 1 (mostly associated with oral lesions) and 2 (mainly genital lesions) can be distinguished, and although cross-reactivity between the variants is prominent, some minor antigenic variations have been observed. The genome structures of the two HSV subtypes are similar and the overall sequence homology between HSV-1 and HSV-2 is about 50%[13]. Restriction endonuclease analysis of viral DNA can distinguish between the two subtypes and among strains of each subtype[14].

The viral envelope appears to fuse with the cells' plasma membrane, permitting the viral nucleocapsid to enter directly into the cytoplasm. Intact viruses may also enter into phagocytic vacuoles, from which they are released by similar viral envelope membrane fusion. In the cytoplasm, the capsid separates from the viral core, which enters the nucleus and initiates viral multiplication. The virion can replicate itself within 5–6 hr and in cell culture each cell has made 10^4–10^5 particles within 17 hr of infection. The biochemical events responsible for viral replication are similar to those of CMV and other DNA viruses. The formation of viral particles correlates with development of basophilic nuclear inclusion bodies. Assembly of the complete virus is accomplished by a coat (capsid) around the DNA, and thus the envelope is acquired from the nuclear membrane or cytoplasmic membrane as the viral particles egress into the cytoplasm. The envelope contains virus-specific sub-units (glycoproteins) as well as host cell material. The basophilic intranuclear inclusion is converted into an eosinophilic inclusion body in the cytoplasm, burnt out remnants of the viral factory with no specific viral antigens. Man is the natural host for HSV, but a relatively wide range of animals are also susceptible, including mice, guinea pigs, hamsters, rabbits, and chick embryos.

The laboratory diagnosis of HSV infection is best confirmed by isolation of the virus by culture or by demonstration of HSV antigen or DNA in lesions or tissues. Antigen detection in asymptomatic subjects from cervical or salivary secretions, however, is only 50% as sensitive as viral isolation[13]. PCR techniques appear to be more sensitive than viral isolation in late lesions and central nervous system involvement.

Acute and convalescent-phase serum can be useful in primary HSV infection, but only 5% of patients with recurrent mucocutaneous disease have fourfold or greater rise in titer[13]. Type-specific assays to identify carriers of HSV-1 or HSV-2 infection are available[15], but are usually used mainly for research purposes.

7.2.3. Epidemiology of Cytomegalovirus and Herpes Simplex Virus

Infection with CMV is common in all populations, reaching 60–70% in urban US cities and nearly 100% of underdeveloped countries, such as in Africa! Most patients never have recognized clinical disease but occasionally present with acute CMV mononuclear syndrome, congenital disease, or reactivation from latent state after immunosuppression.

HSV also has a universal distribution with more than 90% of adults having antibodies to HSV-1 by the fifth decade of life[13]. In the United States, antibodies to HSV-1 were detected in about 50% of higher and 80% of lower socioeconomic groups by age 30, whereas, HSV-2 seroprevalence in adults was about 22%[13].

7.3. ASSOCIATION OF CYTOMEGALOVIRUS AND CARDIOVASCULAR DISEASE

Evidence of association between atherosclerotic complications (cardiovascular disease and stroke) and CMV have been examined by seroepidemiological and pathological evidence of CMV infection. Studies have been performed in three groups of subjects:

1. Patients with native coronary heart disease (CHD);
2. Patients who have undergone percutaneous transluminal coronary angioplasty (PTCA), with or without stenting;
3. Recipients of cardiac transplantation.

7.3.1. Epidemiological Association of Cytomegalovirus in Native Coronary Heart Disease

There have been at least 18 cross-sectional or retrospective case-control studies on the association between CMV serology and CHD or carotid artery disease, see Table 7.1. Some studies used high CMV titers ($>$1:800) but others did not. Five of these studies assessed intima media thickness (IMT) or stenosis of the carotid artery (two included femoral and or popliteal arteries as well)[16–20]. Only two of these five studies showed a positive correlation with CMV antibody and increased evidence of atherosclerosis (odds ratio [OR] 1.2–2.3)[18,20].

Six studies assessed the relationships of CMV serology and CHD by coronary angiogram, mainly using $>$50% to $>$60% stenosis as significant CHD[21–26]. Of these six studies, only one showed a significant association of CHD with CMV antibody[22].

Six other studies using clinical endpoints for CHD or need for vascular surgery or PTCA assessed the association with past CMV infection and cardiovascular disease[27–32], and another study used pathological findings from explanted hearts from cardiac transplant recipients[33]. Four of these studies showed an overall positive association with CMV antibodies and CHD, and another study found significant association only in young patients (OR 3.6)[33]. Thus, overall only 7/18 ($\approx$39%) of the cross-sectional or case control studies found an association of CMV with CHD or carotid artery disease.

There have been at least 15 prospective, longitudinal studies on CMV infection and cardiovascular or cerebrovascular disease, see Table 7.2. Follow up varied from 6 months to 15 years, with a mean follow up of 5.5 years. Fourteen of these studies assessed clinical end points (myocardial infarction, need for revascularization, cardiovascular death, or stroke)[34–47], and one study assessed progress of carotid atherosclerosis by ultrasound[48]. One study used the presence of CMV DNA in peripheral blood mononuclear cells, besides serology[47]. In all, only 3 of the 15 studies showed a significant positive association with CHD or carotid artery disease and CMV infection, including the

Table 7.1

Retrospective and Cross-sectional Studies on Atherosclerosis and
Cytomegalovirus Seropositivity

Study	Subjects (cases/controls)	Measure of atherosclerosis	Result	Comments
Adams et al. 1987[27]	113/113 men	Vascular surgery for atherosclerosis	OR = 3.5 (1.45–5.6)	Controls had high LDL but developed no clinical CHD during 7-year follow up
Sorlie et al. 1994[16]	340/340	Asymptomatic carotid wall thickness	OR = 1.36 ($p = 0.24$)	Subjects with cardiovascular disease were excluded
Dummer et al. 1994[33]	314 transplant candidates	CHD at autopsy	OR = 3.6 (1.4–8.9) for young patients	No association overall or in the 3 older quartiles
Lindberg et al. 1997[17]	267/267	Asymptomatic carotid wall thickness	OR = 1.2 (0.7–2)	Subjects with cardiovascular disease were excluded
Adler et al. 1998[21]	900 having coronary angiogram	>50% coronary stenosis	OR = 1.18 (0.82–1.7)	IgG levels to CMV whole cell and to CMV glycoprotein B studied
Blum et al. 1998[22]	65/65	Single coronary lesion	OR = 6.03 (2.63–13.85)	Cutoff: IgG > 1/800. Also found prospective association with restenosis after angioplasty
Anderson et al. 1998[23]	219/126	>60% coronary stenosis	OR = 1.19 (0.7–1.2)	Controls had <10% stenosis
Kafton et al. 1999[28]	150/160	CHD	OR = 3.62 (1.93–6.76)	Difference found only when IgG >1/800 considered
Tiran et al. 1999[29]	112/112	Need for PTCA	OR = 3.3 (0.9–15) for anti-CMV, +6 (1.3–38) for anti-pp150	High titers considered. Controls were mostly blood donors
Rothenbacher et al. 1999[25]	312/479	>50% coronary stenosis	OR = 1.21 (0.84–1.75)	Controls were blood donors

Table 7.1

(continued)

Study	Subjects (cases/controls)	Measure of atherosclerosis	Result	Comments
Sepulveda et al. 1999[26]	321/113 having coronary angiogram	Lesions in coronary arteries	OR = 0.62 (0.13–2.93)	Cutoff titer 6 by EIA—97–98% of the population was positive
Zhu et al. 2000[24]	238 having coronary angiogram	Coronary arteries not smooth	OR = 1.83 (0.86–3.87)	OR = 41.8 (4.12–423) for the 87 women of the study
Espinola-Klein et al. 2000[18]	504	High carotid IMT plus stenosis	OR = 2.3 (1.1–4.9)	Patients with known cerebrovascular diseases were excluded
Mayr et al. 2000[19]	826	Carotid and femoral IMT	OR = 1.01 (0.91–1.12)	Population-based study
Smieja et al. 2001a[32]	107/107	Angina, MI	OR = 0.7 (0.4–1.3)	Controlled only for age and sex
Gattone et al. 2001[30]	120/120 <50 y old	MI	OR = 2.9 (1.5–5.8)	
Burian et al. 2001[31]	248/53	>50% coronary stenosis	OR = 1.08 (0.57–2.04)	Ab to immediate-early—1 CMV antigen assessed. Controls free of CHD
Espinola-Klein et al. 2002[20]	246/61	Coronary plus carotid or leg arteries atherosclerosis	OR = 1.2 (1.01–1.37)	Prospective association with "pathogen burden" also found

Note. CHD, coronary heart disease; MI, myocardial infarction; OR, odds ratio; RR, relative risk; CMV, cytomegalovirus; IMT, intimal medial thickness; EIA, enzyme immunoassay; Ab, antibody; y, years; mo: months; PTCA, percutaneous transluminal coronary angioplasty; HR, hazards ratio.

study assessing carotid IMT[48] (OR ranged from 0.71 to 5.3 for all the studies).

Eight studies assessed the relationships between restenosis after PTCA and CMV seropositivity[49–57], see Table 7.3. The process involved in restenosis, fibromuscular hyperplasia, is not quite the same as atherosclerosis. It has been postulated that CMV infection of smooth-muscle cells inactivates the tumor suppressive protein p53, thus allowing unchecked smooth-muscle proliferation[58]. The initial report by Zhou et al.[49] showed a strong association with CMV and restenosis 6 months after PTCA (OR 12.9, 95% CI, 2.3–71.1). However, only three of the eight studies showed an association of restenosis

Table 7.2

Prospective Studies on Atherosclerosis and Cytomegalovirus Seropositivity

Study	Subjects	Follow up	End point	Results	Comments
1. Nieto et al. 1996[48]	150/150	13–15 y	Carotid IMT	OR = 5.3 (1.5–18) for high titer	Graded relation between odds for IMT and titers ($p = 0.013$)
2. Ossewaarde et al. 1998[34]	54/108	5 y	CHD event	RR = 0.95 (0.78–1.16)	
3. Ridker et al. 1998[35]	643/643 men	12 y	MI, ischemic stroke	RR = 0.72 (06–0.9)	
4. Ridker et al. 1999[36]	122/244 women	3 y	CHD event, stroke	RR = 1.0 (06–1.7)	
5. Danesh et al. 1999[37]	288/704	4 y	CHD	OR = 1.4 (0.96–2.05)	Adjusted for childhood social class
6. Fagerberg et al. 1999[38]	152 men cohort	3.5 y	Cardiovascular, cerebrovascular events	RR = 0.63 (0.18–2.21)	Some serology results were cross-sectional
7. Haider et al. 1999[39]	1503 men cohort	10 y	MI, CHD death, atherothrombotic stroke	HR = 0.88 (0.64–1.12)	
8. Roivainen et al. 2000[40]	241/241 men	8.5 y	MI, CHD death	RR = 0.96 (0.83–1.11)	Comparison between 1–2nd vs. 4th quartile
9. Sorlie et al. 2000[41]	221/515	5 y	CHD event	RR = 1.89 (0.98–3.67) for high titer	Marked increase of RR with diabetes
10. Siscovick et al. 2000[42]	213/405	3.5–5.5 y	MI, CHD death	OR = 1.2 (0.7–1.9)	Unable to measure titers
11. Mulhestein et al. 2000[43]	985 with CHD	2.7 y	Death	HR = 1.9 ($p < 0.05$)	
12. Choussat et al. 2001[44]	79 with unstable CHD	1 y	CHD event	OR = 0.71 ($p = 0.71$)	
13. Zhu et al. 2001[45]	890 with CHD	3 y	MI, death	RR = 2 (1.4–2.3)	Association with "pathogen burden" in dose-response fashion
14. Smieja et al. 2001b[47]	208 with CHD	6 mo	CHD events or need for revascularization	OR = 0.9 (0.5–1.7)	OR = 1.4 (0.6–3) for CMV DNA in PBMC
15. Rupprecht et al. 2001[46]	1010 with CHD	3.1 y	MI, CHD death	HR = 1.4 (0.7–3.0)	Association with "pathogen burden"

Table 7.3
Studies of Cytomegalovirus Seropositivity and Restenosis after
Percutaneous Transluminal Coronary Procedures

Study	Patients	Follow up	Procedure	Result	Comments
Zhou et al. 1996[49]	75	6 mo	Atherectomy	OR = 12.9 (2.3–71.1)	OR = 8.1 for higher vs. lower IgG titer, no IgM detected
Muhlestein et al. 1997[50]	255	6 mo	Balloon or stent	OR = 0.96 (0.44–2.1)	
Thomas et al. 1997[51]	82	NS	Balloon or atherectomy	No association	
Blum et al. 1998[52]	65	1 y	Balloon	RR = 2.56 (1.56–4.21)	Titers not changed during next 3 months
Manegold et al. 1999[53]	92	6 mo	Balloon	OR = 1.0 (0.48–2.1)	
Carlsson et al. 2000[54]	148	6 mo	Balloon	OR = 0.9 ($p = 0.82$)	
Neumann et al. 2000,[55]	551	30 days	Stent	3% vs. 0% ($p < 0.001$)	End point: death, myocardial infarction, urgent reintervention
Neumann et al. 2001[56]		1 y	Stent	OR = 0.78 (0.52–1.19)	82% of patients followed by angiogram
Schiele et al. 2001[57]	179	6 mo	Stent	OR = 0.44 (0.21–0.89)	Evaluated 3 variables of restenosis by angiogram and intravascular ultrasound. No difference in mean neointimal tissue area

or clinical end points with CMV seropositivity following PTCA. In the largest of these studies, however, involving 551 patients, acute thrombotic events within 30 days of PTCA and stenting was significantly greater in those seropositive for CMV, 3% versus 0%, $p < 0.001$[55]. Further follow up at 1 year, however, showed no significant difference in restenosis in patients with or without CMV antibodies[56].

7.3.2. Epidemiological Association of Cytomegalovirus in Cardiac Transplant

The most compelling data supporting an association of CMV infection with CHD exists for heart transplant recipients, and the subsequent development of allograft vasculopathy. There have been at least 22 studies addressing this issue, summarized in Table 7.4. A total of 2,681 patients have been studied, with follow up varying from 6 months to over 10 years. Three of the studies involved mainly children[59-61], and the other studies were in the adult popluation[62-81]. Twelve of the twenty two (54.5%) showed an overall association of CMV infection with coronary arteriosclerosis. In another study, CMV infection was significantly associated with coronary occlusion at 2 years but not at 4 years post-transplantation[70]; suggesting that CMV infection accelerates the coronary vasculopathy. Furthermore, although there was a greater 6-year mortality in patients with post-transplantation CMV infection than those without (46.0% vs. 26.7%), there was no significant association of post-transplantation graft arteriosclerosis and CMV status in a separate study[68].

7.3.3. Epidemiological Association of Herpes Simplex Virus and Atherosclerotic Disease

There are fewer studies examining the relationships of HSV with cardiovascular or cerebrovascular disease compared to CMV. Six retrospective case-control and cross-sectional studies[16-18,20,27,82] are summarized in Table 7.5. Only one of the six studies showed a small positive association between HSV-2 serology and atherosclerotic changes/stenosis of the coronary, carotid and or peripheral arteries[20].

Eight prospective studies have assessed the association of HSV with CHD or stroke, see Table 7.6[35,36,40-42,45,46,83]. Only two of the eight studies showed a significant association of HSV antibodies and CHD[40,42], with OR of about 2.0.

7.4. PATHOLOGICAL STUDIES

There have been many studies examining arterial tissues for the presence of herpes viruses, predominantly CMV and to a lesser extent HSV. Most of the studies used PCR or in situ hybridization to detect viral nucleic acids, but a few studies have used immunohistochemistry (IHC) or electron microscopy (EM).

Table 7.4
Cytomegalovirus Infection and Cardiac Allograft Vasculopathy in the Cyclosporine Era

Study	Subjects	End point	Result	Comments
Grattan et al. 1989[62]	301	Rejection by >70% biopsy; occlusion by angiogram, CHD	All end points associated at 5 y ($p < 0.05$)	No difference between symptomatic vs asymptomatic or primary vs reinfection
McDonald et al. 1989[63]	102, 1 y+ post	CHD by angiogram	Associated ($p = 0.007$)	
Braunlin et al. 1991[59]	17 children 1 y+ post-transplant	CHD by angiogram	Non significant association ($p = 0.11$)	6 patients with CHD
Sharples et al. 1991[64]	323 first grafts	CHD by angiogram, autopsy	No association	
Everett et al. 1992[65]	129	CHD by angiogram	47 vs. 18% ($p = 0.012$)	Association found only with prolonged (>4 mo) viremia
Koskinen et al. 1993a,b[66,67]	53	CHD by angiogram and biopsy	Associated with 4 histological & angiogram indicators	Histology evolved during first 2 y, angiogram changes followed
Chinnock et al. 1993[60]	207 children	Rejection (non-invasive tests)	Associated	CHD not specified
De Campli et al. 1995[68]	40, 10 y+ post	Death/CHD	6 y mortality RR 1.72 (CI 1.20–2.24)	No association with CHD
McGriffin et al. 1995[69]	200	CHD by angiogram, autopsy	Associated ($p = 0.002$)	CMV serology prior to transplant as measure of infection
Mattila 1995[70]	150	CHD by angiogram and biopsy	Significant ORs for 1st & 2nd y	Result was not sustained after 4 y partial
Mangiavacchi et al. 1995[71]	155, 1 y+ post-transplant	Diffuse coronary lesions by angiogram	37% of infected vs. 15% ($p = 0.029$)	Discrete stenosis was not considered as end point
Hauptman et al. 1995[72]	204	IMT by intravascular U/S	No association	No multivariate analysis considering serum

Table 7.4

(*continued*)

Study	Subjects	End point	Result	Comments
				lipids, prior rejections, HLA matching, etc.
Gao et al. 1996[73]	139, 1 y+ post-transplant	CHD by angiogram	No association	Association with <2 y vs. >2 y onset
Koskinen et al. 1996[74]	72, 1–6 y post-transplant	CHD by angiogram and graft function by U/S	Associated at 6 y ($p < 0.02$)	CMV-associated CHD apparent at 1 y—no difference between primary infection and reactivation
Gamba et al. 1997[75]	163 adult, 1 mo+ post-transplant	CHD by angiogram or autopsy	No association	
Fang et al. 1998[76]	49	CHD progression in 1 y by angiogram	OR = 6.1 (1.3–218.9)	Single CMV Ab measured (positive vs. negative)
Brunner-La Rocca et al. 1998[77]	156	CHD by angiogram and biopsy	OR = 3.21 ($p < 0.05$)	
Dixon et al. 1999[78]	91	CHD by angiogram or autopsy	No association	No other risk factors identified
Esposito et al. 1999[79]	145, 6 mo+ post-transplant	CHD by biopsy or autopsy	100 vs. 12% ($p < 0.001$)	(1) Single CMV Ab measured, (2) association with HCV Ab also found
Pethig et al. 2000[80]	96	CHD progression over 1 y by angiogram	No association	Subjects entered study 0.3–116.4 mo post-transplant
Kuhn et al. 2000[61]	30 children without CHD by intravascular U/S	Maximal intimal thickness by intravascular U/S	Associated in those transplanted as infants or children ($p = 0.04$)	(1) No association when transplanted as neonates, (2) in the cohort, many died before study

Table 7.4

(*continued*)

Study	Subjects	End point	Result	Comments
Bacal et al. 2000[81]	39, 2 y+ post-transplant	CHD by angiogram	No association	Subjects had (1) no angina, MI, heart failure acute rejection; (2) only symptomatic CMV infection

Note. CMV, cytomegalovirus; HCV, hepatitis C virus; CHD, coronary heart disease; Ab, antibody; y, year(s); mo, months; U/S, ultrasound; OR, odds ratio; t, Cox regression coefficient; MI, myocardial infarction; vs. versus.

In general, PCRs have had the highest detection rates but vary from study to study, while the other techniques had lower rates of detection. Arterial samples from various sites have been examined including aorta, coronary, carotid, and femoral arteries.

The results of the various studies are outlined in Table 7.7, and can be divided into three groups: (i) studies involving native atherosclerosis of arteries; (ii) studies on coronary artery restenosis post-PTCA; (iii) and studies on cardiac transplant recipients.

There were 17 studies on native atherosclerosis, and 14 of these analyzed samples for CMV antigens or DNA[84–97], whilst only 8 examined for the presence of HSV[84,85,91,94,98–100] (Table 7.7). A summary of the overall findings from compilation of the data from the studies is shown in Table 7.8. The mean prevalence of CMV was 47.2% in grossly atheromatous arteries and 54.2% in normal arteries, thus suggesting that CMV is a nonspecific finding with no predilection for diseased vessels. This is further supported by the study of Hendrix et al.[90] where CMV was found just as frequently in spleen, pancreas, and other tissues as in the aorta of cadavers.

Although a few studies[91,94] have detected HSV at low rates in atheromatous vessels and none in normal arteries, the overall detection rates were similar, 16.6% and 12.1%, respectively (Table 7.8).

There were only two studies analyzing coronary atherectomy specimens post-PTCA for CMV DNA[58,101]. Both studies detected CMV at a higher rate in restenosis post-PTCA than from native coronary stenosis, overall 47.5% versus 4.2%, respectively (Table 7.8). However, it should be noted that the average prevalence in the restenosis arteries is almost identical to the overall rate in atheromatous arteries from studies on native atherosclerosis (47.2%), and the low detection rates in controls from the restenosis studies are suppressing and difficult to explain. In the initial study by Spier et al.[58], CMV was detected at a much higher rate in samples positive for the tumor surprising

Table 7.5
Retrospective and Cross-sectional Studies of Herpes Simplex and Atherosclerosis

Study	Cases/controls	Virus/method	End point	Result	Comments
Adam et al. 1987[27]	157/157 men	HSV-1, HSV-2, IgG	CHD	OR = 1.26 (0.73–2.17) for HSV-1, =0.96 (0.53–1.72) HSV-2	
Sorlie et al. 1994[16]	340/340	HSV-1, HSV-2, IgG	Carotid wall thickness	OR = 1.21 ($p = 0.45$) for HSV-1, = 0.61 ($p = 0.05$) for HSV-2	Excluded subjects with cardiovascular disease
Lindberg et al. 1997[17]	267/267	HSV-1, HSV-2, IgG	Carotid atherosclerosis	OR = 1.04 (0.61–1.78) for HSV-1, =0.84 (0.49–1.44) for HSV-2	
Espinola-Klein et al. 2000[18]	504	HSV-1, HSV-2 IgG	CHD by angiography	OR = 1.7 (0.77–3.76) for HSV-1, =1.46 (0.82–2.6) for HSV-2	
Zhu et al. 2000[82]	158/75	HSV-1, HSV-2, IgG	CHD by angiography	OR = 2.16 (0.86–5.44) for HSV-1, =1.9 (0.96–3.78) for HSV-2	Association with "pathogen burden" (HSV, CMV, HAV, Cpn)
Espinola-Klein et al. 2002[20]	246/326	HSV-1, HSV-2, EBV IgG	Coronary and carotid and/or femoral-popliteal stenosis	RR = 1.01 (0.84–1.19) for HSV-1, =1.28 (1.05–1.52) for HSV-2, =1.03 (0.88–1.28) for EBV	"Pathogen burden" (HSV, EBV, CMV, Cpn, Mpn, Hpyl) associated with advanced atherosclerosis

Note. HSV, Herpes simplex virus; CMV, cytomegalovirus; EBV, Epstein–Barr virus; Cpn, *Chlamydia pneumoniae*; Mpn, *Mycoplasma pneumoniae*; HPYL, *Helicobacter pylori*; HAV, Hepatitis A virus; CHD, coronary heart disease; RR, relative risk; OR, odds ratio; MI, myocardial infarction.

Table 7.6
Prospective Studies of Herpes Simplex and Atherosclerosis

Study	Virus/ method	Cases/ controls	End point	Result	Comments
Sorlie et al. 2000[41]	High IgG to HSV-1	221/515 men	CHD event	RR = 0.77 (0.36–1.92)	Adjusted for years of education among others
Roivainen et al. 2000[40]	High IgG to HSV-1	241/241	MI, CHD death	OR = 2.07 (1.2–3.56)	No association with adenovirus or enterovirus antibodies
Zhu et al. 2001[45]	IgG to HSV-1, HSV-2	890 with CHD	MI, death	RR = 1.6 (0.9–2.8) for HSV-1, =1.5 (1.0–2.2) for HSV-2	Higher RRs for CMV, HAV, and "pathogen burden"
Havlik et al. 1989[83]	Self-reported herpes manifestations	658 men 919 women	CHD	RR = 1.5 (1.0–2.1) for women	No association overall or in men
Ridker et al. 1998[35]	IgG to HSV-1+2	643/643 men	MI, ischemic stroke	RR = 0.94 (0.7–1.2)	No association with CMV
Ridker et al. 1999[36]	IgG to HSV-1+2	122/244 post-menopausal women	CHD event, stroke	RR = 1.2 (0.6–2.1)	"Pathogen burden" also not associated
Siscovick et al. 2000[42]	IgG to HSV-1	213/405	MI, CHD death	OR = 2.0 (1.1–3.6)	Subjects older than 65
Rupprecht et al. 2001[46]	IgG to HSV-1, HSV-2, IgA to EBV	Cohort of 1010 with CHD	MI, CHD death	HR = 3 (0.4–22.4) for HSV-1, =2 (1.01–4) for HSV-2, =2.8 (1.5–5) for EBV	HR = 5.1 for 6–8 pathogens vs. 0–3, mainly due to herpesviridae

protein, p53, than in specimens negative for p53, 11 of 13 versus 3/11, respectively. It was thus postulated by the investigators that the smooth-muscle cell proliferation seen after post-PTCA stenosis may be due to the CMV gene product, IE 84, binding to and inactivating the p53 gene product. Further studies in this area clearly need to be done as the pathological data is not very convincing.

Table 7.7
Pathological Studies of Herpes Viruses in Blood Vessels

Study	Methods	Virus	Proportion of arteries involved			Significant
			Atheroma	Min. changes	Normal	
Native atherosclerosis						
1. Melnick et al. 1983[84]	IMF, IHC, EM of cultured SMC	CMV HSV	7/26 0/26	— —	4/6 0/6	Not greater in atherosclerosis
2. Yamashiroya et al. 1988[85]	IHC, in situ hybridization	CMV HSV	1/7 3/8	4/24 4/24	1/9 4/9	NS
3. Hendrix et al. 1989[86]	Dot blot and in situ hybrid	CMV	19/44	—	22/30	Not greater in atherosclerosis
4. Hendrix et al. 1990[87]	PCR, dot blot, and in situ hybrid	CMV	27/30	18/34	—	OR = 8 (95% CI, 2.03–31.48) $P = 0.0021$
5. Hendrix et al. 1991[88]	PCR, dot blot	CMV	55/58	—	17/19	NS
6. Melnick et al. 1994[89]	PCR	CMV	58/82	—	45/53	NS
7. Hendrix et al. 1997[90]	PCR, IHC, in situ hybrid	CMV	Various organs 12/12 spleen, 6/8 pancreas		9/12 aorta	Not specific for vasculature
8. Chiu et al. 1997[91]	IHC	CMV HSV-1	27/76 8/76	— —	0/20 0/20	$p < 0.001$ NS
9. Daus et al. 1998[92]	PCR	CMV	0/29 Coronary atherectomy	—	—	Negative
10. Bartels et al. 1999[93]	PCR	CMV	0/38 Coronary vein grafts	—	0/20	Negative

Study	Method	Virus				Result
11. Chiu 1999[94]	IHC	CMV / HSV-1	14/33 / 3/33		0/15 / 0/15	$p = 0.002$ / $p = 0.54$
12. Pampou et al. 2000[95]	IHC, in situ hybrid	CMV	16/18 aorta		6/8	NS
13. Qavi et al. 2000[96]	PCR	CMV	9/17 carotid art.		—	—
14. Rassu et al. 2001[97]	PCR	CMV	3/72 various		—	Low
15. Benditt et al. 1983[98]	in situ hybrid	HSV	10/60—		—	No controls
16. Gyorkey et al.1984[99]	EM	Herpes group, not specified		10/68 aortas	—	Mainly nonatheromas
17. Raza-Ahmad et al. 1995[100]	EM, in situ hybrid	HSV-1 / HSV-2	1/31 / 14/31		— / —	No controls
Restenosis post PTCA (coronary artery)			*Restenosed*	*Native stenosis*		
1. Spier et al. 1994[58]	PCR	CMV / p53+ / p53–	11/13 / 3/11	0/11		$p < 0.0001$ / $p = 0.21$
2. Radke et al. 2001[101]	PCR	CMV	5/16	2/37		OR = 7.95 (95% CI, 1.35–46.9) $p = 0.02$
Cardiac transplants			*Graft atheriosc.*	*No graft atheriosc.*	*Native CHD*	
1. Wu et al. 1992[103]	in situ hybrid	CMV	8/19	—	—	
2. Skowronski, et al. 1993[102]	PCR	CMV	0/7	1/8	—	NS

Table 7.7
(*continued*)

| Study | Methods | Virus | Proportion of arteries involved | | | Significant |
			Atheroma	Min. changes	Normal	
3. Berry et al. 1993[104]	in situ hybrid	CMV EBV	1/15 0/15	— —	0/?	Negative
4. Gulizia et al. 1995[105]	PCR, in situ hybrid	CMV	4/41	—	1/22	OR = 2.7 (95% CI, 0.24–21.66) $p = 0.65$
5. Baas et al. 1996[106]	in situ hybrid, IHC for WAFI	CMV	6/13	—	—	
6. Sambiase et al. 2000[107]	PCR, IHC, in situ hybrid	CMV	1/9	1/21 (minimal changes)	—	OR = 1.75 (95% CI, 0.39–7.788) $p = 0.52$

Note. ART, artery(ies); IMF, immunofluorescence; IHC, immunohistochemistry; SMC, smooth-muscle cell; PCR, polymerase chain reaction; CMV, cytomegalovirus; HSV, herpes simplex virus; PTCA, percutaneous transluminal coronary angioplasty; NS, not statistically significant; OR, odds ratio; MIN, minimal.

Table 7.8

Summary of Pathological Studies—Prevalence of CMV and HSV in Vasculature

Virus	Atheromas	Min. atherosclerosis	Normal arteries	Significance
Native atherosclerosis				
CMV+	236/53 (47.2%)	22/58 (37.9%)	104/192 (54.2%)	OR = 1.35 (95% CI, 0.97–1.89) $p = 0.08$
Post-PTCA				
		Coronary restenosis	*Native CAD*	
CMV+		19/40 (47.5%)	2/48 (4.2%)	OR = 20.81 (95% CI, 4.43–97.6) $p < 0.0001$
Cardiac transplant				
	Graft arterioscler.	*No graft arterioscler.*		
CMV+	20/119 (16.8%)	2/29 (6.9%)	1/22 (4.5%)	OR = 2.72 (95% CI, 0.6–12) and 4.2 (95% CI, 0.56–33.38) $p = 0.2$
Herpes virus				
	Atheroma	*Min. atherosclerosis*	*Normal arteries*	
HSV+	39/234 (16.6%)	4/24 (16.8%)	11/116 (12.1%)	OR = 1.90 (95% CI, 0.94–3.88) $p = 0.07$

Note. CMV, cytomegalovirus; HSV, Herpes simplex virus; CAD, coronary artery disease; Arterioscler., arteriosclerosis; PTCA, percutaneous coronary angioplasty; EM, electron microscopy; Hybrid., Hybridization; IHC, immunohistochemistry; PCR, polymerase chain reaction; CI, confidence interval; OR, odds ratio.

Cardiac graft arteriosclerosis has been associated with CMV infection as mentioned in the previous section on epidemiological association. There were six studies[102–107] assessing atherectomy or autopsy samples from cardiac graft recipient and controls for CMV nucleic acid with varying results—0–42%. However, several of these studies did not include controls from arteries without graft arteriosclerosis or native CHD. The overall results show a greater rate of detection of CMV in arteries with graft arteriosclerosis than in those without or with native CHD (see Table 7.8). However, again the detection of CMV was unusually low for the controls with native CHD (4.5%), and the prevalence in graft arteriosclerosis (16.8%) is actually lower than the overall rate in native atherosclerosis (47.2%).

The large variations and discrepancies in these results may be due to several possible methodologic reasons. These include difference in technique and lack of standardization for the PCR and in situ hybridization methods, including primer and probe selections, sampling error from small atherectomy specimens and possible tissue inhibitors (calcified areas), or contamination.

7.5. BIOLOGICAL MECHANISMS

Interest in the viral cause of atherosclerosis has continued for nearly over 30 years initiated by the early works of Benditt and Benditt[108] and Fabricant et al.[109] Endothelial injury is important in the pathogenesis of atherosclerosis and thrombosis, and there is evidence that several common viruses can infect cultures of endothelial cells obtained from human umbilical vein or bovine thoracic aorta[110]. HSV-1, adenovirus Type 7, measles virus, and parainfluenza virus Type 3 infected both endothelial cell lines but CMV failed to grow in either cell culture[110]. However, there is more recent evidence that CMV can infect human umbilical vein endothelial cells and produce a rapid procoagulant response[111]. Furthermore, infection of the endothelium with CMV in vitro results in increased adherence of polymorphonuclear leukocytes (PMN), which can potentially induce damage of the endothelium[112]. It has also been shown in vitro that CMV infected monocytes can lead to interaction and infection of neighboring endothelial cells and smooth-muscle cells[113]. HSV is also capable of inducing arterial injury, and HSV-infected endothelial cells express adhesion molecule GMP 140 (also known as PADGEM or CD 62), which may be an important pathophysiological mechanism in virus-induced cell injury and inflammation[114].

A critical factor in the development of vasculopathy (post-PTCA stenosis) or atherosclerosis is vessel narrowing caused by infiltration/proliferation of smooth-muscle cells into the vessel intima. Both HSV and CMV can infect vascular smooth cells[115,116] and CMV can initiate viral replication within coronary smooth-muscle cells[117]. Vascular cells generate reactive oxygen species in response to stress, and this may lead to increased transcription of atherosclerosis related cellular and viral genes and to reactivation of latent viral infection. Interestingly, ASA (aspirin) can directly and indirectly attenuate this augmented gene expression[117].

Although, HCMV does not induce cellular proliferation in infected cells in vitro[118], potential mechanism involves smooth-muscle cell proliferation and migration in response to the release of growth factors and cytokines from macrophages and endothelial cells in response to injury. For example, HCMV increases the expression of platelet-derived growth factor (PDGF) receptor, which may induce proliferation and migration of smooth-muscle cells[119]. Moreover, HCMV infection of arterial smooth-muscle cells results in significant cellular migration mediated by the chemokine receptor, US28, in the presence of chemokines including regulated on activation normal T expressed and secreted (RANTES) or monocyte chemoattractant protein-1 (MCP-1)[120].

Another mechanism by which HCMV may contribute to the pathogenesis of smooth-muscle proliferation and restenosis is by the ability of the immediate early (IE) gene product of HCMV, IE 2-84, to bind to p53 and inhibit its transactivational activity[58,121]. Since p53 transcriptionally regulates gene products such as the cyclin-dependent kinase inhibitor p21, which in turn regulates cell cycle progression[122], the inhibitory effect of IE 2-84 on p53 could increase smooth-muscle cell proliferation and accumulation. There is also evidence that HCMV IE protein antagonizes p53-mediated apoptosis which could contribute to smooth-muscle cell accumulation and restenosis[123].

Viral infection of vascular smooth-muscle cells may also contribute to the pathogenesis of atherosclerosis or unstable plaque by alteration of extracellular matrix proteins. In vitro HSV-1 infection of bovine smooth-muscle cells results in suppression of fibronectin and collagen types I and III synthesis, thus altering extracellular matrix synthesis[124].

7.5.1. Effect on Cholesterol and Lipoproteins

The accumulation of cholesterol ester or low-density lipoprotein (LDL) in macrophages and smooth-muscle cells of the intima is the hallmark of atherosclerosis. Avian herpes viruses were shown to enhance cholesterol and cholesterol ester accumulation in cultured arterial smooth-muscle cells[125], due, in part to decreased cholesteryl ester hydrolysis, increased de novo synthesis of cholesterol and decreased excretion of free cholesterol[126]. Human HSV-1 infection of arterial smooth-muscle cells also enhances LDL binding and uptake[127]. The reduced cholesterol ester hydrolysis and cholesterol efflux is related to increased viral-induced protein kinase[127].

Previous investigation indicated that the immune system participates in atherosclerosis, as evidenced by the accumulation of monocytes and T-lymphocytes and cytokines in atheromas[128]. Viral infection could induce mediator release from immune and hematopoetic cells, which may cause phenotypic changes in vascular cells. Cytokines such as TNF can mediate specific biologic effects such as modulation of cholesterol metabolism. In vitro CMV induces macrophages to increase the expression of specific RNAs for interleukin-1β (IL-1β), TNF and colony stimulating factor[129]. It has also been shown that TNF and IL-1 enhance the lipoxygenase product, 12-HETE production which in turn affect both cyclic AMP levels and cholesterol ester hydrolysis[130]. Further studies have shown that HSV infection causes a forty fold increase in cholesterol ester accretion in arterial smooth cells, primarily by decreased acid cholesterol hydrolase synthesis and activity[131]. HSVs accomplish this function by degradation of host mRNA and mediate the cessation of host protein synthesis[131].

The lipid accumulation in foam cells, derived from lipid-laden macrophages and smooth-muscle cells, is the earliest event in plaque forma-tion in the development of atherosclerosis. The lipid accumulation that occurs depends upon the uptake of oxidized LDL (OX-LDL), a process in which the scavenger receptor has been postulated to play an important role. It has recently been shown that HCMV infection of human smooth-muscle cells increases modified LDL uptake and stimulates Class A scavenger receptor gene (SR-A) mRNA expression[132]. In addition, infection of rat smooth-mus-cle cells with HCMV, which causes IE gene expression (IE72/IE84), but no cytopathic effects, also increases uptake of OX-LDL and acetylated LDL[132].

7.5.2. Viral Infection and the Coagulation Cascade

The coagulation system and fibrinolysis play an intricate role in the pathogenesis of atherosclerosis and development of ischemic events, on the basis of thrombotic processes, at the level of the endothelium. HSV-infected endothelium, as well as endothelium exposed to TNF or IL-1, binds platelets[133], granulocytes[134], and expresses tissue factor to a greater extent than it does to noninfected cells[135]. Glycoproteins expression stimulated by HSV genome[136] may play a role on the function of the endothelium through molec-ular mimicry[137]. For example, glycoprotein E can function as an Fc receptor[138] and glycoprotein C can also serve as a complement (C3b) receptor[136].

Infection of the endothelium promotes monocytes adhesion through interaction with virally encoded cell surface glycoprotein C and thrombin[139]. Glycoprotein C bound and promoted activation of Factor X on infected endothelial cells, thus contributing to thrombin generation. Thrombin itself can elicit a variety of cellular events, such as monocyte and neutrophil adhe-sion, release of cytokine and platelet activation on damaged endothelium[139]. In addition, viral injury by HSV-1 to vascular endothelial cells induces secre-tion of von Willebrand factor which mediates enhanced platelet adhesion to these cells[140]. von Willebrand factor, stored in endothelial cells, is an adhesive glycoprotein critical to normal hemostasis.

Cytomegalovirus infection of vascular cells also induces expression of proinflammatory adhesion molecules (adhesion molecule-1 and E-selectin) by paracrine action of secreted IL-1β[141]. Furthermore, CMV-infected human umbilical vein endothelial cells result in a rapid procoagulant response induced by inflammatory mediators[142]. This was related to a facilitated interaction of coagulation factors on the surface of the infected cells, due to membrane perturbations and internalization of Factor X and/or Xa after interaction with the endothelial cell surface[142]. See Figure 7.9 for hypothetical model of viral-induced atherosclerosis.

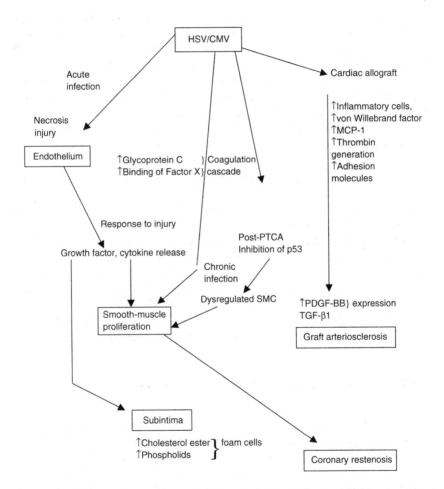

Figure 7.9. A schematic outline for the hypothetic model for development of atherosclerosis, and post-PTCA coronary stenosis or graft arteriosclerosis is shown. PTCA, percutaneous transluminal coronary angioplasty; SMC, smooth-muscle cell; MCP-1, monocyte chemoattractant protein-1; PDGD, platelet-derived growth factor; TGF-β1, transforming growth factor beta-1.

7.6. ANIMAL MODELS

Viruses were first suspected to cause vascular lesions in chickens in the 1940s[143], and the concept that herpes viruses could play a role in the pathogenesis of atherosclerosis was supported by induction of coronary sclerosis in chickens by an infectious agent in 1950[144], and subsequent observation of intracellular cholesterol accumulation in cell cultures infected with feline herpes virus[109].

Further studies with an avian herpes virus that causes Marek's disease (results in malignant T-cell lymphomas in animals), produced atherosclerosis in specific pathogen-free chickens closely resembling human atherosclerotic lesions[145,146]. Coronary arteries, the aorta and its branches were affected, resulting in fatty or fatty-proliferative-type lesions[146]. It was subsequently shown that the aortic tissue of the infected normocholesterolemic chickens had higher concentration of free and esterified cholesterol, and phospholipids than did the uninfected controls[147]. Furthermore, immunization with the antigenically related herpes virus of turkeys prevented the Marek's disease virus-induced atherosclerosis[147,148].

Studies with CMV in the rat model have also resulted in the development of early atherosclerotic lesions[149]. CMV-infected normocholesterolemic male Wistar rats resulted in minimal endothelial cell damage with increased leukocyte adhesion and lipid accumulation in the endothelium. However, infection of hypercholesterolemic rats did not enhance this effect although it resulted in increased migration of the leukocytes into the subendothelial space[149]. Recently it has also been shown that CMV infection of the apolipoprotein E (apoE) deficient mice results in enhancement of atherosclerosis seen in the noninfected hypercholesterolemic mice[150]. In addition, the serum of these infected mice induces MCP-1 expression by endothelial cells[151] and these changes in endothelial function could worsen atherogenesis.

7.6.1. Animal Models of Allograft Arteriosclerosis

Since CMV has been implicated in cardiac transplant graft arteriosclerosis, investigations in this area with animal models have also been performed. CMV infection of rats with aortic allografts demonstrated enhanced generation of allograft arteriosclerosis[152]. Infection was associated with an early inflammatory proliferation in the allograft adventita, and increased proliferation of smooth-muscle cells and alterations in the intima[152]. The same investigators further explored the mechanism of CMV-enhanced graft arteriosclerosis in the rat aortic allograft model, and attributed these changes to enhancement of mRNA expression of PDGF BB and transforming growth factor-beta I with CMV infection[153].

In a different type of rodent model, acute CMV infection was induced in immunocompetent and immunocompromised rats after injury to the common carotid artery by a balloon atheterization[154]. Active CMV infection was shown in the neointima of the injured arteries, mainly affecting neointimal smooth-muscle cells accompanied by inflammatory infiltration of predominantly mononuclear cells[154]. Absence of endothelium and immunosuppression were necessary conditions for arterial CMV infection. CMV infection resulting in subendothelial inflammation of rat aortic allograft consisting of mostly T-lymphocytes and monocytes, were also found to be similar to cardiac allograft arteriosclerosis of patients[155].

In a more recent study, Lemström et al.[156] induced CMV infection in a rat cardiac allograft model (using intra-abdominal heterotopic cardiac allograft), and demonstrated accelerated allograft arteriosclerosis, particularly in small intramyocardial arterioles mediated by inflammatory responses in the vascular wall and perivascular space. It is of interest that ganciclovir (an antiviral agent with activity against CMV and HSV) prophylaxis for 14 days, starting one day after aortic allograft transplantation in rats, significantly delayed and reduced CMV enhanced allograft arteriosclerosis in the rodent model[157].

7.7. CLINICAL TRIAL IN TRANSPLANT ATHEROSCLEROSIS

A recent, small randomized trial was reported to determine the effect of prophylactic ganciclovir on the development of transplant athersclerosis[158]. One hundred and forty-nine consecutive patients undergoing cardiac transplantation were randomized to receive ganciclovir or placebo during the initial 28 days after transplantation, and mean follow up was 4.7 ± 1.3 years. The incidence of transplantation coronary arteriosclerosis appeared to be lower in patients treated with ganciclovir who did not receive calcium channel blockers, $p < 0.03$[158]. This study, however, was limited by its small sample size and by post hoc analysis.

In another pilot study, 80 patients (27 heart transplant and 53 heart-lung transplant recipients) received a combination of ganciclovir plus CMV hyperimmune globulin (CMVIG), and were compared to match historical controls undergoing transplantation within the preceding 2–3 years, but received ganciclovir alone[159]. The patients treated with CMVIG had higher disease-free incidence of CMV, higher survival rate, and lower prevalence and degree of coronary artery intimal thickening compared with patients treated with ganciclovir alone[159].

7.8. CONCLUSION AND FUTURE DIRECTIONS

The epidemiological and pathological data do not support a significant role of CMV or HSV in the pathogenesis of native atherosclerosis in humans. However, the studies on biological mechanisms and animal models suggest that these viruses are potential candidates in the development of atherogenesis. The strongest data in the viral-induced vasculopathy exists for cardiac transplant graft arteriosclerosis, and to a lesser extent for coronary restenosis post-PTCA.

Currently there are no large clinical interventional trials to prove the role of viruses in these vasculopathy. The two potential areas for such studies would be in cardiac transplant recipients with anti-CMV antibodies or CMV negative recipients with positive CMV donor, and in post-PTCA subjects seropositive for CMV antibodies. The availability of an effective oral antiviral agent for treatment of CMV infection, (valganciclovir), should now facilitate the ease of performing these studies. Valganciclovir is an orally administered product that is rapidly hydrolyzed to ganciclovir, and was recently shown to be just as effective as intravenous ganciclovir for induction therapy of CMV retinitis in patients with AIDS[160]. However, a recent in vitro study demonstrated that neither ganciclovir nor foscarnet was able to attenuate the inflammatory response or T-cell activation of allogeneic CMV-infected endothelial cells[161]. Thus, CMVIG plus valganciclovir may best be used in future studies.

Before embarking on a large therapeutic trail to prevent coronary restenosis after PTCA, however, we would warrant further pathological studies from patients with and without coronary restenosis to confirm the results of the two previous reports of the presence of CMV.

REFERENCES

1. Crumparker, C. S. (2000) Cytomegalovirus, in G. L. Mandell, J. E. Bennett, & R. Dolin (Eds.), *Principles and practice of infectious diseases* (5th ed., pp. 1586–1599), Philadelphia, PA: Churchill Livingstone.
2. Chee, M. S., Bankier, A. T., Beck, S., Bohni, R., Brown, C. M., Cerny, R., Hutchinson, C. A. 3rd, Kovzarides, T., & Martiqnetti, J. A. (1990) Analysis of the protein-coding content of the sequence of human cytomegalovirus strain, AD 169, *Curr. Top. Microbiol. Immunol, 154,* 125–169.
3. Crumparker, C. S. (1996) Ganciclovir, *N. Eng. J. Med., 335,* 721–729.
4. Beersma, M. F., Bijlemaker, M. J., & Ploegh, H. L. (1993) Human cytomegalovirus down regulates HLA class I, expression by reducing the stability of class IH chains, *J. Immunol., 15,* 4455–4464.

5. Shuster, E. A., Beneke, J. S., Tegtmeier, G. E., Pearson, G. R., Gleavo, C. A., Wold, A. D., & Smith, T. F. (1985) Monoclonal antibody for rapid laboratory detection of cytomegalovirus infections: characterization and diagnostic application, *Mayo Clin. Proc.*, *60*, 577–585.
6. Fetterman, G. H. (1952) A new laboratory aid in the clinical diagnosis of inclusion disease of infancy, *Am. J. Clin. Pathol.*, *22*, 424–425.
7. Rinaldo, C. R., Black, P. H., & Hirsch, M. S. (1997) Interactions of cytomegalovirus with leukocytes from patients with mononucleosis due to cytomegalovirus, *J. Infect. Dis.*, *136*, 667–678.
8. Vander Bij, W., Schirm, J., Torensma, R., van Son, W. J., Tegzess, A. M., & The, T. H. (1988) Comparison between viremia and antigenemia for detection of cytomegalovirus in *J. Clin. Microbiol.*, *26*, 2531–2535.
9. Wolf, D. G., & Spector, S. A. (1992) Diagnosis of human cytomegalovirus central nervous system disease in AIDS patients by DNA amplification from cerebrospinal fluid, *J. Infect. Dis.*, *166*, 1412–1415.
10. Montgomery, R. I., Warner, M. S., Lum, B. J., & Spear, P. G. (1996) Herpes simplex virus-I entry into cells mediated by a novel member of the TNF/NGF receptor family, *Cell*, *87*, 427–436.
11. Krummenacher, C., Nicola, A. V., Whitbeck, J. C., Lou, N., Hou, W., Lambris, J. D., Geraghty, R. J., Spear, P. G., Cohen, G. N., & Eisenberg, R. J. (1998) Herpes simplex virus glycoprotein D can bind to polio virus receptor-related protein I of herpes virus entry mediator, two structurally unrelated mediators of virus entry, *J. Virol.*, *72*, 7064–7074.
12. Stevens, J. G., Haar, L., Porter, D. D., Cook, M. L., & Wagner, E. R. (1998) Prominence of the herpes simplex virus latency-associated transcript in trigeminal ganglia from seropositive humans, *J. Infect. Dis.*, *158*, 117–123.
13. Corey, L. (2000) Herpes simplex virus, in G. L. Mandell, J. E. Bennett, & R. Dolin (Eds.), *Principles and practice of infection diseases* (5th edn, pp. 1564–1580), Philadelphia, PA: Churchill, Livingston.
14. Buchman, T. G., Roizman, B., Adams, G., & Stover, B. N. (1978) Restriction endonuclease finger-printing of herpes simplex virus DNA: a novel epidemiological tool applied to a nosocominal outbreak, *J. Infect. Dis.*, *138*, 488–498.
15. Ashley, R. L., Militoni, J., Lee, F., Nahmias, A., & Corey, L. (1988) Comparison of Western bolt (immunoblot) and glycoprotein G-specific immunoblot enzyme assay for detecting antibodies to herpes simplex virus types I and 2 in human sera, *J. Clin. Microbiol.*, *26*, 662–667.
16. Sorlie, P. D., Adam, E., Melnick, S. L., Folsom, A., Skelton, T., Chambless, L. E., Barnes, R., & Melnick, J. L. (1994) Cytomegalovirus/herpesvirus and carotid atherosclerosis: the ARIC study, *J. Med. Virol.*, *42*, 33–37.
17. Lindberg, G., Rastram, L., Lundblad, A., Sorlie, P. D., & Folsom, A. R. (1997) The association between serum sialic acid and asymptomatic carotid atherosclerosis is not related to antibodies to Herpes type viruses or *Chlamydia pneumoniae*, *Int. J. Epidemiol.*, *26*, 1386–1391.
18. Espinola-Klein, C., Rupprecht, H. J., Blankenberg, S., Bickel, C., Kopp, H., Rippin, G., Hafner, G., Pfeifer, U., & Meyer, J. (2000) Are morphological or functional changes in the carotid artery wall associated with *Chlamydia*

pneumoniae, Helicobacter pylori, cytomegalovirus, or herpes simplex virus infection? *Stroke, 31*, 2127–2133.

19. Mayr, M., Kiechl, S., Willeit, J., Wick, G., & Xu, Q. (2000) Infections, immunity, and atherosclerosis: associations of antibodies to *Chlamydia pneumoniae, Helicobacter pylori*, and cytomegalovirus with immune reactions to heat shock protein 60 and carotid or femoral atherosclerosis, *Circulation, 102*, 833–839.

20. Espinola-Klein, C., Rupprecht, H. J., Blankenberg, S., Bickel, C., Kopp, H., Rippin, G., Hafner, G., Pfeifer, U., & Meyer, J. (2002) Impact of infectious burden on extent and long term prognosis of atherosclerosis, *Circulation, 105*, 15–21.

21. Adler, S. P., Hir, J. K., Wang, J. B., & Vetrovec., G. W. (1998) Prior infection with cytomegalovirus is not a major risk factor for angiographically demonstrated coronary artery atherosclerosis, *J. Infect. Dis., 177*, 209–212.

22. Blum, A., Giladi, M., Weinberg, M., Kaplan, G., Pasternack, H., Laniado, S., & Miller, H. (1998) High anti-cytomegalovirus (CMV) IgG antibody titer is associated with coronary artery disease and may predict post-coronary balloon angioplasty restenosis, *Am. J. Cardiol., 81*, 866–868.

23. Anderson, J. L., Carlquist, J. F., Muhlestein, J. B., Horne, B. D., & Elmer, S. P. (1998) Evaluation of C-reactive protein, and inflammatory marker, and infectious serology as risk factors for coronary artery disease and myocardial infarction, *J. Am. Coll. Cardiol., 32*, 35–41.

24. Zhu, J., Shearer, G. M., Norman, J. E., Pinto, L. A., Marincola, F. M., Prasad, A., Waclawiw, M. A., Csako, G., Quyyumi, A. A., & Epstein, S. E. (2000) Host response to cytomegalovirus infection as a determinant of susceptibility to coronary artery disease: sex based differences in inflammation and type of immune response, *Circulation, 102*, 2491–2496.

25. Rothenbacher, D., Hoffmeister, A., Bode, G., Wanner, P., Koenig, W., & Brenner, H. (1999) Cytomegalovirus infection and coronary heart disease: results of a German case control study, *J. Infect. Dis., 179*, 690–692.

26. Sepulveda, M. A., Moreu, J., Canton, T., Pajin, F., & Rodriquez, L. (1999) Prevalence of IgG antibodies with angiographically demonstrated coronary atherosclerosis, *Enferm. Infecc. Microbiol. Clin., 17*, 386–389.

27. Adam, E., Probtsfield, J. L., Burek, J., McCollum, C. H., Melnick, J. L., Petrie, B. L., Bailey, K. R., & De Bakey, M. E. (1987) High levels of cytomegalovirus antibody in patients requiring vascular surgery for atherosclerosis, *Lancet, 2*, 291–293.

28. Kafton, H. A., Kafton, O., & Kilic, M. (1999) Markers of chronic infection and inflammation. Are they important in cases with chronic heart disease? *Jpn. Heart J., 40*, 275–280.

29. Tiran, A., Tio, R. A., Oostenveld, E., Harmsen, M. C., Tiran, B., Den Heijier, P., Monnink, S. H., Wilders-Truschnig, M. M., & The, T. H. (1999) Humoral immune response to human cytomegalovirus in patients undergoing transluminal coronary angioplasty, *Clin. Diag. Lab. Immunol., 8*, 45–49.

30. Gattone, M., Jacoviello, L., Colombo, M., Di Castelnuovo, A., Soffiantino, F., Gramoni, A., Picco, D., Benedetta, M., & Giannuzzi, P. (2001) *Chlamydia pneu-*

moniae and cytomegalovirus seropositivity, inflammatory markers, and the risk of myocardial infarction at a young age, *Am. Heart J.*, *142*, 633–640.

31. Burian, K., Kis, Z., Virok, D., Endresz, V., Prohaszka, Z., Duba, J., Berencsi, K., Boda, K., Horvath, L., Romics, L., Fust, G., & Conczol, E. (2001) Independent and joint effect of antibodies to human heat shock protein 60 and *Chlamydia pneumoniae* infection in the development of coronary atherosclerosis, *Circulation*, *103*, 1503–1508.

32. Smieja, M., Cronin, L., Levine, M., Goldsmith, C. H., Yusuf, S. L., & Mahony, J. B. (2001a) Previous exposure to *Chlamydia pneumoniae, Helicobacter pylori* and other infections in Canadian patients with ischemic heart disease, *Can. J. Cardiol.*, *17*, 270–276.

33. Dummer, S., Lee, A., Breinig, M. K., Kormos, R., Ho, M., & Griffith, B. (1994) Investigation of cytomegalovirus infection as a risk factor for coronary atherosclerosis in explanted hearts of patients undergoing heart transplantation, *J. Med. Virol.*, *44*, 305–309.

34. Ossewaarde, J. M., Feskens, E. J. M., De Vries, A., Vallinga, C. E., & Kromhout, D. (1998) *Chlamydia pneumoniae* is a risk factor for coronary heart disease in symptom-free elderly men, but *Helicobacter pylori* and cytomegalovirus are not, *Epidemiol. Infect.*, *120*, 93–99.

35. Ridker, P. M., Hennekens, C. H., Stampfer, M. J., & Wang, F. (1998) Prospective study of herpes simplex virus, cytomegalovirus, and the risk of future myocardial infarction and stroke, *Circulation*, *98*, 2796–2799.

36. Ridker, P. M., Hennekens, C. H., Buring, J. E., Kundsin, U., & Shih, J. (1999) Baseline IgG antibody titers to *Chlamydia pneumoniae, Helicobacter pylori*, herpes simplex virus and cytomegalovirus and the risk for cardiovascular disease in women, *Ann. Intern. Med.*, *131*, 573–577.

37. Danesh, J., Wong, Y., Ward, M., & Muri, J. (1999) Chronic infection with *Helicobacter pylori, Chlamydia pneumoniae*, or cytomegalovirus: population based study of coronary heart disease, *Heart*, *81*, 245–247.

38. Fagerberg, B., Gnarpe, J., Gnarpe, H., Agewall, S., & Wikstrand, J. (1999) *Chlamydia pneumoniae* but not cytomegalovirus antibodies are associated with future risk of stroke and cardiovascular disease, *Stroke*, *30*, 299–305.

39. Haider, A. W., Wilson, P. W. F., Larson, M. G., Sutherland, P., Evans, J. C., O'Donnell, C. J., Wolf, P. A., Michelson, E. L., & Levy, D. (1999) *Chlamydia, H. pylori* and cytomegalovirus seropositivity and risk of cardiovascular disease: the Framingham heart study, *J. Am. Coll. Cardiol.*, *33*(Suppl A) [Abstract no. 892-6] 314A.

40. Roiviainen, M., Vick-Kajander, M., Palosuo, T., Toivainen, P., Leinonen, M., Saikku, P., Tenkanen, L., Manninen, V., Hovi, T., & Manttari, M. (2000) Infections, inflammation and the risk of coronary heart disease, *Circulation*, *101*, 252–257.

41. Sorlie, P. D., Nieto, F. J., Adam, E., Folsom, A. R., Shalnar, A., & Massing, M. (2000) A prospective study of cytomegalovirus, herpes simplex virus I, and coronary heart disease, *Arch. Intern. Med.*, *160*, 2027–2032.

42. Siscovick, D. S., Schwartz, S. M., Corey, L., Grayston, J. T., Ashley, R., Wang, S. P., Psaty, B. M., Tracy, R. P., Kuller, L. H., & Kronmal, R. A. (2000) *Chlamydia*

pneumoniae, herpes simplex virus type I, and cytomegalovirus and incident myocardial infarction and coronary heart disease in older adults, *Circulation, 102*, 2335–2340.

43. Muhlestein, J. B., Horne, B. D., Carlquist, J. F., Madsen, T. E., Pearson, R. R., & Anderson, J. L. (2000) Cytomegalovirus seropositivity and C reactive protein have independent and combined predictive valve for mortality in patients with angiographically demonstrated coronary artery disease, *Circulation, 102*, 1917–1923.

44. Choussat, R., Montalescot, G., Collet, J. P., Jardel, C., Ankri, A., Fillet, A. M., Thomas, D., Raymond, J., Bastard, J. P., Drobinski, G., Orfila, J., Agut, H., & Thomas, D. (2001) Effect of prior exposure to *Chlamydia pneumoniae, Helicobacter pylori*, or cytomegalovirus on the degree of inflammation and one-year prognosis of patients with unstable angina pectoris or non-Q-wave acute myocardial infarction, *Am. J. Cardiol., 86*, 379–384.

45. Zhu, J., Nieto, J., Horne, B., Anderson, J. L., Muhlestein, J. B., & Epstein, S. E. (2001) Prospective study of pathogen burden and risk of myocardial infarction or death, *Circulation, 103*, 45–51.

46. Rupprecht, H. J., Blankenberg, S., Bickel, C., Rippin, G., Hafner, G., Prellwitz, W., Schlumberger, W., & Myer, J. (2001) Impact of viral and bacterial infectious burden on long-term prognosis in patients with coronary heart disease, *Circulation, 104*, 25–31.

47. Smieja, M., Chong, S., Natarajan, M., Petrich, A., Rainen, L., & Mahony, J. B. (2001b) Circulating nucleic acid of *Chlamydia pneumoniae* and cytomegalovirus in patients undergoing coronary angioplasty, *J. Clin. Microbiol., 39*, 596–600.

48. Nieto, F. J., Adam, E., Sorlie, P., Farzadegan, H., Melnick, J. L., Comstock, G. W., & Szklo, M. (1996) Cohort study of cytomegalovirus infection as a risk factor for carotid intimal medial thickening, a measure of subclinical atherosclerosis, *Circulation, 94*, 922–927.

49. Zhou, Y. F., Leon, M. B., Waclawiw, M. A., Popma, J. J., Yu, Z. X., Finkel, T., & Epstein, S. E. (1996) Association between prior cytomegalovirus infection and the risk of restenosis after coronary atherectomy, *N. Engl. J. Med., 335*, 624–630.

50. Muhlestein, J. B., Carlquist, J. F., Horne, B. D., King, G. J., Elmer, S. P., Trehan, S., & Anderson, J. L. (1997) No association between prior cytomegalovirus infection and the risk of clinical restenosis after percutaneous coronary interventions, *Circulation, 96*(Suppl. I), I-650 [Abstract 3638].

51. Thomas, W., Lele, S., Adler, S., Goudreau, E., Cowley, M., & Vetrovec, G. (1997) Lack of evidence for a relationship between cytomegalovirus status in coronary angiographic restenosis, *Circulation, 96*(Suppl I), I-650 [Abstract 3637].

52. Blum, A., Giladi, M., Weinberg, M., Kaplan, G., Pasternack, H., Laniado, S., Miller, H. (1998) High anti-cytomegalovirus (CMV) IgG antibody titer is associated with coronary artery disease and may predict post-coronary balloon angioplasty restenosis, *Am. J. Cardiol., 81*, 866–868.

53. Manegold, C., Alwazzeh, M., Jablonowski, H., Adams, O., Medve, M., Seidlitz, B., Heidlard, U., Haussinger, D., Strauer, B. E., & Heintzen, M. P. (1999) Prior cytomegalovirus infection and the risk of restenosis after percutaneous transluminal coronary balloon angioplasty, *Circulation, 99*, 1290–1294.

54. Carlsson, J., Miketick, S., Brom, J., Ross, R., Bachmann, H., & Tebbe, U. (2000) Prior cytomegalovirus, *Chlamydia pneumoniae* or *Helicobacter pylori* infection and the risk of restenosis after percutaneous transluminal coronary angioplasty, *Int. J. Cardiol.*, *73*, 165–171.
55. Neumann, F. J., Kastrati, A., Miethke, T., Pogatsa-Murray, G., Seyfarth, M., & Schomig, A. (2000) Previous cytomegalovirus infection and risk of coronary thrombotic events after stent placement, *Circulation*, *101*, 11–13.
56. Neumann, F. J., Kastrati, A., Meithke, T., Mehilli, J., Pogatsa-Murray, G., Koch, W., Seyfarth, M., & Schomig, A. (2001) Previous cytomegalovirus infection and restenosis after coronary stent placement, *Circulation*, *104*, 1135–1139.
57. Schiele, F., Batur, M. K., Seronde, M. F., Meneveau, N., Sewoke, P., Bassignot, A., Couetdu, C., Caulfield, F., & Bassard, J. P. (2001) Cytomegalovirus, *Chlamydia pneumoniae*, and *Helicobacter pylori* IgG antibodies and restenosis after stent implantation: an angiographic and intravascular ultrasound study, *Heart*, *85*, 304–311.
58. Spier, E., Modali, R., Huang, E. S., Leon, M. B., Shawl, L. F., Finkel, T., & Epstein, S. E. (1994) Potential role of human cytomegalovirus and p53 interaction in coronary restenosis, *Science*, *265*, 391–394.
59. Braunlin, E. A., Hunter, D. W., Carter, C. E., Gutiernez, F. R., Ring, W. S., Olivari, M. T., Titus, J. L., Spray, T. L., & Bolman, R. M. 3rd (1991) Coronary artery disease in pediatric cardiac transplant recipients receiving triple-drug immunosuppression, *Circulation*, *84*(Suppl 5), III303–309.
60. Chinnock, R. E., Baum, M. F., Larsen, R., & Bailey, L. (1993) Rejection management and long-term surveillance of the pediatric heart transplant recipient: the Loma Linda experience, *J. Heart Lung Transplant.*, *12*, S255–S264.
61. Kuhn, M. A., Jutzy, K. R., Deming, D. D., Cephus, C. E., Chinnock, R. E., Johnston, J., Bailey, L. L., & Larsen, R. L. (2000) The medium-term findings in coronary arteries by intravascular ultrasound in infants and children after heart transplantation, *J. Am. Coll. Cardiol.*, *36*, 250–254.
62. Gratton, M. T., Moreno-Cabral, C., Starnes, V. A., Oyer, P. E., Stinson, E. B., & Shumway, N. E. (1989) Cytomegalovirus infection is associated with cardiac allograft rejection and atherosclerosis, *JAMA*, *261*, 3561–3566.
63. McDonald, K., Rector, T. S., Braunlin, E. A., Kubo, S. N., & Olivari, M. T. (1989) Association of coronary artery disease in cardiac transplant recipients with cytomegalovirus infection, *Am. J. Cardiol.*, *64*, 359–362.
64. Sharples, L. D., Caine, N., Mullins, P., Scott, J. P., Solis, E., English, T. A., Large, S. R., Schofield, P. M., & Wallwork, J. (1991) Risk factor analysis for the major hazards following heart transplantation—rejection, infection, and coronary occlusion disease, *Transplantation*, *52*, 244–252.
65. Everett, J. P., Hershberger, R. E., Norman, D. J., Chou, S., Ratkovec, R. M., Cobanoglu, A., Oh, G. Y., & Hosenpud, J. D. (1992) Prolonged cytomegalovirus infection with viremia is associated with development of cardiac allograft vasculopathy, *J. Heart Lung Transplant.*, *11*, S133–S137.
66. Koskinen, P. K., Nieminen, M. S., Krogerus, L. A., Lemstrom, K. B., Mattila, S. P., Hayry, P. J., & Lautenschlager, I. T. (1993a) Cytomegalovirus infection accelerates cardiac allograft vasculopathy: correlation between angiographic and endomyocardial biopsy findings in heart transplant patients, *Transplant. Int.*, *6*, 341–347.

67. Koskinen, P. L., Lemstrom, K., Mattila, S., Hayry, P. J., & Lautenschlager, I. T. (1993b) Cytomegalovirus infection and accelerated cardiac allograft vasculopathy in human cardiac allografts, *J. Heart Lung Transplant.*, *12*, 724–729.

68. De Campli, W. M., Luikart, H., Hunt, S., & Stinson, E. B. (1995) Characteristics of patients surviving more than ten years after cardiac transplantation, *J. Thorac. Cardiovasc. Surg.*, *109*, 1103–1114.

69. McGriffin, D. C., Savuren, T., Kriklin, J. K., Naftel, D. C., Bourge, R. C., Paine, T. D., White-Williams, C., Sisto, T., & Early, L. (1995) Cardiac transplant coronary artery disease: a multivirate analysis of pretransplatation risk factors for disease development and morbid events, *J. Thorac. Cardiovasc. Surg.*, *109*, 1081–1088.

70. Mattila, S. P. (1995) Discussion of: cardiac transplant coronary artery disease, *J. Thorac. Cardiovasc. Surg.*, *109*, 1088 [at the end of the article by McGriffin et al.].

71. Mangiavacchi, M., Frigerio, M., Gronda, E., Danzi, G. B., Bonacina, E., Mascicco, G., Olivia, F., De Vita, C., & Pellegrini, A. (1995) Acute rejection and cytomegalovirus infection: correlation with cardiac allograft vasculopathy, *Transplant. Proc.*, *27*, 1960–1962.

72. Hauptman, P. J., Davis, S. F., Miller, L., & Yeung, A. C. (1995) The role of non-immune risk factors in the development and progression of graft arteriosclerosis: preliminary insights from a multicenter intravascular ultrasound study, *J. Heart Lung Transplant.*, *14*, S238–242.

73. Gao, S. Z., Hunt, S., Schroeder, J. S., Alderman, E. L., Hill, I., & Stinson, E. B. (1996) Early development of accelerated graft coronary artery disease: risk factors and course, *J. Am. Coll. Cardiol.*, *28*, 673–679.

74. Koskinen, P. K., Lemstrom, K., Matilla, S., Hayry, P. J., Nieminen, M. S. (1996) Cytomegalovirus infection associated heart allograft arteriosclerosis may impair the late function of the graft, *Clin. Transplant.*, *10*, 487–493.

75. Gamba, A., Manprin, F., Fiocchi, R., Senni, M., Troise, G., Ferrazzi, P., Ferrara, R., & Corbetta, G. (1997) The risk of coronary artery disease after heart transplantation is increased in patients receiving low-dose cyclosporine, regardless of blood cyclosporine levels, *Clin. Cardiol.*, *20*, 767–772.

76. Fang, J. C., Kinlay, S., Kundsin, R., & Ganz, P. (1998) *Chlamydia pneumoniae* infection is frequent but not associated with coronary arteriosclerosis in cardiac transplant recipients, *Am. J. Cardiol.*, *82*, 1479–1483.

77. Brunner-La Rocca, H. P., Schneider, J., Kurzli, A., Turina, M., & Kiowksi, W. (1998) Cardiac allograft rejection late after transplantation is a risk factor for graft coronary artery disease, *Transplantation*, *65*, 538–543.

78. Dixon, S. R., Ruygrok, P. N., Agnew, T. M., Lund, M., Aldersley, P. F., Gibbs, H. C., Whitlock, R. M., Haydock, D. A., & Coverdale, H. A. (1999) Cardiac allograft vasculopathy: the Green Lane hospital experience 1987–1998; *N. Z. Med. J.*, *112*, 417–420.

79. Esposito, S., Renzulli, A., Agozzino, L., Thomopoulos, K., Piccolo, M., Maiello, C., Della Corte, A., & Cotrufo, M. (1999) Late complications of heart transplantation: an 11 year experience, *Heart Vessels*, *14*, 272–276.

80. Pethig, K., Klauss, V., Heublen, B., Mudra, H., Westphal, A., Weber, C., Theisen, K., & Haverich, A. (2000) Progression of cardiac allograft vascular disease as assessed by serial intravascular ultrasound: correlation to immunological and non-immunological factors, *Heart, 84*, 494–498.

81. Bacal, F., Veiga, V. C., Fiorelli, A. I., Bellotti, G., Bocchi, E. A., Stolf, N. A., & Ramirez, J. A. (2000) Analysis of the risk factors for allograft vasculopathy in asymptomatic patients after cardiac transplantation, *Arq. Bras. Cardiol., 75*, 421–428.

82. Zhu, J., Quyyumi, A. A., Norman, J. E., Csako, G., Waclawiw, M. A., Shearer, G. M., Epstein, S. E. (2000) Effects of total pathogen burden on coronary artery disease risk and C-reactive protein levels, *Am. J. Cardiol., 85*, 140–146.

83. Havlik, R. J., Blackwelder, W. C., Kaslow, R., & Castelli, W. (1989) Unlikely association between clinically apparent herpesvirus infection and coronary incidence at older ages: the Framingham heart study, *Arteriosclerosis, 9*, 877–880.

84. Melnick, J. L., Petrie, B. L., Dreesman, G. R., Burek, J., McCollum, C. H., & DeBakey, M. E. (1983) Cytomegalovirus antigen within human arterial smooth muscle cells, *Lancet, 2*, 644–647

85. Yamashiroya, H. M., Ghosh, L., Yang, R., & Robertson, A. L. (1988) Herpesviridae in the coronary arteries and aorta of young trauma victims, *Am. J. Pathol., 130*, 71–79.

86. Hendrix, M. G. R., Dormans, P. H. J., Kitslaar, P., Bosman, F., & Bruggerman, C. A. (1989) Presence of cytomegalovirus nucleic acids in arterial walls of atherosclerotic and nonatherosclerotic patients, *Am. J. Pathol., 134*, 1151–1157.

87. Hendrix, M. G. R., Salimans, M. M. M., van Boven, C. P. A., & Bruggeman, C. A. (1990) High prevalence of latently present cytomegalovirus in arterial walls of patients suffering from grade III atherosclerosis, *Am. J. Pathol., 136*, 23–28.

88. Hendrix, M. G. R., Daemen, M., & Bruggeman, C. A. (1991) Cytomegalovirus nucleic acid distribution within the human vascular tree, *Am. J. Pathol., 138*, 563–657.

89. Melnick, J. L., Hu, C., Burek, J., Adam, E., & DeBakey, M. E. (1994) Cytomegalovirus DNA in arterial walls of patients with atherosclerosis, *J. Med. Virol., 42*, 170–174.

90. Hendrix, M. G. R., Wagenaar, M., Slobbe, C. A., & Bruggeman, C. A. (1997) Widespread presence of cytomegalovirus DNA in tissues of healthy trauma victims, *J. Clin. Pathol., 50*, 59–63.

91. Chiu, B., Viira, E., Tucker, W., & Fong, I. W. (1997) *Chlamydia pneumoniae*, cytomegalovirus, and herpes simplex virus in atherosclerosis of the carotid artery, *Circulation, 96*, 2144–2148.

92. Daus, H., Ozbek, C., Saage, D., Scheller, B., Schieffer, H., Pfreundschuh, M., & Gause, A. (1998) Lack of evidence for a pathogenic role of *Chlamydia pneumoniae* and cytomegalovirus infection in coronary atheroma formation, *Cardiology, 90*, 83–88.

93. Bartels, C., Maass, M., Bein, G., Malisius, R., Brill, N., Bechtel, J. F., Sayk, F., Feller, A. C., & Sievers, H. H. (1999) Detection of *Chlamydia pneumoniae* but not cytomegalovirus in occluded saphenous vein coronary artery bypass grafts, *Circulation, 99*, 879–882.

94. Chiu, B. (1999) Multiple infections in carotid atherosclerotic plaques, *Am. Heart J.*, *138*, S534–S536.

95. Pampou, S. Y., Gnedoy, S. N., Bystrevskaya, V. B., Smirnov, V. N., Chazov, E. I., Melnick, J. L., & DeBakey, M. E. (2000) Cytomegalovirus genome and the immediate-early antigen in cells of different layers of human aorta, *Virchows Arch.*, *436*, 539–552.

96. Qavi, H. B., Melnick, J. L., Adam, E., & DeBakey, M. E. (2000) Frequency of coexistence of cytomegalovirus and *Chlamydia pneumoniae* in atherosclerotic plaques, *Central Eur. J. Public Health*, *8*, 71–73.

97. Rassu, M., Cazzavillan, S., Scagnelli, M., Peron, A., Bevilacqua, P. A., Facco, M., Bertoloni, G., Lauro, F. M., Zambello, R., & Bonoldi, E. (2001) Demonstration of *Chlamydia pneumoniae* in atherosclerotic arteries from various vascular regions, *Atherosclerosis*, *158*, 73–79.

98. Benditt, E. P., Barrett, T., & McDougal, J. K. (1983) Viruses in the etiology of atherosclerosis, *Proc. Nat. Acad. Sci. USA*, *80*, 6386–6389.

99. Gyorkey, F., Melnick, J. L., Guinn, G. A., Gyorkey, P., & DeBakey, M. E. (1984) Herpesviridae in the endothelial and smooth muscle cells of the proximal aorta in arteriosclerotic patients, *Exp. Mol. Pathol.*, *40*, 328–339.

100. Raza-Ahmad, A., Klassen, G. A., Murphy, D. A., Sullivan, J. A., Kinely, C. E., Landymore, R. W., & Wood, J. R. (1995) Evidence of type 2 herpes simplex infection in human coronary arteries at the time of coronary bypass surgery, *Can. J. Cardiol.*, *11*, 1025–1029.

101. Radke, P. W., Merkelbach-Bruse, S., Messmer, B. J., von Dahl, J., Dorge, H., Naami, A., Vogel, G., Handt, S., & Hanrath, P. (2001) Infectious agents in coronary lesions obtained by endatherectomy; pattern of distribution, coinfection and clinical findings, *Coron. Artery Dis.*, *12*, 1–6.

102. Skowronski, E. W., Mendoza, A., Smith, S. C., & Jaski, B. E. (1993) Detection of cytomegalovirus in paraffin-embedded postmortem coronary artery specimens of heart transplant recipients by the polymerase chain reaction: implications of cytomegalovirus association with graft atherosclerosis, *J. Heart Lung Transplant.*, *12*, 717–723.

103. Wu, T. C., Hruban, R. H., Ambinder, R. F., Pizzorno, M., Cameron, D. E., Baumgartner, W. A., Reitz, B. A., Hayward, F. S., & Hutchins, G. M. (1992) Demonstration of cytomegalovirus nucleic acids in the coronary arteries of transplanted hearts, *Am. J. Pathol.*, *140*, 739–747.

104. Berry, G. J., Rizeq, M. N., Weiss, L. M., & Billingham, M. E. (1993) Graft coronary disease in pediatric heart and combined heart-lung transplant recipients: a study of fifteen cases, *J. Heart Lung Transplant.*, *12*, S309–S319.

105. Gulizia, J. M., Kandolf, R., Kendall, T. J., Thieszen, S. L., Wilson, J. E., Radio, S. J., Costanzo, M. R., Winters, G. L., Miller, L. L., & McManus, B. M. (1995) Infrequency of cytomegalovirus genome in coronary arteriopathy of human heart allografts, *Am. J. Pathol.*, *147*, 461–475.

106. Baas, I. O., Offerhaus, G. J. A., El-Deiry, W. S., Wu, T. C., Hutchins, G. M., Kasper, E. K., Baughman, K. L., Baumgartner, W. A., Chou, C. I., Hayward, G. S., & Hruban, R. H. (1996) The WAFI-mediated p53 growth-suppressor pathway is intact in the coronary arteries of heart transplant recipients, *Hum. Pathol.*, *27*, 324–329.

107. Sambiase, N. V., Higuchi, M. L., Nuovo, G., Gutierrez, P. S., Fiorelli, A. I., Uip, D. E., & Ramires, J. A. (2000) CMV and transplant-related coronary atherosclerosis: an immunohistochemical, in situ hybridization, and polymerase chain reaction in situ study, *Mod. Pathol.*, *13*, 173–179.

108. Benditt, E. P., & Benditt, J. M. (1973) Evidence for a monoclonal origin of human atherosclerotic plaques, *Proc. Natl. Acad. Sci. USA*, *70*, 1753–1755.

109. Fabricant, C. G., Krook, L., & Gillespie, J. H. (1973) Virus induced cholesterol crystals, *Science*, *181*, 566–567.

110. Friedman, H. M., Macarak, E. J., MacGregor, R. R., Wolfe, J., & Kefalides, N. A. (1981) Virus infection of endothelial cells, *J. Infect. Dis.*, *143*, 266–273.

111. van Dam-Mieras, M. C., Muller, A. D., van Hinsberg, V. W., Mullers, W. J., Bomans, P. H., & Bruggeman, C. A. (1992) The procoagulant response of cytomegalovirus infected endothelial cells, *Thromb. Haemost.*, *68*, 364–370.

112. Span, A. H., Van Boven, C. P., & Bruggeman, C. A. (1989) The effect of cytomegalovirus infection on the adherence of polymorphonuclear leucocytes to endothelial cells, *J. Clin. Invest.*, *19*, 542–548.

113. Guetta, E., Guetta, V., Shibutani, T., & Epstein, S. E. (1997) Monocytes harbouring cytomegalovirus: interactions with endothelial cells, smooth muscle cells, and oxidized low-density lipoprotein. Possible mechanisms for activating virus delivered by monocytes to sites of vascular injury, *Circ. Res.*, *81*, 8–16.

114. Etingin, O. R., Silverstein, R. L., & Hajjar, D. P. (1991) Identification of a monocyte receptor on herpes virus-infected endothelial cells, *Proc. Natl. Acad. Sci. USA*, *88*, 7200–7203.

115. Datta, S. K., Tumilowicz, J. J., & Trentin, J. J. (1993) Lysis of human arterial smooth muscle cells infected with herpes viridae by peripheral blood mononuclear cells: implications for atherosclerosis, *Viral Immunol.*, *6*, 153–160.

116. Tumilowicz, J. J. (1990) Characteristics of human arterial smooth muscle cell cultures infected with cytomegalovirus, *In Vitro Cell Dev. Biol.*, *26*, 1144–1150.

117. Speir, E., Yu, Z. X., & Ferrans, V. J. (1998) Infectious agents in coronary artery disease: viral infection, aspirin and gene expression in human coronary smooth muscle cells, *Rev. Port Cardiol.*, *17*(Suppl 2); II3–9.

118. Lu, M., & Shenk, T. (1996) Human cytomegalovirus infection inhibits cell cycle progression at multiple points, including the transition from GI to S, *J. Virol.*, *70*, 8850–8857.

119. Zhou, Y. F., Yu, Z. X., Wanishsawad, C., Shou, M., & Epstein, S. E. (1999) The immediate early gene products of human cytomegalovirus increase vascular smooth cell migration, proliferation, and expression of PDGF β-receptor, *Biochem. Biophys. Res. Commun.*, *256*, 608–613.

120. Streblow, D. N., Soderberg-Naucler, C., Viera, J., Smith, P., Wakabayashi, E., Ruchti, F., Mattison, K., Altschuler, Y., & Nelson, J. A. (1999) The human cytomegalovirus chemokine receptor US28 mediates vascular smooth cell migration, *Cell*, *99*, 511–520.

121. Zhou, Y. F., Yu, Z. X., Shou, M., & Epstein, S. E. (1999) Expression of human cytomegalovirus immediate early genes increases rat smooth muscle cell proliferation, *J. Am. Coll. Cardiol.*, *33*, 311A [Abstract].

122. el-Deiry, W. S., Tokins, T., Velcwescu, V. E., Levy, D. B., Parsons, R., Trent, J. M., Lin, D., Mercer, W. E., Kinzler, K. W., & Vogelstein, B. (1993) WAFI, a potential mediator of p53 tumor suppression, *Cell*, *4*, 817–825.
123. Tanaka, K., Zou, J. P., Takeda, K., Ferrans, V. J., Sandford, G. R., Johnson, T. M., Finkel, T., & Epstein, S. E. (1999) Effects of human cytomegalovirus immediate early proteins on p53 mediated apoptosis in coronary artery smooth muscle cells, *Circulation*, *99*, 1656–1659.
124. Lashgari, M. S., Friedman, H. M., & Kefalides, N. A. (1987) Suppression of matrix protein synthesis by herpes simplex virus in bovine smooth muscle cells, *Biochem. Biophys. Res. Commun.*, *143*, 145–151.
125. Fabricant, C. G., Hajjar, D. P., Minick, C. R., & Fabricant, J. (1981) Herpes virus infection enhances cholesterol and cholesteryl ester accumulation in cultured arterial smooth muscle cells, *Am. J. Pathol.*, *105*, 176–184.
126. Hajjar, D. P., Falcone, D. J., & Fabricant, C. G., Fabricant, J. (1985) Altered cholesteryl ester cycle is associated with lipid accumulation in herpes virus-infected arterial smooth muscle cells, *J. Biol. Chem.*, *260*, 6124–6128.
127. Hsu, H. Y., Nicholson, A. C., Pomerantz, K. B., Kaner, R. J., & Hajjar, D. P. (1995) Altered cholesterol trafficking in herpes virus infected arterial cells, *J. Biol. Chem.*, *270*, 19630–19637.
128. Ross, R. (1981) Atherosclerosis: a problem of the biology of arterial wall cells and their interactions with blood components, *Atherosclerosis*, *1*, 293–311.
129. Dudding, L., Haskill, S., Clark, B. D., Auron, P. E., Sporn, S., & Huang, E. S. (1989) Cytomegalovirus infection stimulates expression of monocyte associated mediator genes, *J. Immunol.*, *143*, 3343–3352.
130. Etingin, O. R., & Hajjar, D. P. (1990) Evidence for cytokine regulation of cholesterol metabolism in herpes virus-infected arterial cells by the lipoxygenase pathway, *J. Lipid Res.*, *31*, 299–305.
131. Hajjar, D. P., Nicholson, A. C., Hajjar, K. A., Sando, G. N., & Summers, B. D. (1989) Decreased messenger RNA translation in herpes virus-infected arterial cells: effects on cholesterol ester hydrolase, *Proc. Natl. Acad. Sci. USA*, *86*, 3366–3370.
132. Zhou, Y. F., Guetta, E., Yu, Z. X., Finkel, T., & Epstein, S. E. (1996) Human cytomegalovirus increases modified low density lipoprotein uptake and scavenger receptor mRNA expression in vascular smooth muscle cells, *J. Clin. Invest.*, *98*, 2129–2138.
133. Visser, M. R., Tracy, P. B., Vercellotti, G. M., Goodman, J. L., White, J. G., & Jacob, H. S. (1988) Enhanced thrombin generation and platelet binding on herpes simplex virus infected endothelium, *Proc. Natl. Acad. Sci. USA*, *85*, 8227–8230.
134. MacGregor, R. R., Friedman, H. M., Macarack, E. J., & Kefalides, N. A. (1980) Virus infection of endothelial cells increases granulocyte adherence, *J. Clin. Invest.*, *65*, 1469–1477.
135. Key, N. S., Vercelloti, G. M., Winkelmann, J. C., Moldow, C. F., Goodman, J. L., Esmon, N. L., Esmon, C. T., & Jacob, H. S. (1990) Infection of vascular endothelial cells with herpes virus enhances tissue factor activity and reduces thrombomodulin expression, *Proc. Natl. Acad. Sci. USA*, *87*, 7095–7099.

136. Friedman, H. M., Cohen, G. H., Eisenberg, R. J., Seidel, C. A., & Cines, D. B. (1984) Glycoprotein C of herpes simplex-1 acts as a receptor for the C3b complement component of infected cells, *Nature*, *309*, 633–635.

137. Hajjar, D. P. (1991) Viral pathogenesis of atherosclerosis, impact of molecular mimicry and viral genes, *Am. J. Pathol.*, *139*, 1195–1211.

138. Cines, D. B., Lyss, A. P., Bina, M., Corkey, R., Kefalides, N. A., & Friedman, H. M. (1982) FC and C3 receptors induced by herpes simplex virus on cultured human endothelial cells, *J. Clin. Invest.*, *69*, 123–128.

139. Etingin, O. R., Silverstein, R. L., Friedman, H,.M., & Hajjar, D. P. (1990) Viral activation of the coagulation cascade: molecular interaction at the surface of infected endothelial cells, *Cell*, *61*, 657–662.

140. Etingin, O. R., Silverstein, R. L., & Hajjar, D. P. (1993) von Willebrand factor mediates platelet adhesion to virally infected endothelial cells, *Proc. Natl. Acad. Sci. USA*, *90*, 5153–5156.

141. Dengler, T. J., Raftery, M. J., Werle, M., Zimmermann, R., & Schonrich, G. (2000) Cytomegalovirus infection of vascular cells induces expression of pro-inflammatory adhesion molecules by paracrine action of secreted interleukin-1 beta, *Transplantation*, *69*, 1160–1168.

142. van Dam-Mieras, M. C., Muller, A. D., van Hinsberg, V. W., Mullers, W. J., Bomans, P. H., & Bruggeman, C. A. (1992) The procoagulant response of cytomegalovirus infected endothelial cells, *Thromb. Haemost.*, *68*, 364–370.

143. Patterson, J. C., Mitchell, C. A., & Wallace, A. L. (1949) Experimental coronary sclerosis II. The role of infection in coronary sclerosis of cockerels, *Arch. Pathol.*, *47*, 335–339.

144. Patterson, J. C., & Cottral, G. E. (1950) Experimental coronary sclerosis: III lymphomatosis as a cause of coronary sclerosis in chickens, *Arch. Pathol.*, *49*, 699–707.

145. Fabricant, C. G., Fabricant, J., Litrenta, M. M., & Minick, C. R. (1978) Virus induced atherosclerosis, *J. Exp. Med.*, *148*, 335–340.

146. Minick, C. R., Fabricant, C. G., Fabricant, J., & Litrenta, M. M. (1979) Atherosclerosis induced by infection with a herpes virus, *Am. J. Pathol.*, *96*, 673–706.

147. Hajjar, D. P., Fabricant, C. G., Minick, C. R., & Fabricant, J. (1986) Virus induced atherosclerosis: herpes virus infection alter aortic cholesterol metabolism and accumulation, *Am. J. Pathol.*, *122*, 62–70.

148. Fabricant, C. G., Fabricant, J., Minick, C. R. & Litrenta, M. M. (1983) Herpes virus induced atherosclerosis in chickens, *Fed. Proc.*, *42*, 2476–2479.

149. Span, A. H. M., Yrauls, G., Bosman, F., van Boven, C. P. A., & Bruggeman, C. A. (1992) Cytomegalovirus infection induces vascular injury in the rat, *Atherosclerosis*, *93*, 41–52.

150. Burnett, M. S., Gaydos, C. A., Madico, G. E., Glad, S. M., Paigen, B., Quinn, T. C., & Epstein, S. E. (2001) Atherosclerosis in apoE knockout mice infected with multiple pathogens, *J. Infect. Dis.*, *183*, 226–231.

151. Rott, D., Zhu, J., Burnett, M. S., Zhou, Y. F., Wasserman, A., Walker, J., & Epstein, S. E. (2001) Serum of cytomegalovirus-infected mice induces monocyte chemoattractant protein-1 expression by endothelial cells, *J. Infect. Dis.*, *184*, 1109–1113.

152. Lemstrom, K. B., Bruning, J. H., Bruggeman, C. A., Lautenschlager, I. T., & Hayry, P. J. (1993) Cytomegalovirus infection enhances smooth muscle cell proliferation and intimal thickening of rat aortic allografts, *J. Clin. Invest.*, *92*, 549–558.

153. Lemstrom, K. B., Aho, P. T., Bruggeman, C. A., & Hayry, P. J. (1994) Cytomegalovirus infection enhances mRNA expression of platelet-dervied growth factor BB and transforming growth factor-beta I in rat allografts. Possible mechanisms for cytomegalovirus-enhanced graft arteriosclerosis, *Arterioscler. Thromb.*, *14*, 2043–2052.

154. Persoons, M. C., Daemen, M. J., Brunning, J. H., & Bruggeman, C. A. (1994) Active cytomegalovirus infection of arterial smooth muscle cells in immunocompromised rats. A clue to herpesvirus-associated atherogenesis, *Circ. Res.*, *75*, 214–220.

155. Koskinen, P., Lemstrom, K., Bruggeman, C., Lautenschlager, I., & Hayry, P. (1994) Acute cytomegalovirus infection induces a subendothelial inflammation (subendotheliatis) in the allograft vascular wall. A possible linkage with enhanced allograft arteriosclerosis, *Am. J. Pathol.*, *144*, 41–50.

156. Lemström, K., Koskinen, P., Krogerus, L., Daemen, M., Bruggeman, C., & Hayry, P. (1995) Cytomegalovirus antigen expression, endothelial cell proliferation, and intimal thickening in rat cardiac allografts after cytomegalovirus infection, *Circulation*, *92*, 2594–2604.

157. Lemström, K. B., Koskinen, P. K., Bruning, J. H., Bruggeman, C. A., Lautenschlager, I. T., & Hayry, P. J. (1994) Effect of ganciclovir prophylaxis on cytomegalovirus enhanced allograft arteriosclerosis, *Transplant. Int.*, *7*(Suppl 1), S383–S384.

158. Valantine, H. A., Gao, S. Z., Menon, S. G., Renlund, D. G., Hunt, S. A., Oyer, P., Stinson, E. B., Brown, B. W. Jr., Merigan, T. C., & Schroeder, J. S. (1999) Impact of prophylactic immediate post-transplant ganciclovir on development of transplant atherosclerosis: a post hoc analysis of a randomized, placebo-controlled study, *Circulation*, *100*, 61–66.

159. Valantine, H. A., Luikart, H., Doyle, R., Theodore, J., Hunt, S., Oyer, P., Robbins, R., Berry, G., & Reitz, B. (2001) Impact of cytomegalovirus hyperimmune globulin on outcome after cardiothoracic transplantation: a comparative study of combined prophylaxis with CMV hyperimmune globulin plus ganciclovir versus ganciclovir alone, *Transplantation*, *72*, 1647–1652.

160. Martin, D. F., Sierra-Madero, J., Walmsley, S., Wolitz, R. A., Macey, K., Georgiou, P., Robinson, C. A., & Stempien, M., for the Vanciclovir Study Groups (2002) A controlled trial of valganciclovir as induction therapy for cytomegalovirus retinitis, *N. Engl. J. Med.*, *346*, 1119–1126.

161. Waldman, W. J., Le Claire, J. D., & Knight, D. A. (2002) T-cell activation response to allogeneic CMV-infected endothelial cells is not prevented by ganciclovir or foscarnet: implication for transplant vascular sclerosis, *Transplantation*, *73*, 314–318.

8

Miscellaneous Infections and Atherosclerosis: Cardiovascular and Cerebrovascular Disease

8.1. INTRODUCTION

There are several other infections besides *Chlamydia pneumoniae*, periodontitis, and the herpes viruses (including cytomegalovirus [CMV]) which have been implicated or associated with cardiovascular and cerebrovascular diseases over the years. However, the accumulative data to support such associations have been much less and even more conflicting than the three major infectious diseases previously discussed in chapters 5–7. A new paradigm has been proposed by S. Epstein and his collaborators[1] on the "pathogen burden" of infectious agents that may play a greater role than individual microorganisms in the pathogenesis of atherosclerosis. This new concept and other miscellaneous infections, such as *Helicobacter pylori*, influenza, and Coxsackie virus, will be discussed in this chapter.

8.2. *HELICOBACTER PYLORI* AND THE CARDIOVASCULAR SYSTEM

8.2.1. Microbiology and Epidemiology

H. pylori (formerly known as *Campylobacter pylori* or *pyloridis*) was first isolated from humans in 1981[2]. It is a highly motile, gram negative rod that lives within the mucus overlying the gastric and occasionally the duodenal epithelium[3]. Chronic colonization of *H. pylori* in the stomach, which is commonly present, is associated with cellular infiltrate in the lamina propria of the gastric antrum and fundus[4]. It is now well established and accepted that *H. pylori* is a cause of peptic ulcers, and it is strongly associated with gastric carcinoma and gastric lymphomas (mucosa-associated lymphoid tumors)[5].

H. pylori has been isolated from persons all over the world and similar organisms are present in primates, but not other animals. Humans are the major or only reservoir for *H. pylori* and the incidence of colonization is highest in countries and settings of suboptimal sanitary conditions, suggesting fecal-oral transmission[5]. The prevalence of *H. pylori* colonization is mainly related to age and geographic location, but is similar for the sexes[6,7]. In developing countries, 70% by age 10 carry *H. pylori* and by age 20 nearly everyone would have been colonized[5]. In developed countries such as the United States, colonization is uncommon in childhood but gradually increases over the years and by age 60 or more, 50–60% of the population would have been colonized.

8.2.2. Pathogenicity of *Helicobacter pylori*

H. pylori can survive and multiply in the acid environment of the stomach through several mechanisms, including protection within the mucus gel and urease activity with generation of ammonium ions that buffer gastric acidity[8]. *H. pylori* only colonizes gastric type but not intestinal type or other epithelial cells. Most of the bacteria are free living in the mucus layer but some are adherent to the epithelial cells by adhesions[5]. An inflammatory infiltrate composing of mononuclear cells and neutrophils to a lesser extent is usually present in the lamina propria and in the epithelium, and epithelial glands are affected and have less mucus.

The mechanisms of tissue injury are not clear; *H. pylori* does not appear to invade tissues, but may be related to extracellular products. *H. pylori* has little lipopolysaccharide (or endotoxin[9]) but the presence of the bacteria in the mucosa is able to activate the epithelium to produce proinflammatory cytokines, adhesion molecules, and superoxide[10]. Ammonia produced by the bacteria may also be toxic to cells and may stimulate neutrophil-induced injury, and the urease shed by *H. pylori* is a chemoattractant and activator of host phagocytic cells[11].

There is also evidence that 50% of *H. pylori* strains produce a protein (Vac A product) that in vitro produces vacuolation of epithelial cells[12]. Strains from patients with ulcers more often produce Vac A in vitro than strains from patients with gastritis only[12]. In addition, about 60% of the *H. pylori* in the

United States and most strains in the Orient possess a CagA gene that encodes a highly antigenic protein of 120–128 kDa[13], and nearly all patients with duodenal ulceration are infected with CagA positive strains.

8.2.3. Diagnosis of *Helicobacter pylori* Infection

The presence of *H. pylori* colonization or infection can be made either invasively by endoscopy and biopsy or noninvasively by serology or the urease breath test. Each of these procedures' diagnostic accuracy approaches 95% or more[5]. Biopsy specimens may be cultured for *H. pylori* on antibiotic containing media, by special selective Skirrou's medium or nonselective chocolate medium. The procedure is laborious and requires 2–5 days incubation in a moist microaerophilic environment and is not performed by most routine microbiology laboratories. Most laboratories depend on visualization of the typical comma or S-shaped organisms seen on histologic sections stained with Gram, Silver, Giemsa, or Acridine orange stains or by immunofluorescence or immunoperoxidase methods[14]. A rapid urease test can also be done on tissue to detect *H. pylori*.

Serology may be a more sensitive method to detect colonization as it is not prone to sampling error as a small biopsy specimen. Nearly all *H. pylori* colonized persons develop high stable IgG responses and, less frequently, IgA responses[14]. Antibody levels decline over 3–6 months after effective antimicrobial therapy and high antibody titer persists with ineffective therapy[15]. IgM seroconversion occurs after initial infection/colonization and, then returns to baseline but may increase again with recurrences.

The urease breath test utilizes the high urease activity of *H. pylori* and corresponds to the number of urease producing *H. pylori* present. The test can be falsely negative soon after therapy for *H. pylori* without eradication, but a negative test 1–3 months after therapy usually indicates eradication of the organism. The test procedure involves ingestion of a meal containing ^{13}C or ^{14}C-urea after fasting and over the next hour the subject's breath is examined for $^{13}CO_2$ or $^{14}CO_2$[16].

8.3. EPIDEMIOLOGICAL ASSOCIATION OF *HELICOBACTER PYLORI* AND CARDIOVASCULAR DISEASE

H. pylori has been associated with coronary heart disease (CHD) and cerebrovascular disease in some studies but not in others; most of the studies showing a positive association were small and did not adjust for potential confounders[17]. Twenty larger studies with proper control groups tended to show no or weaker associations[17]. Since 1997 one large case control and several small retrospective and cross-sectional studies have tended to show a positive association of *H. pylori* with stroke or CHD[18–21], but larger prospective studies have failed to show significant association[22–25]. In a meta-analysis of five prospective studies published in 1999, the combined odds ratio (OR) for association with CHD was only 1.13 (95% CI, 0.93–1.38)[26]. It has been suggested that the discordant findings with regard to the association of *H. pylori* and CHD may be dependent on the genetic heterogeneity of the organism and the association may be restricted to CagA bearing strain of *H. pylori*, as found in some studies[27]. However, other studies failed to find any association of CHD and CagA seropositivity[28,29].

   To date there have been 18 prospective, longitudinal studies[22–25,30–44] assessing the association between *H. pylori* past infection and CHD or stroke, see Table 8.1. The OR for association with cardiovascular disease varied from 0.9 to 2.6, but only one of the 18 studies (5.5%) showed a positive association with IgG antibodies OR 2.5 (95% CI, 1.4–4.4), and another study showed a trend, OR 2.6 ($p = 0.08$). Two studies that specifically measured the antibodies to the virulence factor CagA found no association with CHD or cardiovascular mortality.

8.3.1. Pathological Association of *Helicobacter pylori* and Atherosclerosis

   There is no good evidence that *H. pylori* enters the systemic circulation to cause bacteremia, or even cause invasion of the tissues (mucosa) of the stomach or duodenum. However, a few studies have examined atheromatous tissue of various arteries for the presence of *H. pylori* (nucleic acid) primarily by polymerase chain reaction (PCR) techniques with mixed results. There are seven studies[45–51] the results of which are summarized in Table 8.2 that have addressed this issue, and four of the seven studies failed to detect *H. pylori* or could not exclude contamination in one sample. However, three studies[48–50] reported detection of *H. pylori* in atheromatous vessels but not in control arteries, from 22% to 52.6%. The marked discrepancies in these studies may reflect techniques in the PCR methods and size or proportion of tissue samples used. At present, no validated commercialized or standardized PCR techniques are available. Therefore, the results of the positive studies cannot be confirmed or accepted as proven until further studies are published with validated, standardized methods. It is not clear whether centers reporting positive

Table 8.1

H. pylori and Atherosclerosis Prospective Studies

Study	Subjects	Follow up (years)	Endpoint	Results (95% CI)	Comments
1. Whincup et al. 1996[30]	272/136 men	11–13	MI, stroke for MI, =0.96 (0.46–2) for stroke	OR = 1.31 (0.7–2.4)	Heavily confounded by other risk factors
2. Aromaa et al. 1996[31]	441/842 men	9–12	MI	OR = 1.29 (0.96–1.73)	Association with stomach cancer confirmed
3. Wald et al. 1998[22]	648/1296 men	15.6	CHD death	OR = 1.06 (0.86–1.31)	
4. Ossewaarde et al. 1998[23]	54/108 elderly men	5	CHD death	No association	
5. Strachan et al. 1998[32]	1796 men cohort	13	CHD death	OR = 1.52 (0.99–2.34)	Adjustment for childhood social class did not change ORs
6. Regnstrom et al. 1998[33]	92 young men with MI	5	CHD events or progression	No association	
7. Folsom et al. 1998[24]	217/281	3.3	CHD	OR = 1.03 (0.68–1.57)	
8. Danesh et al. 1999[34]	246/642	4	CHD	OR = 1.28 (0.93–1.75)	Adjusted for childhood social class
9. Ridker et al. 1999[35]	122/244 women	3	CHD event	RR = 0.9 (0.6–1.4)	No association with "pathogen burden"
10. Roivainen et al. 2000[36]	241/241	8.5	MI, CHD death	No association	
11. Whincup et al. 2000[37]	505/1025	16	CHD	OR = 1.3 (0.88–1.9)	Before adjustment for childhood social class OR = 1.5 (1.1–2). No association with CagA antibodies
12. Choussat et al. 2000[38]	81 with unstable CHD	1	CHD events	OR + 2.6 (*p* = 0.08)	

Table 8.1
(continued)

Study	Subjects	Follow up (years)	Endpoint	Results (95% CI)	Comments
13. Mayr et al. 2000[39]	826, cohort 40–79 years old	5	Carotid/femoral atherosclerosis	Non-stenotic OR = 1.01 (0.88–1.17) Stenotic OR = 1.14 (0.93–1.38)	NS, part of Branek study
14. Zhu et al. 2001[40]	890 with CHD	3	MI, death	RH = 1.12 (0.81–1.54)	RH = 1.98 (1.18–3.31) for MI, but 0.76% (0.5–1.14) for death. Association with "pathogen burden" found
15. Rupprecht et al. 2001[41]	1010 with CHD	3.1	MI, CHD death	OR = 2.5 (1.4–4.4) for IgA	Association with "pathogen burden" found
16. Stone et al. 2001[42]	172/172 case control	10	MI or death	OR = 1.13 (0.61–2.07)	Assessed CagA seropositivity
17. Ridker et al. 2001[43]	445/445 case control men	8.9	MI	OR = 0.96 (0.7–1.3)	NS
18. Zhu et al. 2002[44]	929 with CHD	3	MI, death	OR = 1.12 (0.81–1.54)	

Note. OR, odds ratio; RH, relative hazard; CHD, coronary heart disease; MI, myocardial infarction; RR, rate ratio; CagA, product of cytotoxin associated gene A.

Table 8.2

Helicobacter pylori in Arteries

Study	Method	Vessels involved diseased	Control	Comment
1. Blasi et al. 1996[45]	PCR	0/51 AAAs		47 seropositive for *H. pylori*
2. Danesh et al. 1999[46]	PCR	1/39 carotid		Contamination could not be excluded
3. Malnick et al. 1999[47]	PCR	0/10 carotid		
4. Farsak et al. 2000[48]	PCR	17/46 various arteries	0/39 various arteries	
5. Rassu et al. 2001[49]	PCR	4/18 various arteries	0/22 various arteries	
6. Ameriso et al. 2001[50]	PCR, IHC	20/38 carotid	0/7 carotid	Good correlation of methods
7. Radke et al. 2001[51]	PCR	0/53 coronary		Controls not mentioned
Total	Any	42/255 (16%)	0/68 (00%)	

Note. AAA, abdominal aortic aneurysm; PCR, polymerase chain reaction; IHC, immunohistochemistry.

findings could be the result of contamination or not. The failure of previous pathological studies to detect such a large organism by electron microscopy leads to further questions on credibility of these few reports.

8.3.2. Biological Mechanisms for *Helicobacter pylori*

There are few data to support the theory that *H. pylori* plays a role in the pathogenesis of cardiovascular disease or atherosclerosis. Only a few studies have been performed to address this issue. Hypothetical mechanisms include stimulation of an autoimmune reaction to human endogenous heat shock protein (HSP) 60 by *H. pylori* HSP, and an indirect effect of systemic inflammatory mediators by local mucosal inflammation, which may affect homeostasis[52].

In a recent study[39], antibody levels to *C. pneumoniae* and *H. pylori* correlated significantly with antibodies to mycobacterial HSP 65 (mHSP65) ($p = 0.03$ and $p = 0.001$, respectively). Increased concentrations of anti-mHSP65 were sustained in subjects with carotid atherosclerosis in a 5-year follow-up study[53]. However, in another recent report, high antibodies to *H. pylori* HSP60 was not an independent risk factor for CHD in a German population aged 40–68 years[54]. Yet in a study of 136 men undergoing coronary angiography, anti-mHSP65 titer correlated with the severity and extent of coronary atherosclerosis ($p = 0.012$); and in 100 patients with active *H. pylori* infection, successful eradication of *H. pylori* led to a significant fall in anti-mHSP65 titer from a mean of 256.4 to 137.5 $AU \cdot ml^{-1}$, $p = 0.033$[55].

Two small studies suggesting that people who are seropositive for *H. pylori* have an increased concentration of inflammatory or procoagulant markers have not been confirmed by larger studies[54,56–59]. *H. pylori* causes platelet aggregation and induces procoagulant activity in experimentally infected mice[60], and has been associated with increased fibrinogen in a couple of studies[61,62], thus, could potentiate acute thrombus formation and lead to ischemic events theoretically. However, other studies have not found increased fibrinogen associated with *H. pylori* seropositivity[38,59] and the presence of *H. pylori*, as determined by histological and microbiological investigation, a rapid urease test, and a ^{13}C urea breath test was not associated with increased circulating levels of fibrinogen, Factor VII: C, Factor VIII: C or von Willebrand factor in 103 subjects undergoing endoscopy for dyspepsia[63].

Hyperhomocystinemia has been strongly implicated in atherothrombosis and cardiovascular disease, and the atherogenic propensity may result from endothelial dysfunction and injury followed by platelet activation and thrombus formation[64]. It has been proposed that *H. pylori* infection can cause changes in gastric juice by inducing gastritis, which could lead to reduced folate absorption and thus result in folate deficiency, with subsequent hyperhomocystinemia from the reduced methionine synthase activity (which is folate dependent)[65]. In type 2 diabetics infected with *H. pylori* (documented by ^{13}C urea breath test) homocysteine levels were found to be significantly higher than those without *H. pylori* (14.0 ± 6.5 vs. 10.6 ± 4.7 mmol/L, respectively, $p < 0.01$), without differences in vitamin B_{12}, folate or genetic polymorphism of methylenetetrahydrofolate reductase[66]. However, in another study of subjects undergoing coronary angiography lower vitamin B_{12} but not folate levels were found in patients seropositive for *H. pylori* CagA compared to CagA negative cases (209.6 ± 104.2 vs. 252.9 ± 109.8 pmol/L, respectively, $p = 0.023$)[67]. Although higher homocysteine levels were found in subjects with CHD in this study, there were no significant differences in any of the parameters studied between *H. pylori* seropositive and seronegative groups.

It has been suggested that the association of cardiovascular disease with *H. pylori* may be partly due to metabolic risk factors for CHD, secondary to low grade inflammation caused by infections. In a recent study, 245 subjects with combined serology for *H. pylori* and *C. pneumoniae* were compared to 57 controls without any positive serology, the group with positive serology had greater body mass index (BMI) (27.3 vs. 25.8 kg/m^2, $p < 0.05$), higher fasting insulin levels (12.7 vs. 11.6 pmol/L, $p < 0.05$), but this did not remain significant after adjustment for age and BMI, and lower socioeconomic class[68]. However, there was no difference in levels of glucose and lipids. In another study of 116 patients with CHD and 116 matched controls, those who were *H. pylori* seropositive among the controls had higher triglycerides than those who were seronegative ($p = 0.03$), and among the cases the trend was similar but nonsignificant[69]. The concentration of high-density lipoprotein (HDL) cholesterol also tended to be lower in those who were *H. pylori* positive than those who were *H. pylori* negative, among both the cases and controls[69].

8.3.3. Animal Models for *Helicobacter pylori*

A mouse model exists using CDI and BALB/C mice that mimics human disease of the gastric mucosa, when infected repeatedly with clinical isolates of *H. pylori* that express the vacuolating cytotoxin (VACA) and the cytotoxin associated antigen (CagA)[70]. Other animal models for *H. pylori* gastric colonization/infection include germ-free animals[71], nude mice[72], primates (chimpanzee)[73], and Mongolian gerbils[74]. In gerbils chronically infected with *H. pylori* for up to 5 months, there is predominately superficial inflammation of the antral mucosa and in addition deep gastric wall inflammation (reaching beyond the muscularis mucosae), which is in contrast to *H. pylori* induced gastric inflammation in humans. In parallel with the deep inflammation, *H. pylori* organisms were seen in the glandular lumina, in contrast to their usual confinement to the surface epithelium and gastric pits in humans[74]. However, no deep invasion of tissues with *H. pylori* are found in any animal models to suggest possible systemic inoculation.

Recently there is one reported animal experiment with *H. pylori* on enhancing atherosclerosis in C57/B16 and LDL-receptor deficient mice fed a high cholesterol diet. No effect of *H. pylori* infection was found on athero-sclerosis in either genotype mouse[75]. However, only 8 mice per group was studied; thus the study may not be powered to show a 20–30% increase in atherosclerosis. Furthermore, the animals were kept for only 12 weeks which may be too short a duration, as in C57BL/CJ mice on high diet it took over 15 weeks to demonstrate enhancement with *C. pneumoniae* infection[76].

8.3.4. Clinical Trials in *Helicobacter pylori* Infection and Cardiovascular Disease

There are a few preliminary studies assessing treatment specific for *H. pylori* and assessing the effect on surrogate markers and cardiovascular endpoints. In a study involving 84 patients with CHD and antibodies to *H. pylori* or *C. pneumoniae*, or both, 43 treated patients had significantly lower fibrinogen levels at 6 months than the untreated controls[62]. However, the reduction in fibrinogen may have been related primarily to the effect of clarithromycin on *C. pneumoniae* infection.

Although there is no epidemiological or pathological evidence to suggest an association with post-percutaneous transluminal coronary angioplasty (PTCA) coronary restenosis, one small study has assessed the benefits of *H. pylori* treatment. In a group of 40 patients undergoing PTCA for single vessel disease with *H. pylori* infection (confirmed by ^{13}C urea breath test and serology), treatment was randomized equally to triple anti-*H. pylori* therapy or placebo[77]. After 6 months the reduction in coronary artery lumen was significantly less in the treated group versus placebo, 22% and 44%, respectively, $p < 0.05$[77].

In a preliminary report of the STAMINA trial, 324 patients with acute myocardial infarction or unstable angina were randomized to receive 1 week of azithromycin plus metronidazole and omeprezole, or 1 week of amoxicillin plus metronidazole and omeprezole, or placebo[78]. Both treatment regimens, which were targeting *H. pylori* but only the former targeting *C. pneumoniae*, reduced cardiac events compared to placebo by 37% after 3 months or 1 year[78]. This study suggests that *H. pylori* or periodontal pathogens (which would be affected by both regimens) could contribute to acute cardiac events. However, more detailed information is needed regarding *H. pylori* infection status in the groups, as this was not provided in the abstract.

8.4. VIRUSES (OTHER THAN HERPES VIRUSES) ASSOCIATED WITH ATHEROSCLEROTIC CARDIOVASCULAR DISEASE

8.4.1. Coxsackie virus

Coxsackie viruses are well-established causes of myocarditis and pericarditis, but small series have suggested a role of Coxsackie B virus in acute myocardial infarction[79]. However, controlled studies with relatively small sample sizes have yielded conflicting results[80–86]. Also some of the cases diagnosed as acute myocardial infarction may actually be focal myocarditis[87].

8.4.2. Influenza Virus

Influenza infections and seasonal outbreaks have been associated with excess morbidity and mortality in elderly people from cardiac and pulmonary complications. However, most of these complications are considered to be secondary to bacterial pneumonia, or direct lung involvement, or precipitation of heart failure and rarely secondary myocarditis. However, in epidemics of influenza in the early part of the 20th century, excess mortality was attributed to causes other than influenza and pneumonia, including heart disease[88]. A few retrospective studies[89–91] and one prospective study[92] have suggested that acute respiratory infection might trigger myocardial infarction. Influenza vaccine has been shown to reduce the risk of acquiring influenza and of hospitalization and death, particularly in the elderly[93]. In a recent case–control study of 218 patients (109 with acute myocardial infarction and 109 controls with stable CHD), vaccination against influenza was associated with reduced risk of new myocardial infarction in the same season (OR 0.33, 95% CI, 0.13–0.82, $p = 0.017$)[94]. In another case–control study of 270 subjects during an influenza epidemic period, 90 consecutive patients older than 60 years admitted with brain infarction and 180 population-based, age and sex-matched controls were analyzed for influenza vaccination[95]. After adjustment for age, traditional risk factors, and recent use of antibiotics, the risk of stroke was reduced in subjects vaccinated during the year of the study and in those vaccinated during the last 5 years, with an OR of 0.50 (95% CI, 0.26–0.94, $p = 0.033$) and 0.42 (95% CI, 0.21–0.81, $p = 0.009$), respectively[95]. Similar associations were observed in cases and controls free of previous cardiovascular history.

Acute phase proteins such as C-reactive protein (CRP) and serum amyloid A (SAA) elevations have been associated with increased risk of atherosclerotic events, and have been shown to be markers of current and future cardiovascular disease. In a recent study these acute phase proteins were measured during and 4 weeks after influenza illness in 7 young persons, 15 elderly out patients, and 36 hospitalized adults[96]. Striking elevations were seen in mean SAA and CRP levels in all groups, but hospitalized patients had the highest levels (SAA, 503 vs. 310 μg/mL [$p = 0.006$]; CRP, 120 mg vs. 34 μg/mL [$p < 0.001$])[96]. Thus, it is possible that direct effects of CRP may exacerbate preexisting atherosclerotic lesions, or may precipitate a thrombus on an unstable plaque, and may help explain cardiovascular events associated with acute influenza.

8.4.3. Hepatitis A Virus

Hepatitis A virus (HAV), the commonest cause of sporadic hepatitis does not produce chronic or persistent liver disease, and is not known to reside or produce disease in other tissues. HAV is usually eliminated from the body within a month, although lifelong immunity and antibodies usually persist[97]. Most infections are subclinical and 40–70% of the population in developed countries develop antibodies by adulthood, whereas virtually all adults in developing countries show evidence of past infection[97]. Theoretically, if infections play a role in atherogenesis, they would more likely occur in situations where the microorganisms exists intracellularly in a chronic, persistent, or latent state. Certainly, HAV would not be considered a candidate agent with this model. However, two recent studies from the same group have raised the possibility of HAV playing a role in the pathogenesis of atherosclerosis. In their first study, Zhu et al.[1] studied the role of multiple pathogens in atherosclerotic disease in a cohort of 238 individuals, and found a strong association between HAV and CHD. In a follow-up study, the original cohort was increased to 391 subjects and an in-depth analysis of the relationship between HAV and CHD was performed[98]. The prevalence of CHD was 74% in HAV seropositive and 52% in HAV seronegative patients ($p < 0.001$), significance persisted after correction for traditional risk factors and serologies for other infections. In addition, the CRP levels were significantly higher in the HAV seropositive than in HAV seronegative patients ($p = 0.013$)[98]. The biological mechanisms by which HAV infection may predispose to atherosclerosis has been suggested to relate to the inflammatory and immune responses evoked by all pathogens[98]. However, these mechanisms would only have been transiently increased or stimulated during the acute infectious episode. It is more likely that the association of HAV and atherosclerotic vascular diseases is a spurious one or an epiphenomenon.

8.4.4. Human Immunodeficiency Virus (HIV)

Prior to highly active antiretroviral therapy (HAART) for HIV infection, lipidemia and hypertriglyceridemia were seen commonly in patients with uncontrolled infection or acquired immunodeficiency syndrome (AIDS). This was attributed to excessive cytokine activation (particularly TNF-α), and excessive fasting triglycerides was used as a surrogate marker for cytokine stimulation[99]. Excessive cardiovascular mortality or morbidity was not a concern then as patients were dying prematurely of opportunistic infections or neoplastic complications. With the advent of HARRT and markedly improved survival of HIV-infected patients, there has been increasing reports of cardiovascular events in young adults with HIV infection. HIV infection and resulting complications from the immunosuppression can lead to dilated cardiomyopathy, pericarditis and pericardial effusion, myocarditis, pulmonary hypertension, neoplastic invasion, and secondary endocarditis[100]. However, with better control of HIV infection with combination of new agents, these complications are becoming rare, but increasing morbidity and mortality from CHD have now become a concern[101,102]. Recent case control studies indicate that HIV-infected patients with the metabolic syndrome characterized by lipodystrophy, profound insulin resistance and hyperlipidemia are mainly at risk for cardiovascular events[102], and ischemic CHD events in HIV-infected persons are commonly associated with traditional risk factors such as cigarette smoking, hypertension, family history of CHD, and hypercholesterolemia[103].

The exact causes of the lipodystrophy and metabolic syndrome in HIV-infected persons are not well established, but studies have linked these abnormalities to the HAART itself, particularly the protease inhibitors[104,105] but also to the nucleoside analogs which have been associated with mitochondrial toxicity[106,107]. Thus, at the present time the increased risk for CHD in HIV-infected persons appears to be multifactorial, with a major component attributed to the drug therapy and there is no evidence that the increased cardiovascular events are related to the HIV infection itself or other infectious agents. However, there is a paucity of data addressing the issue of concomitant infections, such as *C. pneumoniae*, CMV, or periodontitis, in this population and possible association with atherosclerotic vascular disease.

8.5. *MYCOPLASMA PNEUMONIAE* AND CARDIOVASCULAR/CEREBROVASCULAR DISEASE

M. pneumoniae, a primary respiratory pathogen, has been reported to cause pericarditis[108] and rarely endocarditis[109]. However, there are several case reports of cerebral infarctions, occurring in young adults[110,111] and young children[112-114] associated with acute *M. pneumoniae* infections. Although there is one report of detecting *M. pneumoniae* with *C. pneumoniae* in thrombosed ruptured atheromas of three patients who died of acute myocardial infarction[115], it is likely that rare cases of stroke associated with *M. pneumoniae* infarction (especially in children) are probably related to vasculitis of the cerebral arteries. In the rabbit model, repeated infection with *M. pneumoniae* does not result in any atherosclerotic changes but some animals develop evidence of periaortitis of the abdominal aorta which may represent early changes of vasculitis[116].

8.6. PATHOGEN BURDEN AND ATHEROSCLEROTIC VASCULAR DISEASE

The concept that infections can influence development of atherosclerosis mediated through alterations of circulating cytokines or by immune response to infection, or by an autoimmune mechanism(s) suggests that multiple pathogens even at distant sites could play a role in atherogenesis[117]. Molecular mimicry, a mechanism requiring that the infecting pathogen contain peptides homologous to those present in human host protein, is one of the mechanisms responsible for infection-induced autoimmune related disease (such as rheumatic fever, myocarditis and Guillin Barré syndrome, etc.). Such a mechanism does not require the presence of the candidate pathogen within the atherosclerotic vessel.

The paradigm that molecular mimicry by an autoimmune mechanism could contribute to atherogenesis is supported by studies that have identified auto-antibodies to HSPs in patients with atherosclerosis[118,119]. These ubiquitous intracellular proteins are normally present in low concentrations, increase in response to stress, and become accessible to the immune system after being transported to the cell membrane. Peptides derived from HSP may reach the cell surface of stressed endothelial cells, and result in complement mediated lytic effects of anti-HSP antibodies[120,121]. Normally, the amount of such peptides presenting on the cell surface may be insufficient to stimulate an immune response in persons with low or absent levels of specific auto-antibodies or auto-aggressive T-cells. However, an infection with a pathogen bearing homologous peptides may stimulate the immune response resulting in high levels of cross-reactive antibodies or auto-aggressive T-cells that lead to an autoimmune disease.

Since HSPs are highly conserved and all bacteria encode for HSPs, with high homology between prokaryotic and mammalian HSP, then HSP would be a candidate homologous pathogen/host peptide that could cause infection-induced autoimmune response of the arterial wall leading to atherosclerosis. Although viruses generally do not encode for HSPs, they incorporate the host HSP into their envelopes when budding from host cells[122]. Although most studies investigating the relationship between infection and atherosclerotic related disease concentrate on the effect of single individual pathogens, a few studies have examined the effect of multiple pathogen burden. It has been postulated that the aggregate pathogen burden, through molecular mimicry and cytokine stimulation, may have a greater effect on atherogenesis than a single or individual pathogen[117].

A few cross-sectional studies have examined the effect of individual pathogens versus aggregate pathogen burden and the risk for cardiovascular disease. In one study, for example, serologies to either *C. pneumoniae* or *H. pylori* alone did not predict the risk for CHD but seropositivity to both organisms correlated with increased risk of CHD (OR 2.6, $p = 0.02$)[123]. Also, Zhu et al.[1] in a cross-sectional study demonstrated that whereas several individual pathogens (CMV, *C. pneumoniae*, herpes simplex virus (HSV) types I and II, and HAV) were variably associated with the risk of CHD, it was the aggregate pathogen burden that most significantly related infection to atherosclerotic vascular risks. A similar finding was reported in 218 patients who underwent coronary angiography and assessed serologic markers for six infectious pathogens[124]. Whereas seropositivity for a single pathogen was not a predictor risk for CHD, individuals exposed to four or more pathogens correlated with prevalence of CHD, $p = 0.02$[124].

A few prospective studies[125–129] addressing the issue of pathogen burden and atherosclerotic vascular complications are summarized in Table 8.3. Four of the five studies found greater association of cardiovascular events with serologies to multiple pathogens than a single organism or even three or less pathogens.

8.6.1. Pathological Evidence of Multiple Organisms in Atheroma

Multiple pathogens have been identified in atheromatous plaques in a few studies by immunohistochemical stains or PCR. Examination of 76 carotid endarterectomy specimens by immunostain using specific monoclonal antibodies for *C. pneumoniae*, CMV and HSV-1, we were able to detect two microorganisms in 12 (23.7%), three microorganisms in 6 (7.9%), but mainly single pathogen in up to 77%[130]. However, although the presence of *C. pneumoniae* or CMV was associated with a fresh thrombus ($p = 0.038$ and $p = 0.007$, respectively), the presence of three pathogens was not ($p = 0.12$)[130]. In a smaller study of 17 carotid endarterectomy sample analyzed for CMV and *C. pneumoniae* DNA by PCR, 4 of 17 (24%) specimens contained both microorganism, whereas either pathogen was detected in 12 of 17 (71%) carotid plaques[131]. The presence of both CMV and *C. pneumoniae* together in large coronary specimens have been detected at lower rates by PCR in one study of 53 patients; two organisms together were detected in 5 of 106 (5%) lesions or 5 of 53 (9%) coronary arteries, whereas individually CMV and *C. pneumoniae* were detected in 30% and 32% of the samples, respectively[51].

Chiu[132] examined 33 carotid endarterectomy specimens for multiple pathogens including CMV, HSV-1, *C. pneumoniae* (using monoclonal antibodies for immunostain) and oral pathogens (*Porphyromonas gingivalis* and *Streptococcus sanguis* by polyclonal antibodies). From one to four organisms were found in the same specimen with two or three in 24% and 21%, and four pathogens in 6%. The use of polyclonal antibodies for immunostain for oral bacteria raises the issue of nonspecificity or false positive results.

As previously mentioned in Chapter 6, two studies by the same group have detected multiple oral bacteria in carotid endarterectomy specimens using PCR for 16S ribosomal RNA[133,134]; however, these results need to be

Table 8.3
Prospective Studies of Pathogen Burden and Atherosclerosis

Study	Subjects	Follow up (years)	Pathogens	End point	Results	Comments
Ridker et al. 1999[125]	122/244 women	3	Cp, Hp, HSV, CMV	CHD events or procedures, stroke	RR = 1.2 (0.7–2.2)	
Roivainen et al. 2000[126]	241/241	8.5	Cp, HSV-1	MI, CHD death	OR = 4.1 (1.88–8.98)	Cp alone did not reach statistical significance
Zhu et al. 2001[127]	890	3	CMV, HSV-1, HSV-2, HAV	MI, death	RH = 7.61 (1.04–55.7)	No association with Cp and Hp individually
Rupprecht et al. 2001[128]	1014 with CHD	3.1	Cp, Hp, Mp, Hi, HSV-1, HSV-2, EBV CMV	Cardiovascular events	HRR = 5.1 (1.4–18.3) for 0–3 vs. >5 pathogens	Only viral pathogen burden statistically significant
Espinola-Klein et al. 2002[129]	570 with CHD	3.2	Cp, Hp, Mp, Hi, HSV-1, HSV-2, EBV CMV	Cardiovascular death	HR = 2.9 (1.2–9.6) for 0–3 vs. >5 pathogens	Also cross-sectional association with extent of atherosclerosis

Note. RR, rate ratio; HRR, hazard risk ratio; OR, odds ratio; RH, relative hazard; HR, hazards ratio; CHD, coronary heart disease; MI, myocardial infarction; Cp, *Chlamydia pneumoniae*; HP, *Helicobacter pylori*; Mp, *Mycoplasma pneumoniae*; Hi, *Haemophilus influenza*; HSV, herpes simplex virus; CMV, cytomegalovirus; EBV, Epstein–Barr virus; HAV, hepatitis A virus.

confirmed by other centers. Also, *H. pylori* and *C. pneumoniae* DNA have detected together in 6 of 46 (13%) endarterectomy specimens[48], and in 6 of 90 (7.6%) arteries (various) and CMV and *C. pneumoniae* together in 3 of 90 (3.3%), and all three microorganisms in 1 of 90 (1.1%) arteries[49]. However, the presence of *H. pylori* in atheromas has not been validated and these findings may be questioned.

8.6.2. Biological Mechanisms and Animal Model for Multiple Pathogens in Atherosclerosis

Beside the theoretical hypothesis that an aggregate of pathogens may more likely cause an autoimmune response or greater cytokine stimulation than an individual microorganism, thus greater role in atherogenesis, there is little in vitro data on biological mechanisms to support this concept. CMV is believed to exist in host tissues in a latent state with periodic reactivation, and a recent in vitro study demonstrated that co-infection of HeLa cells with *C. pneumoniae* resulted in increased transactivation of the major immediate early promoter of CMV (which is essential for viral gene expression and viral replication)[135]. These results suggest that CMV and *C. pneumoniae* could synergistically contribute to development of atherosclerosis.

However, in an animal model using apoê knockout mice, murine CMV alone or *C. pneumoniae* alone increased atherosclerotic lesion size by 84% ($p < 0.001$) and 70% ($p < 0.001$), respectively; but the combination of the two pathogens increased lesion size only by 45% ($p < 0.01$)[136]. Thus, this model did not confirm that multiple pathogens increase progression of atherosclerosis to a greater extent than seen with a single infection.

8.7. CONCLUSION AND FUTURE DIRECTIONS

With respect to the viral infections association with atherosclerotic vascular diseases, the data on Coxsackie virus and HAV is weak and lacks convincing biological plausible explanation. The emerging relationships of HIV infection and cardiovascular disease appear to be strong but largely due to the effects of medications compounded by lifestyle risk factors. The correlation of reduction of cardiovascular events with influenza vaccination is most intriguing and merits further investigation. It is quite feasible that persons with a critical coronary artery stenosis or vulnerable plaque, on developing influenza infection are prone to acute coronary thrombosis from distant effects of the release of proinflammatory cytokines and activation of tissue factor leading to a procoagulant environment. On the other hand, the effect of influenza infection may be just another nonspecific stressful event (such as shoveling snow) in subjects with unstable plaque or critical narrowing of the artery.

Future investigations of the effect of influenza seasons or outbreaks need to be performed in prospective studies. Randomized placebo controlled studies would be unethical where influenza vaccine is clearly indicated (in most elderly subjects or those with chronic cardiopulmonary, metabolic, and immunosuppressive diseases). However, controlled trials could be performed in subjects younger than 65 years with otherwise stable CHD.

The overall data on *H. pylori* and association with cardiovascular or cerebrovascular disease are weak. The few studies demonstrating *H. pylori* DNA in plaques are suspect as numerous studies in human subjects with peptic ulcer disease or dyspepsia have been unable to demonstrate invasion of the bacteria into the mucosa or submucosa; thus, the bacteria is unlikely to enter the systemic circulation. A single report of *H. pylori* infecting an abdominal aneurysm[136] cannot be substantiated or verified as no detailed microbiological data was provided. A remote effect by stimulation of local cytokines cannot be excluded, but future studies in humans should determine whether the proinflammatory cytokines are increased in the circulation in persons with active peptic ulcer disease secondary to *H. pylori*. Testing the theory of exacerbating atherosclerosis with *H. pylori* in a murine model or other animals prone to this infection would be the next step, with larger samples of animals and longer duration than the single previous report[75].

The accumulating epidemiological data on pathogen burden and atherosclerotic complications are fairly good, but future studies need to expand on biological mechanisms for aggregate infection versus single infection. Furthermore, studies on animal models should be expanded using other animals such as rabbits, guinea pigs, and mini-pigs with various combination of infectious agents (i.e., *C. pneumoniae*, periodontal pathogens and CMV or *H. pylori* singly and in combination).

REFERENCES

1. Zhu, J., Quyyumi, A. A., Norman, J. E., Csako, G., Waclawiw, M. A., Shearer, G. M., & Epstein, S. E. (2000) Effects of total pathogen burden on coronary artery disease risk and C-reactive protein levels, *Am. J. Cardiol., 85,* 140–146.

2. Marshall, B. J. (1989) History of the discovery of *Campylobacter pylori*, in M. J. Balser (Ed.) Campylobacter pylori *in gastritis and peptic ulcer disease* (pp. 7–23), New York: Igaku Shoin.

3. Hazell, S. L., Lee, A., Brady, L., & Hennessy, W. (1986) *Campylobacter pyloridis* and gastritis: association with intracellular spaces and adaptation to an environment of mucus as important factors in colonization of the gastric epithelium, *J. Infect. Dis., 153*, 658–663.

4. Paull, G., & Yardley, J. H. (1989) Pathology of pylori-associated gastric and esophageal lesions, in M. J. Blaser (Ed.) Campylobacter pylori *in gastritis and peptic ulcer disease* (pp. 73–98), New York: Igaku Shoin.

5. Blaser, M. J. (2000) *Helicobacter pylori* and related organisms, in G. L. Mandell, J. E. Bennett, & R. Dolin (Eds.) *Principles and practice of infectious diseases* (5th ed., Vol. 2, pp. 2285–2293), Philadelphia: Churchill Livingstone.

6. Taylor, D. N., & Blaser, M. J. (1991) The epidemiology of *Helicobacter pylori* infections, *Epidemiol. Rev., 13*, 42–59.

7. Dooley, C. P., Fitzgibbons, P. L., Cohen, H., Bauer, M., Appleman, M. D., Perez-Perez, G. I., & Blaser, M. J. (1989) Prevalence of *Helicobacter pylori* infection and histologic gastritis in asymptomatic person, *N. Engl. J. Med., 321*, 1562–1566.

8. Perez-Perez, G. I., Olivares, A. Z., Cover, T. L., & Blaser, M. J. (1992) Characteristics of *Helicobacter pylori* variants selected for urease deficiency, *Infect. Immun., 60*, 3658–3663.

9. Perez-Perez, G. I., Shepherd, V. L., Morrow, J. D., & Blaser, M. J. (1995) Activation of human THP-I cells and rat bone marrow-derived macrophages by *Helicobacter pylori* lipopolysaccharide, *Infect. Immun., 63*, 1183–1187.

10. Sharma, S. A., Tummuru, M. K. R., Miller, G. G., & Blaser, M. J. (1995) Interleukin-8 response of gastric epithelial cell lines to *Helicobacter pylori* stimulation in vitro, *Infect. Immun., 63*, 1681–1687.

11. Mai, U. E., Perez-Perez, G. I., Allen, J. B., Wahl, S. M., Blaser, M. I., & Smith, P. D. (1992) Surface proteins from *Helicobacter pylori* exhibit chemotactic activity for human leucocytes and are present in gastric mucosa, *J. Exp. Med., 175*, 517–525.

12. Cover, T. L. (1996) The vacuolating cytotoxin of *Helicobacter pylori, Mol. Microbiol., 20*, 241–246.

13. Covacci, A., Censini, S., Bugnoli, M., Petracca, R., Burroni, D., Macchia, G., Massone, A., Papini, E., Xiang, Z., & Figura, N. (1993) Molecular characterization of the 128 kDa immunodominant antigen of *Helicobacter pylori* associated with cytotoxicity and duodenal ulcer, *Proc. Natl. Acad. Sci. USA, 90*, 5791–5795.

14. Dunn, B. E., Cohen, H., & Blaser, M. J. (1997) *Helicobacter pylori, Clin. Microbiol. Rev., 10*, 720–741.

15. Kosunen, T. U., Seppala, K., Sarna, S., & Sipponen, P. (1992) Diagnostic value of decreased IgG, IgA and IgM antibody titers after eradication of *Helicobacter pylori, Lancet, 339*, 893–895.

16. Marshall, B. J., & Surveyor, I. (1988) Carbon-14 urea breath test for the diagnosis of *Campylobacter pylori*-associated gastritis, *J. Nucl. Med., 29*, 11–16.

17. Danesh, J., Collins, R., & Peto, R. (1997) Chronic infections and coronary heart disease: is there a link? *Lancet, 350*, 430–436.

18. Ossei-Gerning, N., Moayyedi, P., Smith, S., Braunholtz, D., Wilson, J. I., Axon, A. T., & Grant, P. J. (1997) *Helicobacter pylori* infection is related to atheroma in patients undergoing angiography, *Cardiovasc. Res.*, *35*, 120–124.
19. de Luis, D. A., Lahera, M., Canton, R., Boixeda, D., San Roman, A. L., Aller, R., & de La Calle, H. (1998) Association of *Helicobacter pylori* infection with cardiovascular and cerebrovascular disease in diabetic patients, *Diabetes Care*, *21*, 1129–1132.
20. Markus, H. S., & Mendall, M. A. (1998) *Helicobacter pylori* infection: a risk factor for ischaemic cerebrovascular disease and carotid atheroma, *J. Neurol. Neurosurg. Psychiatry*, *64*, 104–107.
21. Danesh, J., Youngman, L., Clark, S., Parish, S., Peto, R., & Collins, R. (1999) *Helicobacter pylori* infection and early onset myocardial infarction: case control and sibling pairs study, *BMJ*, *319*, 1157–1162.
22. Wald, N. J., Law, M. R., Morris, J. K., & Bagnall, A. M. (1997) *Helicobacter pylori* and mortality from ischaemic heart disease: negative result from a large prospective study, *BMJ*, *315*, 1199–1201.
23. Ossewaarde, J. M., Feskens, E. J., De Vries, A., Vallinga, C. E., & Kromhout, D. (1998) *Chlamydia pneumoniae* is a risk factor for coronary heart disease in symptom free elderly men, but *Helicobacter pylori* and cytomegalovirus are not, *Epidemiol. Infect.*, *120*, 93–99.
24. Folsom, A. R., Neito, F. J., Sorlie, P., Chambless, L. E., & Graham, D. Y. (1998) *Helicobacter pylori* seropositivity and coronary heart disease incidence. Atherosclerosis risk in communities (ARIC) study investigators, *Circulation*, *98*, 845–850.
25. Khurshid, A., Fenske, T., Bajwa, T., Bourgevis, K., & Vakil, N. (1998) A prospective controlled study of *Helicobacter pylori* seroprevalence in coronary artery disease, *Am. J. Gastroenterol.*, *93*, 717–720.
26. Danesh, J. (1999) Coronary heart disease, *Helicobacter pylori*, dental disease, *Chlamydia pneumoniae*, and cytomegalovirus; meta-analyses of prospective studies, *Am. Heart J.*, *138*, S434–S437.
27. Gunn, M., Stephens, J. C., Thompson, J. R., Rathbone, B. J., & Samani, N. K. (2000) Significant association of cag A positive *Helicobacter pylori* strains with risk of premature myocardial infacrtion, *Heart*, *84*, 267–271.
28. Koenig, W., Rothenbacher, P., Hoffmeister, A., Miller, M., Bode, G., Adler, G., Hombach, V., Marz, W., Pepys, M. B., & Brenner, H. (1999) Infection with *Helicobacter pylori* is not a major independent risk factor for stable coronary heart disease: lack of a role of cytotoxin associated protein A positive strains and absence of a systemic inflammatory response, *Circulation*, *100*, 2326–2331.
29. Murrary, L. J., Bamford, K. B., Kee, F., McMaster, D., Cambien, F., Dallongeville, J., & Evans, A. (2000) Infections with virulent strains of *Helicobacter pylori* is not associated with ischemia heart disease: evidence from a population-based case–control study of myocardial infarction, *Atherosclerosis*, *149*, 379–385.
30. Whincup, P. H., Mendall, M. A., Perry, I. J., Strachan, D. P., & Walker, M. (1996) Prospective relations between *Helicobacter pylori* infection, coronary heart disease, and stroke in middle aged men, *Heart*, *75*, 568–672.

31. Aromaa, A., Knekt, P., Reunanen, A., Rautelin, H. I., & Kosunen, T. U. (1996) *Helicobacter infection* and the risk of myocardial infarction, *Gut, 39* (Suppl. 2), A1.

32. Strachan, D. P., Mendall, M. A., Carrington, D., Butland, B. K., Yarnell, J. W., Sweetnam, P. M., & Elwood, P. C. (1998) Relations of *Helicobacter pylori* infection to 13-year mortality and incident ischemic heart disease in the Caerphilly prospective heart disease study, *Circulation, 98,* 1286–1290.

33. Regnstrom, J., Jovinge, S., Bavenholm, P., Ericsson, C. G., De Faire, U., Hamsten, A., Hellenius, M. L., Nilsson, J., & Tornvall, P. (1998) *Helicobacter pylori* seropositivity is not associated with inflammatory parameters, lipid concentrations and degree of coronary artery disease, *J. Intern. Med., 243,* 109–113.

34. Danesh, J., Wong, Y., Ward, M., & Muri, J. (1999) Chronic infection with *Helicobacter pylori, Chlamydia pneumoniae,* or cytomegalovirus: population based study of coronary heart disease, *Heart, 81,* 245–247.

35. Ridker, P. M., Hennekens, C. H., Buring, J. E., Kundsin, R., & Shih, J. (1999) Baseline IgG antibody titers to *Chlamydia pneumoniae, Helicobacter pylori,* herpes simplex virus and cytomegalovirus and the risk of cardiovascular disease in women, *Ann. Intern. Med., 131,* 573–577.

36. Roivainen, M., Viik-Kajander, M., Palosuo, T., Toivainen, P., Leinonen, M., Saikku, P., Tenkanen, L., Manninen, V., Hovi, T., & Manttari, M. (2000) Infections, inflammation, and the risk of coronary heart disease, *Circulation, 101,* 252–257.

37. Whincup, P., Danesh, J., Walker, M., Lennon, L., Thomson, A., Appleby, P., Hawkey, C., & Atherton, J. (2000) Prospective study of potentially virulent strains of *Helicobacter pylori* and coronary heart disease in middle aged men, *Circulation, 101,* 1647–1652.

38. Choussat, R., Montalescot, G., Collet, J. P., Jardel, C., Ankri, A., Fillet, A. M., Thomas, D., Raymond, J., Bastard, J. P., Drobinski, G., Orfila, J., Agut, H., & Thomas, D. (2000) Effect of prior exposure to *Chlamydia pneumoniae, Helicobacter pylori,* or cytomegalovirus on the degree of inflammation and one-year prognosis of patients with unstable angina pectoris or non-Q wave acute myocardial infarction, *Am. J. Cardiol., 86,* 379–384.

39. Mayr, M., Kiechl, S., Willeit, J., Wick, G., & Xu, Q. (2000) Infection, immunity and atherosclerosis. Association of antibodies to *Chlamydia pneumoniae, Helicobacter pylori* and cytomegalovirus with immune reactions to heat shock protein 60 and carotid or femoral atherosclerosis, *Circulation, 102,* 833–839.

40. Zhu, J., Nieto, J., Horne, B. D., Anderson, J. L., Muhlestein, J. B., & Epstein, S. E. (2001) Prospective study of pathogen burden and risk of myocardial infarction or death, *Circulation, 103,* 45–51.

41. Rupprecht, H. J., Blankenberg, S., Bickel, C., Rippin, G., Hafner, G., Prellwitz, W., Schlumberger, W., & Meyer, J. (2001) Impact of viral and bacterial infectious burden on long-term prognosis in patients with coronary artery disease, *Circulation, 104,* 25–31.

42. Stone, A. F., Risley, P., Markus, H. S., Butland, B. K., Strachan, D. P., Elwood, P. C., & Mendall, M. A. (2001) Ischaemic heart disease and CagA strains of *Helicobacter pylori* in the Caerphilly heart disease study, *Heart, 86,* 506–509.

43. Ridker, P. M., Danesh, J., Youngman, L., Collins, R., Stampfer, M. J., Peto, R., & Hennekens, C. H. (2001) A prospective study of *Helicobacter pylori* seropositivity

and the risk for future myocardial infarction among socioeconomically similar US men, *Ann. Intern. Med.*, *135*, 184–188.

44. Zhu, J., Quyyumi, A. A., Muhlestein, J. B., Nieto, F. J., Zalles-Ganley, A., Anderson, J. L., & Epstein, S. E. (2002) Lack of association of *Helicobacter pylori* infection with coronary artery disease and frequency of acute myocardial infarction or death, *Am. J. Cardiol.*, *89*, 155–158.

45. Blasi, F., Denti, F., Erba, M., Cosentini, R., Raccanelli, R., Rinaldi, A., Fagetti, L., Esposito, G., Ruberti, U., & Allegra, L. (1996) Detection of *Chlamydia pneumoniae* but not *Helicobacter pylori* in atherosclerotic plaques of aortic aneurysms, *J. Clin. Microbiol.*, *34*, 2766–2769.

46. Danesh, J., Koreth, J., Youngman, L., Collins, R., Arnold, J. R., Balarajan, Y., McGee, J., & Roskell, D. (1999) Is *Helicobacter pylori* a factor in coronary atherosclerosis? *J. Clin. Microbiol.*, *37*, 1651.

47. Malnick, S. D., Goland, S., Kaftoury, A., Schwarz, H., Pasik, S., Mashiach, A., & Sthoeger, Z. (1999) Evaluation of carotid arterial plaques after endarterectomy for *Helicobacter pylori* infection, *Am. J. Cardiol.*, *83*, 1586–1587.

48. Farsak, B., Yildirir, A., Akyon, Y., Pinar, A., Oc, M., Boke, E., Kes, S., & Tokgozoglu, L. (2000) Detection of *Chlamydia pneumoniae* and *Helicobacter pylori* DNA in human atherosclerotic plaques by PCR, *J. Clin. Microbiol.*, *38*, 4408–4411.

49. Rassu, M., Cazzavillan, S., Scagnelli, M., Peron, A., Bevilacqua, P. A., Facco, M., Bertoloni, G., Lauro, F. M., Zambello, R., & Bonoldi, E. (2001) Demonstration of *Chlamydia pneumoniae* in atherosclerotic arteries from various vascular regions, *Atherosclerosis*, *158*, 73–77.

50. Ameriso, S. F., Fridman, E. A., Leiguarda, R. C., & Sevlever, G. E. (2001) Detection of *Helicobacter pylori* in human carotid atherosclerotic plaques, *Stroke*, *32*, 385–391.

51. Radke, P. W., Merkelbach-Bruse, S., Messmer, B. J., vom Dahl, J., Dorge, H., Naami, A., Vogel, G., Handt, S., & Hanrath, P. (2001) Infectious agents in coronary lesions obtained by endatherectomy: pattern of distribution, coinfection, and clinical findings, *Coron. Artery Dis.*, *12*, 1–6.

52. Montemurro, P., Barbuti, G., Dundon, W. G., Del Giudice, G., Rappuoli, R., Colucci, M., De Rinaldis, P., Montecucco, C., Semeraro, N., & Papini, E. (2001) *Helicobacter pylori* neutrophil activating protein stimulates tissue factor and plasminogen activator inhibition-2 production by human blood mononuclear cells, *J. Infect. Dis.*, *183*, 1055–1062.

53. Xu, Q., Kiechl, S., Mayr, M., Metzler, B., Egger, G., Wick, G., Oberhollenzer, F., & Willeit, J. (1999) Association of serum antibodies to mycobacteria heat shock protein 65 with carotid atherosclerosis: clinical significance found determined in a follow-up study, *Circulation*, *100*, 1169–1174.

54. Rothenbacher, D., Hoffmeister, A., Bode, G., Miller, M., Koenig, W., & Brenner, H. (2001) *Helicobacter pylori* heat shock protein 60 and risk of coronary heart disease: a case control study with focus on markers of systemic inflammation and lipids, *Atherosclerosis*, *156*, 193–199.

55. Birnie, D. H., Holme, E. R., McKay, I. C., Hood, S., McColl, K. E., & Hillis, W. S. (1998) Association between antibodies to heat shock protein 65 and coronary

atherosclerosis. Possible mechanism of action of *Helicobacter pylori* and other bacterial infections in increasing cardiovascular risk, *Eur. Heart J.*, *19*, 387–394.

56. Galante, A., Pietroiusti, A., Carta, S., Franceschelli, L., Piccolo, P., Mastino, A., Fontana, C., Grelli, S., Bergamaschi, A., Magrini, A., & Favalli, C. (2000) Infection with *Helicobacter pylori* and leucocyte response in patients with myocardial infarction, *Eur. J. Clin. Microbiol. Infect. Dis.*, *19*, 298–300.

57. McDonagh, T. A., Woodward, M., Morrison, C. E., McMurray, J. J., Tunstall-Pedoe, H., Lowe, G. D., McColl, K. E., & Dargie, H. J. (1997) *Helicobacter pylori* infection and coronary heart disease in the North Glascow MONICA population, *Eur. Heart J.*, *18*, 1257–1260.

58. Murray, L. J., Bamford, K. B., O'Reilly, D. P. J., McCrum, E. E., & Evans, A. E. (1995) *Helicobacter pylori* infections: relations with cardiovascular risk factors, ischaemic heart disease and social class, *Br. Heart J.*, *74*, 497–501.

59. Regnstrom, J., Jovinge, S., Bavenholm, P., Ericsson, C. G., De Faire, U., Hamsten, A., Hellenius, M. L., Nilsson, J. & Tornvall, P. (1998) *Helicobacter pylori* seropositivity is not associated with inflammatory parameters, lipid concentrations and degree of coronary artery disease, *J. Intern. Med.*, *243*, 109–113.

60. Elizalde, J. I., Gomez, J., Panes, J., Lozano, M., Casadevall, M., Ramirez, J., Pizcueta, P., Marco, F., Rojas, F. D., & Granger, D. N. (1997) Platelet activation in mice and human *Helicobacter pylori* infection, *J. Clin. Invest.*, *100*, 996–1005.

61. Zito, F., Di Castelnuovo, A., D'Orazio, A., Negrini, R., De Lucia, D., Donati, M. B., & Iacoviello, L. (1999) *Helicobacter pylori* infection and the risk of myocardial infarction: role of fibrinogen and its genetic control, *Thromb. Haemost.*, *82*, 14–18.

62. Torgano, G., Cosentini, R., Mandelli, C., Perondi, R., Blasi, F., Bertinieri, G., Tien, T. V., Ceriani, G., Tarsia, P., Arosio, C., & Ranzi, M. L. (1999) Treatment of *Helicobacter pylori* and *Chlamydia pneumoniae* infections decreases fibrinogen plasma levels in patients with ischaemic heart disease, *Circulation*, *99*, 1555–1559.

63. Carter, A. M., Moayyedi, P., Catto, A., Heppell, R. M., Axon, A. T., & Grant, P. J. (1996) The influence of *Helicobacter pylori* status on circulating levels of coagulation factors fibrinogen, von Willebrand factor, Factor VII, and Factor VIII, *Helicobacter*, *1*, 65–69.

64. Welch, G. N., & Loscalzo, J. (1998) Homocysteine and atherothrombosis, *N. Engl. J. Med.*, *338*, 1042–1049.

65. Markle, H. V. (1997) Coronary artery disease associated with *Helicobacter pylori* infection is at least partially due to inadequate folate status, *Medical Hypothesis*, *49*, 289–292.

66. Cenerelli, S., Bonazzi, P., Galeazzi, R., Testa, I., Bonfili, A. R., Sirolla, C., Giunta, S., Galeazzi, L., Fumelli, D., & Testa, R. (2002) *Helicobacter pylori* masks differences in homocysteine plasma levels between controls and Type 2 diabetes patients, *Eur. J. Clin. Invest.*, *32*, 158–162.

67. Aydin, A., Vardar, R., Evrengu, I. H., Ungan, M., Yilmaz, M., & Payzin, S. (2001) Does *Helicobacter pylori* infection have a role in coronary artery disease? *Turkish J. Gastro.*, *12*, 287–293.

68. Ekesbo, R., Nilsson, P. M., Lindholm, L. H., Persson, K., & Wadstrom, T. (2000) Combined seropositivity for *H. pylori* and *C. pneumoniae* in associated with age, obesity and social factors, *J. Cardiovasc. Risk, 7*, 191–195.

69. Niemela, S., Karttunen, T., Karhonen, T., Laara, E., Karttunen, R., Ikaheimo, M., & Kesaniemi, Y. A. (1996) Could *Helicobacter pylori* infection increase the risk of coronary heart disease by modifying serum lipid concentrations? *Heart, 75*, 573–575.

70. Marchetti, M., Arico, B., Burroni, D., Figura, N., Rappuoli, R., & Ghiara, P. (1995) Development of a mouse model of *Helicobacter pylori* infection that mimics human disease, *Science, 267*, 1655–1658.

71. Eaton, K. A., Morgan, D. R., & Krakowka, S. (1989) *Campylobacter pylori* virulence factors in gnotobiotic piglet, *Infect. Immun., 57*, 1119–1125.

72. Tsuda, M., Karita, M., Morshed, M. G., Okita, K., & Nakazawa, T. (1994) A urease-negative mutant of *Helicobacter pylori* constructed by allelic exchange mutagenesis lacks the ability to colonize the nude mouse stomach, *Infect. Immun., 62*, 3586–3589.

73. Hazell, S. L., Eichberg, J. W., Lee, D. R., Alpert, L., Evans, D. G. Evans, D. J., Jr., & Graham, D. Y. (1992) Selection of the chimpanzee over the baboon as a model for *Helicobacter pylori* infection, *Gastroenterology, 103*, 848–854.

74. Wirith, H. P., Beins, M. H., Yang, M., Tham, K. T., & Blaser, M. J. (1998) Experimental infection of Mongolian gerbils with wild-type and mutant *Helicobacter pylori* strains, *Infect. Immun., 66*, 4856–4866.

75. Mach, F., Sukhova, G. F., Michetti, M., Libby, P., & Michetti, P. (2002) Influence of *Helicobacter pylori* infection during atherogenesis in vivo in mice, *Circ. Res., 90*, el (circresaha.org).

76. Blessing, E., Campbell, L. A., Rosefeld, M. E., Choug, L. N., & Kuo, C. C. (2001) *Chlamydia pneumoniae* infection accelerates hyperlipidemia induced atherosclerotic lesion development in C57BL/6J mice, *Atherosclerosis, 158*, 13–17.

77. Kowalski, M., Konturek, P. C., Pieniazek, P., Karczewska, E., Kluczka, A., Grove, R., Kranig, W., Nasseri, R., Thale, J., Hahn, E. G., & Konturek, S. J. (2001) Prevalence of *Helicobacter pylori* infection in coronary artery disease and effect of its eradication on coronary lumen reduction after percutaneous coronary angioplasty, *Dig. Liver Dis., 33*, 222–229.

78. Stone, A. F. M., Mendall, M. A., Kaski, J., Edger, T. M., Gupta, S., Polonieck, J., Camm, A. J., & Northfield, T. C. (2001) The South Thames trail of antibiotics in myocardial infarction and unstable angina (STAMINA trail), *Eur. Heart J., 22*(Abstract suppl), 643 [Abstract p3516].

79. Nicholls, A. C., & Thomas, M. (1977) Coxsackie virus infection in acute myocardial infarction, *Lancet, 1*, 883–884.

80. Wood, S. F., Rogen, A. S., Bell, E. J., & Grist, N. R. (1978) Role of coxsackie B virus in myocardial infarction, *Br. Heart J., 40*, 523–525.

81. Griffiths, P. D., Hannington, G., & Booth, J. C. (1980) Coxsackie B virus infections and myocardial infarction: results from a prospective epidemiologically controlled study, *Lancet, 1*, 1387–1389.

82. Pönkä, A., Jalanko, H., Pönkä, T., & Stenvik, M. (1981) Viral and mycoplasmal antibodies in patients with myocardial infarction, *Ann. Clin. Res.*, *13*, 429–432.
83. Lau, R. C. (1982) Coxsackie B virus infection in acute myocardial infarction and adult heart disease, *Med. J. Aust.*, *2*, 520–522.
84. O'Neill, D., McArthur, J. D., Kennedy, J. A., & Clements, G. (1983) Coxsackie B virus infection in coronary care unit patients, *J. Clin. Pathol.*, *36*, 658–661.
85. Nikoskelainen, J., Kalliomäki, J. L., Lapin Leimu, K., Stenvik, M., & Halonen, P. E. (1983) Coxsackie B virus antibodies in myocardial infarction, *Acta Med. Scand.*, *214*, 29–32.
86. Matilla, K. J. (1987) Viral and bacterial infections in patients with acute myocardial infarction, *J. Intern. Med.*, *225*, 293–296.
87. Miklozek, C. L., Crumpacker, C. S., Royal, H. D., Come, P. C., Sullivan, J. L., & Abelmann, W. H. (1988) Myocarditis presenting as acute myocardial infarction, *Am. Heart J.*, *115*, 768–776.
88. Collins, S. D. (1932) Excess mortality from causes other than influenza and pneumonia during influenza epidemics, *Public Health Rep.*, *47*, 2159–2180.
89. Bainton, D., Jones, G. R., & Hole, D. (1978) Influenza and ischaemic heart disease: a possible trigger for acute myocardial infarction? *Int. J. Epidemiol.*, *7*, 231–239.
90. Zheng, Z. J., Mittleman, M. A., Tofler, G. H., Pomeroy, C., Dampier, C., Wides, B., & Muller, J. E. (1998) Infections prior to acute MI onset, *J. Am. Coll. Cardiol.*, *31*(Suppl. A), 132A.
91. Abinader, E. G., Sharif, D. S., & Omary, M. (1993) Inferior wall infarction preceded by acute exudative pharyngitis in young males, *Israel J. Med. Sci.*, *29*, 764–769.
92. Spodick, D. H., Flessas, A. P., & Johnson, M. M. (1984) Association of acute respiratory symptoms with onset of acute myocardial infarction: a prospective investigation of 150 consecutive patients and matched control patients, *Am. J. Cardiol.*, *53*, 481–482.
93. Gross, P. A., Hermogenes, A. W., Sacks, H. S., Lau, J., & Levandowski, R. A. (1995) The efficiency of influenza vaccine in elderly persons: a meta-analysis and review of the literature, *Ann. Intern. Med.*, *123*, 518–527.
94. Naghavi, M., & Casscells, W. (2000) Association of influenza vaccination and reduced risk of recurrent myocardial infarction, *Circulation*, *102*, 3039–3045.
95. Lavallee, P., Perchaud, V., Gautier-Bertrand, M., Grabli, D., & Amarenco, P. (2002) Association between influenza vaccination and reduced risk of brain infarction, *Stroke*, *33*, 513–518.
96. Falsey, A. R., Walsh, E. E., Francis, C. W., Looney, R. J., Kolassa, J. E., Hall, W. J., & Abraham, G. N. (2001) Response of C-reactive protein and serum amyloid A to influenza A infection in older adults, *J. Infect. Dis.*, *183*, 995–999.
97. Feinstone, S. M., & Gust, I. A. (2000) Hepatitis A virus, in G. L. Mandell, J. E. Bennett, & R., Dolin (Eds.) *Principles and practice of infectious diseases* (5th edn, Vol. 2, pp. 1920–1940), Philadelphia: Churchill Livingstone.
98. Zhu, J., Quyyumi, A. A., Norman, J. E., Costello, R., Csako, G., & Epstein, S. E. (2000) The possible role of Hepatitis A virus in the pathogenesis of atherosclerosis, *J. Infect. Dis.*, *182*, 1583–1587.
99. Dezube, B. J., Pardee, A. B., Chapman, B., Beckett, L. A., Korvick, J. A., Novick, W. J., Chiurco, J., Kasdan, P., Ahlers, C. M., Ects, L. T., Crumpacker,

C. S., & the NIAD AIDS Clinical Trials Group (1993) Pentoxifylline decreases tumor necrosis factor expression and serum triglycerides in people with AIDS, *J. Acquir Immune Defic Syndr.*, *6*, 787–794.

100. Krishnaswamy, G., Chi, D. S., Kelley, J. L., Sarubbi, F., Smith, J. K., & Peiris, A. (2000) The cardiovascular and metabolic complications of HIV infection, *Cardiol. Rev.*, *8*, 260–268.
101. Henry, K., Melroe, H., Huebsch, J., Hermundson, J., Levine, C., Swensen, L., & Daley, J. (1998) Severe premature coronary artery disease with protease inhibitors, *Lancet*, *351*, 1328.
102. Hadigan, C., Meigs, J., Corcoran, C., Rietschel, P., Piecuch, S., Basgoz, N., Davis, B., Sax, P., Stnaley, T., Wilson, P. W. F., D'Agostino, R. B., & Grinspoon, S. (2001) Metabolic abnormalities and cardiovascular disease risk factors in adults with human immunodeficiency virus infection and lipodystrophy, *Clin. Infect. Dis.*, *32*, 130–139.
103. David, M. H., Hornung, R., & Fichtenbaum, C. J. (2002) Ischemic cardiovascular disease in persons with human immunodeficiency virus infection, *Clin. Infect. Dis.*, *34*, 98–102.
104. Carr, A., Samaras, K., Thorisdottir, A., Kaufmann, G. R., Chisholm, D. J., & Cooper, D. A. (1999) Diagnosis, prediction, and natural course of HIV-1 protease inhibitor associated lipodystropy, hyperlipidemia, and diabetes mellitus: a cohort study, *Lancet*, *353*, 2093–2099.
105. Hadigan, C., Corcoran, C., Stanley, T., Piecuch, S., Klibanski, A., & Grinspoon, S. (2000) Fasting hyperinsulinemia in HIV-infected men: relationship to body composition, gonadol function and protease-inhibitor use, *J. Clin. Endocrin. Metab.*, *85*, 35–41.
106. Saint-Marc, T., Partisani, M., Poizot-Martin, I., Bruno, F., Rouviere, O., Lang, J. M., Gastaut, J. A., & Touraine, J. L. (1999) A syndrome of peripheral fat wasting (lipodystrophy) in patients receiving long-term nucleoside analogue therapy, *AIDS*, *13*, 1659–1667.
107. Walker, U. A., Bickel, M., Lütke, Volksbeck, S. I., Ketelsen, U. P., Schöfer, H., Setzer, B., Venhoff, N., Rickerts, V., & Staszewski, S. (2002) Evidence of nucleoside analogue reverse transcriptase inhibitor-associated genetic and structural defects of mitochondria in adipose tissue of HIV infected patients, *J. Acquir. Immune Defic. Syndr.*, *29*, 117–121.
108. Farrj, R. S., McCully, R. B., Oh, J. K., & Smith, T. F. (1997) *Mycoplasma* associated pericarditis [Review], *Mayo Clin. Proceed*, *72*, 33–36.
109. Popat, K., Barnardo, D., & Webb-Peploe, M. (1980) *Mycoplasma pneumoniae* endocarditis, *Br. Heart J.*, *44*, 111–112.
110. Padovan, C. S., Pfister, H. W., Bense, S., Fingerle, V., & Abele-Horn, M. (2001) Detection of *Mycoplasma pneumoniae* DNA in cerebrospinal fluid of a patient with *M. pneumoniae* infection-"associated" stroke, *Clin. Infect. Dis.*, *33*, E119–21.
111. Mulder, L. J., & Spierings, E. L. (1987) Stroke in a young adult with *Mycoplasma pneumoniae* infection complicated by intravascular coagulation, *Neurology*, *37*, 1430–1431.

112. Fu, M., Wong, K. S., Lam, W. W., & Wong, G. W. (1998) Middle cerebral artery occlusion after recent *Mycoplasma pneumoniae* infection, *J. Neurol. Sci., 157,* 113–115.
113. Visudhiphan, P., Chiemchanya, S., & Sirinavin, S. (1992) Internal carotid artery occlusion associated with *Mycoplasma pneumoniae* infection, *Pediatr. Neurol., 8,* 237–239.
114. Parker, P., Puck, J., & Fernandez, F. (1981) Cerebral infarction associated with *Mycoplasma pneumoniae, Pediatrics, 67,* 373–375.
115. Higuchi, M. L., Sambiase, N., Palomino, S., Gutierrez, P., Demarchi, L. M., Aiello, V. D., & Ramires, J. A. (2001) Detection of *Mycoplasma pneumoniae* and *Chlamydia pneumoniae* in ruptured atherosclerotic plaques. *Brazilian J. Med. Biol. Res., 33,* 1023–1026.
116. Fong, I. W., Chiu, B., Viira, E., Jang, D., & Mahony, J. B. (1999) De novo induction of atherosclerosis by *Chlamydia pneumoniae* in a rabbit model, *Infect. Immun., 67,* 6048–6055.
117. Epstein, S. E., Zhu, J., Burnett, M. S., Zhou, Y. F., Vercellotti, G., & Hajjar, D. (2000) Infection and atherosclerosis: potential roles of pathogen burden and molecular mimicry, *Artherioscler. Thromb. Vasc. Biol., 20,* 1417–1420.
118. Xu, Q., Willeit, J., Marosi, M., Kleindienst, R., Oberhollenzer, F., Kiechl, S., Stulnig, T., Luef, G., & Wick, G. (1993) Association of serum antibodies to heat shock protein 65 with carotid atherosclerosis, *Lancet., 341,* 255–259.
119. Xu, Q., Weimam, S., Gupta, R. S., Wolf, H., & Wick, G. (1993) Staining of endothelial cells and macrophages in atherosclerotic lesions with human heat shock protein reactive antisera, *Arterioscler. Thromb., 13,* 1763–1769.
120. Schett, G., Xu, Q., Amberger, A., Van der Zee, R., Recheis, H., Willeit, J., & Wick, G. (1995) Autoantibodies against heat shock protein 60 mediate endothelial cytotoxicity, *J. Clin. Invest., 96,* 2569–2577.
121. Metzlier, B., Kiechl, S., Mayr, M., Willeit, J., Schett, G., Xu, Q., & Wick, G. (1999) Endothelial cytotoxicity mediated by serum antibodies to heat shock proteins of Escherichia coli and *Chlamydia pneumoniae*: immune reactions to heat shock proteins as a possible link between infection and atherosclerosis, *Circulation, 99,* 1560–1566.
122. Zinkernagel, R. M., Cooper, S., Chambers, J., Lazzarini, R. A., Hengartner, H., & Arnheiter, H. (1990) Virus induced autoantibody response to a transgenic viral antigen, *Nature, 345,* 68–71.
123. Anderson, J. L., Carlquist, J. F., Muhlestein, J. B., Horne, B., & Elmer, S. P. (1998) Evaluation of C-reactive protein, an inflammatory marker, and infectious serology as risk factors for coronary artery disease and myocardial infarction, *J. Am. Coll. Cardiol., 32,* 35–41.
124. Auer, J., Berent, R., Weber, T., & Eber, B. (2002) Interleukin-1 receptor antagonist gene polymorphism, infectious burden, and coronary artery disease, *Clin. Infec. Dis., 34,* 1536–1537.
125. Ridker, P. M., Hennekens, C. H., Buring, J. E., Kundsin, U. & Shih, J. (1999) Baseline IgG antibody titers to *Chlamydia pneumoniae, Helicobacter pylori,* herpes simplex virus and cytomegalovirus and the risk for cardiovascular disease in women, *Ann. Intern. Med., 131,* 573–577.

126. Roivainen, M., Viik-Kajander, M., Palosuo, T., Toivainen, M., Leinonen, M., Saikku, P., Tenkanen, L., Manninen, V., Hovi, T., & Manttari, M. (2000) Infections, inflammation, and risk of coronary heart disease, *Circulation, 101*, 252–257.
127. Zhu, J., Nieto, J., Horne, B., Anderson, J. L., Muhlestein, J. B., & Epstein, S. E. (2001) Prospective study of pathogen burden and risk of myocardial infarction or death, *Circulation, 103*, 45–51.
128. Rupprecht, H. J., Blankenberg, S., Bickel, C., Rippin, G., Hafner, G., Prellwitz, W., Schlumberger, W., & Meyer, J. (2001) Impact of viral and bacterial infectious burden on long-term prognosis in patients with coronary artery disease, *Circulation, 104*, 25–31.
129. Espinola-Klein, C., Rupprecht, H. J., Blankenberg, S., Bickel, C., Kopp, H., Rippin, G., Victor, A., Hafner, G., Schlumberger, W., & Meyer, J. (2002) Impact of infectious burden on extent and long term prognosis of atherosclerosis, *Circulation, 105*, 15–21.
130. Chiu, B., Viira, E., Tucker, W., & Fong, I. W. (1997) *Chlamydia pneumonia,* cytomegalovirus and herpes simplex virus in atherosclerosis of the carotid artery, *Circulation, 96*, 2144–2148.
131. Qavi, H. B., Melnick, J. L., Adam, E., & Debakey, M. E. (2000) Frequency of coexistence of cytomegalovirus and *Chlamydia pneumoniae* in atherosclerotic plaques, *Central Eur. J. Public Health, 8*, 71–73.
132. Chiu, B. (1999) Multiple infections in carotid atherosclerotic plaques, *Am. Heart J., 128*, S534–S536.
133. Haraszthy, V. I., Zambon, J. J., Trevisan, M., Zeid, M., & Genco, R. J. (2000) Identification of periodontal pathogens in atheromatous plaques, *J. Periodontal, 71*, 1554–1560.
134. Haraszthy, V. I., Jordan, S. F., Zambon, J. J., Zafiropoulos, G. G., Mastragelopoulos, N., & Genco, R. J. (2001) Periodontal pathogens in atheromas from a German population, *Ann. Periodontal, 6*, 64 [Abstract].
135. Wanishsawad, C., Zhou, Y. F., & Epstein, S. E. (2000) *Chlamydia pneumoniae*-induced transactivation of the major immediate early promoter of cytomegalovirus: potential synergy of infectious agents in the pathogenesis of atherosclerosis, *J. Infect. Dis., 181*, 787–790.
136. Burnett, M. S., Gaydos, C. A., Madico, G. E., Glad, S. M., Paigen, B., Quinn, T. C., & Epstein, S. E. (2001) Atherosclerosis in APOE knockout mice infected with multiple pathogens, *J. Infect. Dis., 183*, 226–231.
137. Hirose, H., & Kugimiya, T. (2000) Abdominal aortic aneurysm infected with *Helicobacter pylori*: a case report, *Angiology, 51*, 867–871.

Index